Vaccination & Homoeoprophylaxis?

A Review of Risk and Alternatives

7th edition

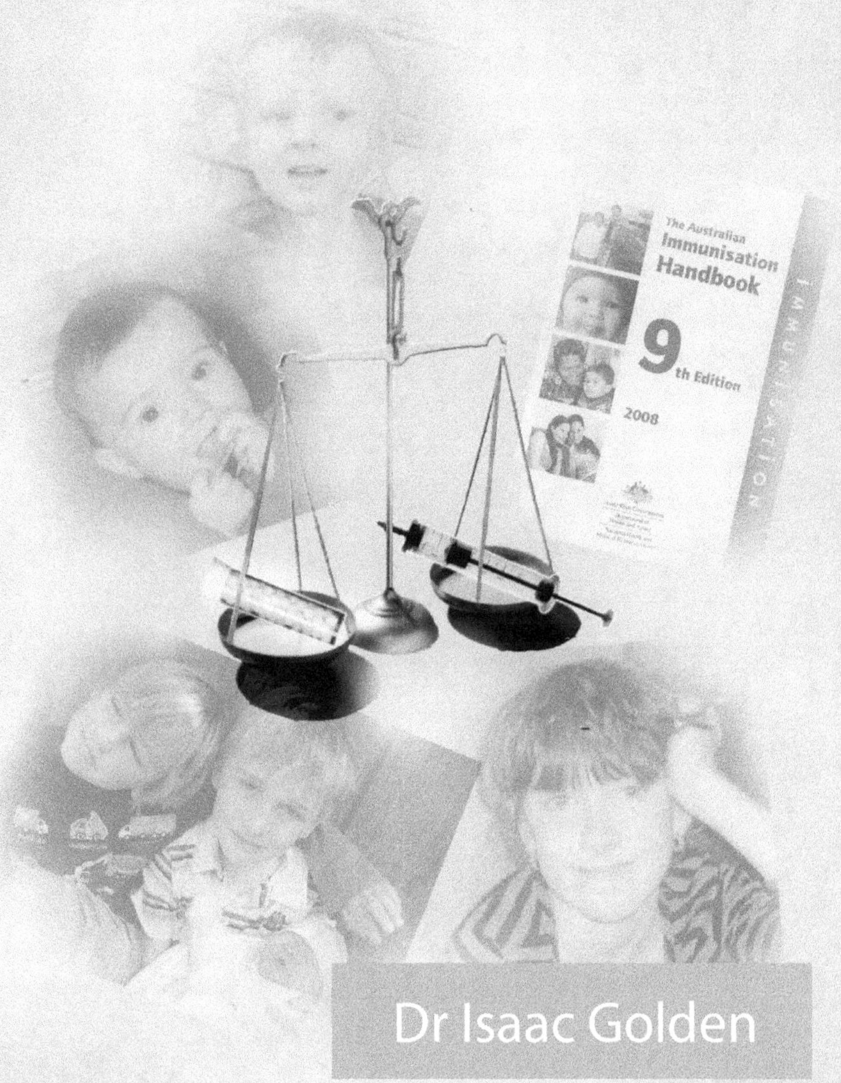
The Australian
Immunisation
Handbook
9th Edition
2008
IMMUNISATION

Dr Isaac Golden

Vaccination & Homœoprophylaxis?

A Review of Risks and Alternatives

7th Edition

Dr Isaac Golden, PhD

7th Edition 2010
6th Edition 2007 (Revised)
6th Edition 2005
5th Edition 1998 (Revised)
5th Edition 1997 (Revised)
5th Edition 1994
4th Edition 1993
3rd Edition 1992 (Revised)
3rd Edition 1991
2nd Edition 1990
1st Edition 1989

Vaccination & Homœoprophylaxis? A Review of Risks and Alternatives - 7th Ed.

Dr Isaac Golden PhD, DHom, ND, BEc (Hon)

Principal, Aurum Healing Centre, 1984 -

Director, Australasian College of Hahnemannian Homoeopathy

Director, Homoeopathy International Online College

Business Manager, Endeavour College of Natural Health, 2009 -

Homoeopathic Coordinator, Melbourne College of Natural Medicine, 1995-2004

President, Australian Homoeopathic Association (Victoria), 1992-1998

Australian Homoeopathic Association, Distinguished Service Award, 13.3.1999

Inquiries: Postal: P.O. Box 695, Gisborne. Victoria. Australia. 3437

Phone: (03) 5427 0880

E-Mail: admin@homstudy.net

Web Pages: www.homstudy.net (link to different pages)

ISBN: 978-0-9578 726-7-7

National Library, Canberra (02) 6262 1434

Other Publications by the Author:

Vaccine Damaged Children – Treatment, Prevention, Reasons, revised 2010
ISBN 0 - 9578 - 726 - 6 - 0

Homœoprophylaxis – A Fifteen Year Clinical Study. 2004.
ISBN 0 - 9578 - 726 - 3 - 1

Vaccination ? - A Review of Risks and Alternatives. 5th ed. 1997
ISBN 0 - 7316 - 8099 - 5

Homœoprophylaxis - A Practical and Philosophical Review. 4th ed. 2007
ISBN 0 - 646 - 19529 - 8

Homœoprophylaxis – A Ten Year Clinical Study. 1997
ISBN 0 – 646 – 32054 - 8

Australian Homoeopathic Home Prescriber - Part 1. 3rd ed. 2007
ISBN 0 - 646 - 15057 - X

Australian Homoeopathic Home Prescriber - Part 2. 2001
ISBN 0 – 9578 - 726 – 0 – 7

Australian Homoeopathic Home Prescriber - Part 3. 2006
ISBN 0 – 9578 - 726 – 5 - 3

Homoeopathic Treatment of the Energy Bodies. 2002
ISBN 0 – 9578 - 726 – 1 - 5

Homoeopathic Body-System Prescribing - A Practical Workbook of Sector Remedies, 2nd ed. 2002
ISBN 0 - 646 - 27292 - 6

Other Publications by the Author

Preface to the 7th Edition

So much has changed since I last revised the 6th edition in 2007 that a 7th edition has become inevitable. The HPV vaccine (marketed as Gardasil in Australia) has been vigorously promoted, the world has been through the first phase of the Swine Flu Pandemic, and most importantly to me, the world has also seen the largest documented use of homeopathic immunisation take place, in Cuba in 2007, 2008, 2009, and 2010.

There has also been a coordinated attack on homeopathy, especially in the United Kingdom, following a meta analysis published in the *Lancet* in 2005 which led the Editors to announce the death of homeopathy. This work has subsequently been discredited, the credibility of the *Lancet* as a truly objective scientific journal of reference has been diminished, and the evidence base of homeopathy has been strengthened. However the international pharmaceutical lobby remains powerful due to the extraordinary amounts of money which it spends annually to buy influence. Homeopathy is constantly under attack from "skeptics", although one of the most prominent has recently been shown to have falsified his homeopathic "credentials".

In my own country, economic realities are causing the forward thinkers in the Federal Government to consider ways to reduce the economically crippling health budget, thus promoting the consideration of safe and inexpensive natural options to expensive drugs and even more expensive medical delivery systems.

So the world has changed, and further change is inevitable.

I will leave the Preface to the 6th edition in place as it describes major aspects of the book.

The first major change in this 7th edition relates to layout. I have been asked to make the material simpler. On the other hand, this is a complex topic and people need facts. So I have tried to do both – retain and expand on all the previous detail, but at the same time restructure the book so that readers can begin with a basic summary and then delve deeper if they wish to learn more about a particular point.

This will give readers the option of reading all the material if they wish, or reading the summary and then going straight to the Sections where they want more information, and setting aside the other parts until they are ready. To reduce the bulk of the early reading I have moved descriptions of the characteristics of individual diseases, and individual vaccines into Section 9 which is a new Appendix to Questions 1 and 3.

There have also been changes and extensive reference updates throughout the book, and **the following new Sections have been added** to the 7th edition:

Overview of the argument and some issues (a simple summary preceding Section 1)

9.1.21	Dengue Fever	9.2.24 Dengue vaccination
9.1.22	Human Papiloma Virus;	9.2.25 HPV vaccination
9.1.23	Leptospirosis;	9.2.26 Leptospirosis vaccination
9.1.24	Rotavirus;	9.2.27 Rotavirus vaccination
9.1.25	Swine Flu;	9.2.28 Swine Flu vaccination

Section 4.2.3: The Cuban experience, which is one of the most important additions to the 7th edition.

Section 3.5.6: Research into vaccine damaged children: This replaces Section 8.4, and has been considerably expanded to include new research which I published in 2008.

Section 5.4: The economics of immunisation options.

But as I sit here contemplating why this book is needed, and why some people will choose to read it and use the information it offers, I keep coming back to the sad but undeniable fact that health authorities and many within the orthodox medical system are, either knowingly or unwittingly, not providing parents of young children with truthful information. People are realising this in the hundreds of thousands and are seeking for truth elsewhere. Pharmaceutical spin has been exposed for what it is. Blind belief is no longer acceptable. "Trust me I'm a doctor" no longer works like it did 50 years ago. We have choices – and this book provides you with the chance to make a choice which will impact on the health of your entire family for the rest of their lives

– may it shine light into a dark place, and bring you peace of mind.

Preface to the 6th Edition

I began writing the first edition of this book in the late 1980's. My hope was that this 6th edition would be the last. However, experience tells me that such hopes often are not realised because there is always something new to add, and we can always do better.

I have changed the book substantially from the previous editions, both in style and content. The aim has been to make it a more valuable and readable reference for parents in particular, but also for practitioners in the different modalities of natural medicine. I also hope a few open-minded orthodox medical practitioners will find it a useful reference, and that it will become a valuable resource for homoeopathic students and practitioners who are learning about homœoprophylaxis.

To achieve this aim I have decided to ask, and answer, six basic questions. They are:

QUESTION 1: Should we attempt to prevent infectious diseases?

QUESTION 2: What is the best overall approach to infectious disease prevention?

QUESTION 3: What are the risks and benefits of the vaccination option?

QUESTION 4: What are the risks and benefits of the homœoprophylaxis option?

QUESTION 5: What are the comparative risks and benefits of the disease-prevention options?

QUESTION 6: Which option is best for my child?

These questions represent the essence of the issues parents must confront when making what is probably their most difficult decision concerning the health of their young child – should they vaccinate or not? The decision is made more difficult because of the unreasonable and uninformed statements made by some advocates on both sides of the debate. It is an area where the scientists often become unscientific, where Government policy is driven by pressure groups with significant vested interests, and where some opponents of vaccination take unsustainable positions in an effort to be heard.

A diagram outlining the decision making process that many parents will have to face is shown following the Preface.

I hope that each question (and therefore each Chapter or Section in the book) will stand alone, so that readers may quickly turn to the relevant Section in the book to find the information they require. I have included most of the material contained in the previous editions of this book, as well as new material generated during my Doctoral research at the Graduate School of Integrative Medicine at Swinburne University. A significant amount of new material from orthodox medical journals and books has also been added.

My 20 year journey with homœoprophylaxis (HP) - the homoeopathic option to vaccination – has been quite a ride! In summary, I can say that the journey has convinced me that HP has a tremendous amount to offer to parents. It is what I eventually used for my own children once I became aware of the method. It is what I now recommend my grandchildren to use. I have felt the considerable opposition to HP from supporters of pharmaceutical medicine, and (for different reasons) from some members of my own profession.

I believe that truth will always win in the end, and that as the years pass and the data collected grows and improves in quality, the real value of HP will become increasingly clear.

My personal view is that it does no harm for healthy children to contract mild infectious diseases, but that there are some potentially devastating diseases that should be prevented if at all possible. I believe that mass vaccination has at times conferred benefits by reducing the likelihood of a child contracting severe diseases, and at times has caused both short-term and long-term damage due to the very nature of the procedure, as well as due to the toxic materials in the vaccines. The appropriate use of the homoeopathic option can, I believe, bring similar benefits without the risk of either short-term or long-term damage.

I believe that the next step forward should be the introduction of a dual national system of immunisation where vaccination and homœoprophylaxis are equally available, and supported by Government health authorities.

I believe that this will:

(i) Improve the national immunisation coverage against potentially serious infectious diseases by ensuring more children are protected

(ii) Lessen the incidence of chronic illness in the community

(iii) Save federal and state governments hundreds of millions of dollars annually,

(iv) Allow an objective scientific comparison of the two methods to be undertaken

Initially, most of the people who would use the homoeopathic option would be those who would not have vaccinated their children anyway, so the orthodox authorities could not claim that children were being endangered by changing immunisation methods. Further, making choice available to all would take a lot of the heat out of the anti-vaccination debate and put Australia at the cutting edge of modern national immunisation policy.

I can imagine many readers shaking their heads at this point, and saying that this will never happen. Maybe it won't, but it is worth serious consideration. All that is needed is a few independently minded politicians to realise the potential benefits of a dual national immunisation system, and who knows what may transpire?

I can also imagine some readers, including some of my friends in the anti-vaccination lobby, shaking their heads and thinking that my advocacy of a dual system that includes vaccination is a sell-out! To be honest, I don't believe that vaccination will be banned in our lifetime due to the huge financial structures that support it. I do believe that it is more realistic to offer it alongside a proven, risk-free alternative. Change will then happen, slowly but surely, and in a cooperative way.

We should all be on the same side here – doctors, governments, homoeopaths, mums and dads, etc. We should all be calling for the best health system possible, including a safe method of protecting the health of our children. We need to put entrenched positions, and vested interests aside, and have an honest and fully informed debate – and let truth decide the outcome, for the benefit of all.

AN EXAMPLE OF THE DECISION MAKING PROCESS
(Note: the numbers shown relate to Section numbers in the book)

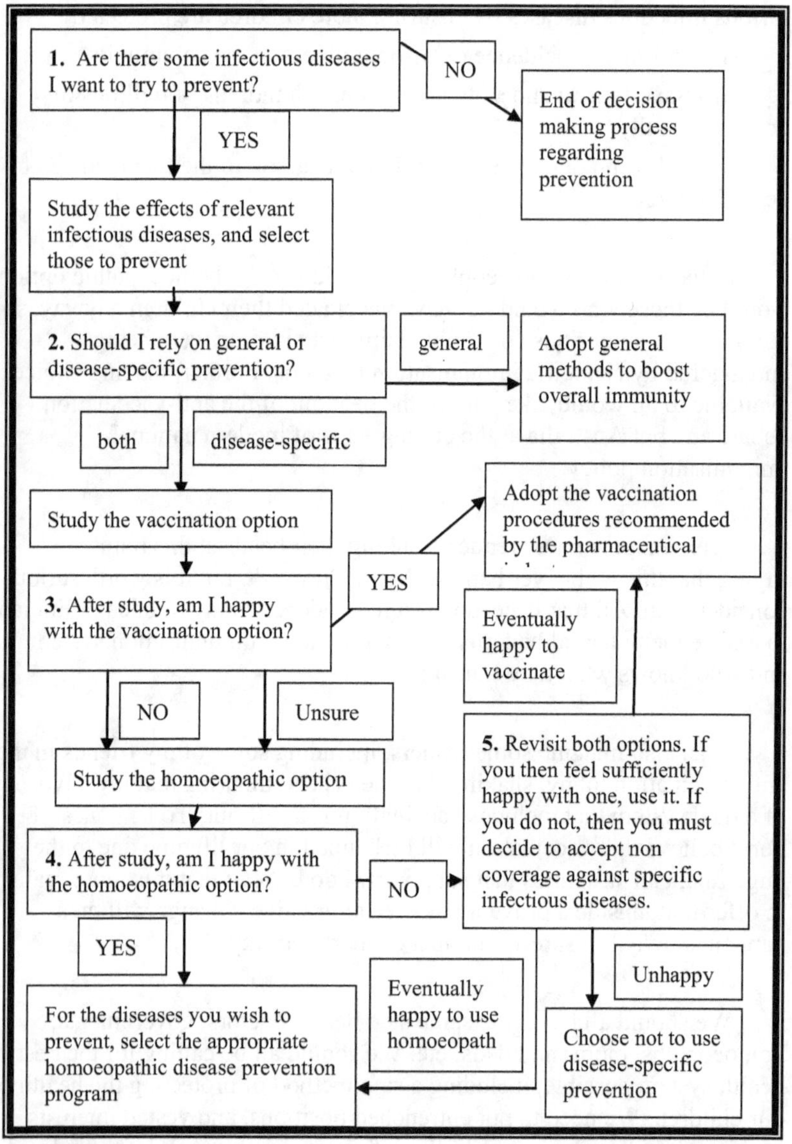
1. Are there some infectious diseases I want to try to prevent?
NO
End of decision making process regarding prevention
YES
Study the effects of relevant infectious diseases, and select those to prevent
2. Should I rely on general or disease-specific prevention?
general
Adopt general methods to boost overall immunity
both
disease-specific
Study the vaccination option
Adopt the vaccination procedures recommended by the pharmaceutical
YES
3. After study, am I happy with the vaccination option?
Eventually happy to vaccinate
NO
Unsure
Study the homoeopathic option
5. Revisit both options. If you then feel sufficiently happy with one, use it. If you do not, then you must decide to accept non coverage against specific infectious diseases.
4. After study, am I happy with the homoeopathic option?
NO
YES
Unhappy
Eventually happy to use homoeopath
For the diseases you wish to prevent, select the appropriate homoeopathic disease prevention program
Choose not to use disease-specific prevention

Style Notes

The following comments may help to make the book more readable:

1. Vaccination and Immunisation

In the book I use the word "vaccination" to mean the administration of legally defined vaccines, either orally or by injection. I use the word "immunisation" to mean any method designed to stimulate immunity against targeted infectious diseases.

So vaccination is one form of immunisation, as is homœoprophylaxis, good diet, and so on.

2. References

In the book I use the Harvard system of referencing, where the author's name and year of publication are shown immediately following the material quoted. The full details of the work are shown in the Bibliography at the end of the book, sorted alphabetically by the surname of the lead author.

3. Chapters or Sections

I have referred to the parts of the book as Sections rather than Chapters.

4. Need for an Index at the End

Because the Table of Contents is so complete, and because I have shown the Sections in the book where different references (shown in the Bibliography at the end) appear, I have decided not to add to the volume of the book by compiling a significant Index at the end. I suggest that you search for different sections by using the Table of Contents.

* * * * * *

Acknowledgements

I would like to gratefully acknowledge the support given me by Professor Avni Sali and Dr Luis Vitetta of the former Graduate School of Integrative Medicine, Swinburne University of Technology. The research undertaken at the University would not have happened without their encouragement and assistance.

I also gratefully acknowledge the assistance of Dr Mary Faeth Chenery and homoeopath Anna Lamaro who made valuable comments on an earlier draft of my doctoral thesis, which has contributed new data for this new edition. Dr Chenery also edited an earlier draft of the 6th edition and made it a better work as a result.

Naturopath Anita DiStasio directed the rewriting of Section 2 of the book, concerning herbal and nutritional supports to the immune system. Her efforts have improved both the readability and the current relevance of this material.

I would like to acknowledge the people who helped me during the very early stages of this work:

- The late Dr Glen Dettman, PhD, for his generous contributions of reference material;
- Dr Harold Buttram, MD, for his communications and encouragement;
- The late Mr Simon Schot, ND, for advice concerning certain herbal remedies;
- Mrs Kara Millar, MSc, for all her time playing devil's advocate, reading various drafts of articles and the final manuscript (1st Edition);
- Ms Alida Veugen, who intercepted the third edition and made it far more readable and presentable than the first two.

I also greatly appreciate the support of the editors of Australia's leading natural health journals, who have not been afraid to publish controversial material on this subject. These high quality publications - *Nature & Health*, *Australian Wellbeing*, *Simply Living*, *Grass Roots*, and

Australasian Health and Healing - all contain worthwhile and interesting material.

I appreciate the practical support of Mr John Feenie, CEO of Endeavour College of Natural Health, for his generosity in supporting my recent visit to Cuba through the College, and for his growing enthusiasm and support for homoeoprophylaxis as an international solution to an issue which has profound health consequences for the planet.

The friendship and cooperation with Dr Concepcion Campa Huergo and especially Dr Gustavo Bracho of the Finlay Institute in Havana Cuba has been a life changing experience for me, as well as changing the face of HP research in the world – they are treasured relationships.

Another new relationship of friendship and support with Dr Simon Floreani and Dr Jennifer Barham-Floreani has been a pleasure both personally, and for the fact that I now see the next generation of people to bring facts and fairness to our health system.

Lastly, I would like to dedicate this book to my children. In many ways it is for them, but they are the ones who have paid the price of my many absences over the years due to work, study, and research. In the end, I can only hope that they will feel that what this work contributes is worth what they have lost.

TABLE OF CONTENTS

Index of Tables

Index of Figures

Definitions

Note: References in brackets show the Section in the book where the term was first used.

Antigen – a substance that the body recognises as being not of itself, thus provoking an immune response. (Section 1)

Antibody – an immunoglobulin (one of 5 classes of protein) produced to protect against an antigen. (Section 1)

The **Effectiveness** of a homoeopathic preventative program is the proportion of those using the program who did not acquire the targeted disease, to the total number of persons using the program. Where possible, the figure for effectiveness is refined by identifying those users of the program who were exposed to the targeted disease, and using that total in the proportion. (Section 2.5.1)

Endemic – present in a community at all times, but occurring in only small numbers of cases. (Section 1)

Epidemic – occurring in a great number of cases in a community at the same time. (Section 1)

The **Genus Epidemicus** is the homoeopathic remedy chosen during an outbreak of an infectious disease that best matches the common symptom picture of the disease. The remedy is selected after analysing the symptoms of a number of patients with the disease. (Section 4)

Homœoprophylaxis (HP) is the use of homoeopathically prepared potentised substances in a systematic manner to prevent the development of the characteristic symptoms of infectious diseases. (Introduction)

An **Isode** is a remedy prepared from the patient's OWN diseased material, e.g., a remedy prepared from a whooping-cough patient's own sputum. (Section 4)

Immunisation is taken to mean any method that reduces the likelihood of the recipient acquiring a targeted infectious disease if exposed to the disease. (Introduction)

The **Law of Similars** states that a substance that is capable of causing a group of symptoms in a healthy person is capable of removing a group of **similar** symptoms in a sick person. (Section 4)

A **Nosode** is a homoeopathic preparation (potency) of diseased tissue, e.g., a remedy prepared from the sputum of a number of patients with whooping cough. (Section 4)

Pandemic – a widespread epidemic, often international. (Section 1)

Potentisation is the method used in homoeopathy to prepare remedies. The original material is subjected to a series of dilutions and succussions (violent shaking of the diluting medium against a firm surface), or triturations (grinding of insoluble substances). (Section 4)

Provings are controlled experiments where doses of the substance being tested (usually in potentised form) are given to healthy volunteers, who record new symptoms produced by taking the substance. The Master Prover (the person supervising the proving) then extracts those symptoms that are common to a number of provers, and this information is entered into the Materia Medica. (Section 4)

Succussion is the process used in the preparation of homoeopathic remedies in liquid form where the container holding the medicinal solution is repeatedly shaken firmly with vertical movements against a firm surface thus violently agitating the medicinal solution. (Section 4)

Trituration is the process used in the preparation of homoeopathic remedies in solid form where the active substance and a medicinally neutral powder, often sugar crystals prepared from maize or milk, are ground together using a mortar and pestle. Usually trituration is used only until the mixture is soluble. (Section 4)

Vaccination is defined as the administration, usually orally or by injection, of attenuated antigenic material together with preservatives and adjuvants to stimulate the production of antibodies in the recipient. (Introduction)

The **Vital Force** is defined by homoeopaths as a person's self-balancing (healing) energy that is present from birth, and which acts to maintain homoeostasis on the mental, emotional and physical levels of the person's being. (Section 4)

Some Thoughts

For parents

"The public surely is entitled to convincing proof, beyond any reasonable doubt, that artificial immunization is in fact a safe and effective procedure, in no way injurious to health, and that the threat of the corresponding natural diseases remain sufficiently clear and urgent to warrant mass inoculation of everyone, even against their will if necessary.

"Unfortunately, such proof has never been given."

Dr R Moskowitz MD. *The Case Against Immunization*

For practitioners

"The salutary eruptive diseases of infancy are responsible for much miasmic elimination, and the unnatural vaccinations which are so extremely contrary to the proper stability of the human race, make the Sycotic condition deeper by suppressing or preventing the miasm from taking an acute form."

Dr P S Ortega. *Notes on the Miasms*

For scientists

"A science which ignores all evidence in order to believe what it prefers is a science not worthy of the name."

Dr L Pascal. *What Happens When Science Goes Bad*

For everyone

All truth goes through three steps:

1. First, it is ridiculed.
2. Second, it is violently opposed.
3. Finally, it is accepted as self-evident

Arthur Schopenhauer (German philosopher, 1788-1860)

"Secrecy is the antithesis of the true scientific method. The scientists should never forget this"

Dr Isaac Golden, July 2005

PART 1: GENERAL DISCUSSION

Overview of the argument, and some issues

Before we commence our detailed study of each of the 6 questions asked (remembering that Sections do not need to be read in order), I would like to present a few pages summarising the book. I know that some readers will always begin at the beginning, and at times don't get to the homeopathic Sections until after the information is needed. For others, the volume of material may be challenging, or time is not available, so a simple summary will be useful.

We all want the best for our children. We want them to be safe and healthy. We would like to protect them from any suffering – mental, emotional or physical. However life is not like that. It is inevitable that we will suffer at times, but it is sensible to try to minimise the frequency and severity of this. At the same time we don't want prevention methods to come at too great a cost, especially hidden long-term costs in terms of debilitating chronic diseases.

There are many infectious diseases circulating in our communities. In Australia, leaving aside seasonal influenza, we are generally free of epidemics. However some potentially lethal diseases are still present such as meningococcal diseases, Hib, and even whooping cough in infants. So it does make sense to prevent, provided the means of prevention does not cause more long-term problems than the condition itself. And this is where the debate commences.

Question 1 looks at the potential severity of the different diseases for which vaccines are available. Most people accept that it is worth preventing at least some diseases, but some are concerned that the most commonly used form of prevention – vaccination – may cause problems.

Question 2 looks at whether general prevention or disease-specific prevention is most appropriate, and concludes that maximum prevention comes from targeting specific diseases with disease-specific remedies. There are two types of disease-specific prevention, and the remainder of the book compares these options.

Question 3 outlines some concerns with vaccines. However the recommendation is not that you should never vaccinate. That is your decision alone, and will be influenced by a variety of facts including family pressures, work requirements, school issues and so on. My position is that you do have a choice between the two methods of disease prevention, neither of which are 100% effective but which are comparably effective, but with very different levels of potential toxicity.

The point of this work is to say to parents that you can actually provide comparably effective prevention against the diseases of greatest concern without risking toxic damage that may result from vaccination.

Much of **Question 4** is devoted to providing evidence of the safety and the effectiveness of the homoeopathic option. There is very little disagreement regarding safety, because homoeopathic medicines are prepared past the point where there are toxic materials present - the main debate quite properly relates to effectiveness.

Your job will be to assess the evidence provided, and there is now a considerable body of evidence quantifying the effectiveness of homoeoprophylaxis. It is both interesting and disappointing to see how many people in orthodox science claim that there is no evidence, whilst at the same time admitting they have never read the existing materials. OF COURSE, if you never examine what is available then you can say that you are not aware of any evidence. But that is a world away from having examined evidence and concluded that it is inadequate.

This is all I ask:– that parents are given the opportunity to freely examine both sides of the argument, to examine all the evidence available, and then be supported in the decision they make.

In practice, some individuals and groups want to suppress free speech for a variety of motives. Some because they genuinely believe that their option is the best (even if others don't realise it); others for simple vested interest (and it is not necessary to speculate about the massive profits big pharma makes from vaccines – this is common knowledge), and others because of some pseudo-scientific herd mentality.

For example, in 2009 I appeared on a local TV channel to debate the immunisation issue with a Professor who was a vaccine manufacturer. I introduced the Cuban material which the Professor was not aware of. Some members of the Skeptics Society saw the debate and viciously attacked the TV Channel and the two presenters, criticising both for allowing any air time to discuss the issue. They wanted the public to be prevented from knowing that 2.4 million people had been successfully immunised using homoeoprophylaxis – not an opinion but a fact.

But the suppression of free speech is the first sign of a lie – if a person is speaking truth then they have no need to suppress discussion. So we often hear it said that anyone who opposes vaccination is threatening the wellbeing of the whole community because they are reducing the herd immunity effect which vaccines bring. But homoeoprophylaxis also brings with it a herd immunity effect. This is not realised simply because people have not studied evidence.

So we are dealing with an issue where emotions and deception often hold more currency than truth. It is the task of each parent to try to see past deception to the facts, and thus make informed decisions.

Question 5 of the book compares the two immunisation options – vaccination and homoeoprophylaxis, and **Question 6** asks – which option is best for my child? It is totally appropriate to begin with these Sections if you wish, and in fact I recommend this for readers who think they might struggle with the volume of material contained in the earlier Sections.

So start by reading Section 5 and then Section 6, and then return to the remainder of the material if you prefer.

The progression of logical reasoning asks -

QUESTION 1: Should we attempt to prevent infectious diseases?
QUESTION 2: What is the best overall approach to infectious disease prevention?
QUESTION 3: What are the risks and benefits of the vaccination option?
QUESTION 4: What are the risks and benefits of the homœoprophylaxis option?
QUESTION 5: What are the comparative risks and benefits of the two disease-prevention options?
QUESTION 6: Which option is best for my child?

But you can pick up the book at any point.

What I have done in the 7th edition is to put the bulk of the writing relating to specific diseases and specific vaccines into Appendices, so even if you start at the beginning, you will gain a comprehensive overview by the time you have read about a third of the book, then you can delve deeper if you so wish.

1 QUESTION 1: Should we attempt to prevent infectious diseases?

To some readers it may seem a silly question – after all, why would we NOT want to prevent possible suffering in our children. However, there is serious debate within both the orthodox and complementary (or natural, or traditional) medical circles concerning the desirability of preventing all infectious diseases.

We shall begin our examination of this question by considering how potentially serious the common infectious diseases really are (individual diseases are now examined in Appendix 9.1). It is always worthwhile remembering that what may be a simple and harmless disease in a healthy person may become lethal in a person whose immune system is seriously compromised. The example of measles in a child suffering from malnutrition is a good example of this. So in a country like Australia, measles is potentially less serious than in a country where a majority of people are starving.

We shall then consider something called the *hygiene hypothesis*, which, stated simply, says that the acquisition of some childhood infectious diseases assists in the normal maturation of a child's immune system. This hypothesis has supporters from all fields of healing.

Finally, we shall consider some of the options that parents have when they come to make their first basic decision – should we attempt to prevent a particular infectious disease in our children?

1.1 The characteristics of common infectious diseases

The focus of this book is on the standard childhood diseases in Australia. This list typically applies in most developed countries. However overseas travel is always a possibility and so some diseases commonly of concern in overseas travel will be considered. Of course, the recommendations made in the book can apply for adults as well as children.

Table 1-1 lists the infectious diseases which shall be examined, as well as summarising some relevant information about incubation and spread of the diseases

Refer to “Definitions” (page xii above) for descriptions of the differences between an epidemic, an endemic, and a pandemic outbreak of disease.

READER’S NOTE: Table 1-1 summarises some of the material now presented in Appendix 9.1. This Section can be skipped if you already have a good idea of the diseases you want prevented, or if you prefer to come back later and study the disease information more carefully. However, a careful look at Table 1-4 at the end of this Section is recommended.

Table 1-1 Infectious Diseases with Summary of Characteristics - I

Section	Disease	Bacterial or Viral	Usual Period of Incubation	Period of Infectivity	Recommended Exclusion Period	Mode of Spread
9.1.1	Chicken Pox	V	11-20 days	1-2 days prior to the rash until 5 days after onset, or while new lesions appear	Until no new lesions appear	Respiratory droplets, or direct contact
9.1.2	Cholera	B	1-5 days	Months if left untreated	Up to 24 hours after last diarrhoea	Contaminated food and water
9.1.3	Diphtheria	B	2-7 days	2-3 weeks if not treated	Until throat swab is negative	Contact with infected nasal, throat, eye and skin discharges
9.1.4	Haemophilis influenzae type b (Hib)	B	Unknown, may develop 5 days after exposure	Unknown	48 hours after treatment started	Respiratory droplets, or direct contact
9.1.5	Hepatitis A	V	15-50 days av. 28 days)	1-2 weeks before, to 1 week after onset of symptoms	5 days from onset of symptoms	Faeces, food, water, blood, with oral ingestion
9.1.6	Hepatitis B	V	45-180 days (av. 60-90 days)	4-6 months after onset; indefinite in carriers	None	Blood. Sexual contact. Through skin and mucus memb. At birth.

Sect-ion	Disease	Bacterial or Viral	Usual Period of Incubation	Period of Infectivity	Recommended Exclusion Period	Mode of Spread
9.1.7	Hepatitis C	V	2-20+ wks (av. 56 days)	2 wks before & during; indefinite in carriers	None	Blood. Sexual contact. Through skin. At birth.
9.1.8	Influenza	V	1-3 days	Unknown	None	Respiratory droplets
9.1.9	Japanese encephalitis	V	Unknown	Unknown		Carried by domestic pigs & wild birds, and spread by mosquitos.
9.1.10	Measles	V	6-19 days	Unknown	5 days from onset of rash	Respiratory droplets
9.1.11	Meningococc-al infections		Unknown	Unknown	48 hours from start of treatment	Respiratory droplets
9.1.12	Mumps	V	15-24 days	3-6 days before, and for 3-9 days after glandular enlargement	5 days from onset of inflammation of glands	Saliva, respiratory droplets, and rarely by urine
9.1.13	Pertussis (Whooping Cough)	B	5-21 days (rarely more than 10 days)	Unknown	At least 3 weeks if untreated., or 5 days following antibiotic	Respiratory droplets

Sect-ion	Disease	Bacterial or Viral	Usual Period of Incubation	Period of Infectivity	Recommended Exclusion Period	Mode of Spread
9.1.14	Pneumococc-al infections	B	1-3 days	Unknown	None	Respiratory droplets or recently soiled handkerchiefs
9.1.15	Polio-myelitis	V	3-35 days	Few days before onset to several weeks after		Mainly faeces. Saliva. Rarely food and water
9.1.16	Rubella	V	15-20 days	Probably before rash	5 days from onset of rash	Respiratory droplets
9.1.17	Tetanus	B	1 day to months	Not contagious	None	Contaminated wound
9.1.18	Tubercu-losis	B	1-12 months	Up to 2 weeks	2 weeks after starting treatment	Respiratory droplets
9.1.19	Typhoid	B	5-34 days	1-3 weeks; indefinite for carriers	Until negative stools obtained	Food and water contaminated by infected faeces or urine
9.1.20	Dengue Fever	V	5-6 days OR 3-14 days	Not contagious between humans	None	Bite of an infected Aedes mosquito.

Sect-ion	Disease	Bacterial or Viral	Usual Period of Incubation	Period of Infectivity	Recommended Exclusion Period	Mode of Spread
9.1.21	Human Papiloma Virus	V	Varies. Months or years	Unknown – probably years	Years. Condome required to prevent spread	Sexual contact
9.1.22	Leptospirosis	P	4-14 days	Not contagious between humans	None	Water contaminated by rodent and other animal urine
9.1.23	Rotavirus	V	1-3 days	Normally 2 weeks	None is protective hygiene	Faecal-oral via contaminated food and water
9.1.24	Swine Flu H1N1	V	1-3 days	Unknown	None	Respiratory droplets

The major references used to develop the following material are:

The National Health & Medical Research Council. *The Australian Immunisation Handbook*, 9th edition, 2008.

The handbook contains a wealth of "scientific" information about diseases and vaccines, and is very thoroughly referenced for those who wish to examine back-up evidence in medical journals and medical texts. Unfortunately I was not able to obtain permission to directly quote from the Handbook when preparing the final draft, so readers who want additional information (all of which is also available publicly elsewhere) may obtain their own copy. The handbook is accessible for free online at www.immunise.health.gov.au.

Davies E G, et al., *Manual of Childhood Infections*, 2nd edition, 2001. W.B. Saunders, London.

A very thorough handbook of many infectious diseases, and how they manifest in children.

Neustaedter R. *Vaccine Guide – Risks and Benefits for Children and Adults*. Revised Edition, 2002. North Atlantic Books, Berkeley, California.

A well known publication among natural therapists interested in the vaccination issue. Very well researched, informative and readable.

Lessell C B. *The World Travellers Manual of Homoeopathy*. 1993. C W Daniel, London.

An excellent reference for the world traveller. He discusses homoeopathic treatment and prevention, as well as giving some great common sense suggestions concerning prevention.

NOTE: The following general structure is used when examining each disease in Appendix 9.1:

1. The Organism
2. Clinical Symptoms
3. Orthodox and Homoeopathic Treatment
4. Summary

PLEASE NOTE: Because point 3 refers to possible treatment options for the diseases examined, I am obliged to repeat the Disclaimer given at the front of the book. Some of these diseases are potentially life threatening, and professional help should be sought to ensure that appropriate treatment is undertaken.

Disclaimer: This book is not intended to replace the services of a qualified practitioner. Any application of the recommendations set forth in the following pages is at the reader's discretion and sole risk.

1.2 The hygiene hypothesis in orthodox and complementary medicine

There is some agreement within both orthodox and traditional medicine that acquiring some infectious diseases may be beneficial to the normal maturation of a child's immune system. For example, Morgan referred to epidemiological studies showing that a typical measles illness "may actually confer non-specific health benefits leading to reduced childhood mortality rates" (Morgan, 2004). Martinez reported that "infants exposed to infections in early life appeared to have fewer allergies later - his study of 1,000 children showed infections might be protective, allowing the immune system to 'develop batteries' against infection" (Herald Sun, 1996). Cookson and Moffatt concluded that "childhood infections may, therefore, paradoxically protect against asthma" (Cookson W O & Moffatt M E, 1997). Traditional Chinese Medicine practitioners certainly believe that a typical measles infection can be very beneficial in maturing the immune system.

The so-called *"hygiene hypothesis"* states that a lower level of exposure to bacteria and viruses, and fewer infectious diseases in childhood, results in an increase in asthma, eczema and allergic diseases in later years. The term was first coined by David P. Strachan in 1989 (Strachan, 1989). The hypothesis is controversial within orthodox medicine, with supporters (Von Mutius E (2007); Matricardi et al, 2002; Braun-Fahrlander et al, 2002; Pawankar R et.al., 2008), and those who question its validity (Dahl et al, 2004).

However, there is little if any evidence that demonstrates that every child needs to acquire **every** disease in order to be healthy. In fact, there is ample evidence that infectious diseases at times create "layers" of distress in otherwise apparently healthy persons, for example, those patients "never well since" measles, glandular fever, pertussis, etc., who are regularly seen in homoeopathic practice.

Further, it can be argued that if the stimulation caused by an infectious disease is beneficial, then the similar stimulation on the subtle level provided by homœoprophylaxis (HP) remedies will be similarly beneficial, but without the risks sometimes associated with either the natural disease, or the vaccine.

Section 4.4 presents the evidence I collected during my doctoral studies which examined the long-term health of children who were vaccinated, who used homœoprophylaxis, who used constitutional prevention, and who used no method of prevention at all. This showed that those who used HP were generally healthier than all other groups, and that the vaccinated group were clearly the least healthy of all.

This reinforces the beliefs of those who support the hygiene hypothesis in regards to the negative effects of vaccination, but suggests that the appropriate use of HP appears to have similar effects as the natural disease when it comes to gently stimulating the immune system and maintaining long-term health.

Further research is of course needed, but if this finding is true, it provides a significant additional reason to support the use of HP.

1.2.1 Some implications of the hygiene hypothesis

Let's make some assumptions in order to explore possible implications of the hygiene hypothesis as it may relate to the link between asthma and vaccination:

Assumption 1. Vaccination against measles reduces the annual deaths from measles by 11-20 per year.

We estimate this by examining in Table 1-2 the trend in deaths prior to the introduction of measles vaccination in Australia in 1970, and by the fact that there has been only 1 death recorded from 1995 to 2008.

Table 1-2 Deaths from Measles Before and After Vaccination in 1970

Year	60	61	62	63	64	65	66	67	68	69
Deaths	16	30	11	13	23	20	17	24	15	36
Year	**70**	71	72	73	74	75	76	77	78	
Deaths	**9**	18	6	6	12	5	11	8	11	

Average 1960 to 1969 = 20.5; Average 1970 to 1978 = 9.6

Assumption 2. Vaccination causes a fivefold increase in the incidence of asthma in vaccinated children.

This assumption is supported by the data collected by myself and others (see Sections 3.6.13.4 and 4.2.3.3 below). There is also research in the orthodox literature demonstrating there is a case to answer regarding the asthma-vaccination link (Enriquez R et.al., 2005).

There were 447 deaths from asthma in Australia in 2008 (NACA, 2010). Seven deaths were in the youngest age groups (0-9 years). Figures from the Asthma Foundation of Victoria show that over 2 million people nationwide have the condition, and that asthma is one of the most common reasons for childhood admissions to hospital.

Economically, the annual cost to the Australian community is estimated to be in excess of $720 million, the cost to companies through absenteeism of those with asthma is $110 million per year, the cost of carer absence is in excess of $120 million per year, and the cost of asthma medication over $110 million per year (Asthma Foundation of Australia, 2004).

So we can compare a saving of at the most 20 deaths a year from fewer measles deaths as a result of vaccination, with a causation of say 320 deaths a year from an increase in asthma as a result of vaccination (assumed to contribute 4/5 of the total deaths).

Comment: This analysis is by no means complete. It does not take into account the many additional variables that would need to be considered to make the analysis complete (such as the costs of measles infections, the costs of other vaccine reactions and long-term side-effects). However, it shows that this type of analysis needs to be done. Whilst the simple comparison of 320 deaths to 20 deaths is "academic", it shows that there is clearly a case to answer, an examination which the orthodox health authorities have neglected and the pharmaceutical industry rigorously avoided.

1.3 Options

Should a particular disease be prevented and, if so, how? are major questions that responsible parents will eventually have to face.

There is no one single answer that will fit every possible situation – the severity of diseases varies considerably, as does the general health of the children who may be infected. What may be a potentially serious disease for some people may be generally benign for others. We are all different, with a unique level of individual susceptibility.

It seems to me, when looking at the diseases examined above, that for an Australian child we can break the diseases into three groups, as shown below in Table 1-3. I emphasise that this list is totally subjective. It is my own opinion. You have every right to hold a different opinion and you should act on your opinion.

It is recommended that parents and other readers prepare their own list. It is of course quite appropriate to have a fourth column –"uncertain". This exercise is part of the required decision making process for any person with a young child.

Table 1-3 Diseases Listed According to Suggested Need for Prevention for an Average, Healthy Australian Child

Prevention not essential	Prevent if travelling to area where disease is active	Prevention recommended in Australian conditions
Chicken Pox	Cholera	Hib
Measles	Diphtheria	Meningococcal disease
Mumps	Hepatitis A	Polio
Rubella (unless in early pregnancy)	Japanese encephalitis	Pneumococcal disease
Tetanus (treat if wounded)	Typhoid	Whooping Cough
Hepatitis B (unless high risk)	Tuberculosis	
Hepatitis C (unless high risk)	Leptospirosis	
Swine Flu	Dengue	
Rotavirus		
Human Papiloma Virus		

It certainly is reasonable to conclude that the material presented in Section 1 indicates that **the prevention of some of the diseases examined is preferable to having to treat the diseases**. We shall therefore now examine which approach to the prevention of specific diseases yields the most certain result.

2 QUESTION 2: What is the best approach to infectious disease prevention – general and/or specific?

We shall now continue for the remainder of the book under the assumption that there are some infectious diseases that we would prefer our children (or ourselves) not to get.

So the next question to be asked, and answered, concerns the two broad options we have in disease prevention – general prevention, or disease-specific prevention.

We shall examine these two options in turn, and finally draw some conclusions.

2.1 General methods to prevent specific diseases

When Dr Archie Kalokerinos undertook his pioneering work with Aboriginal groups in the 1960's, he discovered that severe Vitamin C deficiencies caused sudden infant deaths, as well as contributing to a significant number of fatalities when Vitamin-C-deficient children were vaccinated. At the time, his findings were dismissed by most members of the medical profession (Kalokerinos A, 1974).

Today, the link between immune deficiencies and nutritional status has been 'discovered' by medical science to be true. Research has shown that the malnourished are more susceptible to infections, and that diseases affect them more severely. For example, it has been shown that measles infection will persist in malnourished children, whereas it is relatively quickly resolved in a healthy child (Dossetor et al, 1977, pp. 1633-1635). At the other end of the age spectrum, research has shown that appropriate nutritional supplements will improve immunity in elderly patients (Chandra R K, 1982, pp. 223-232). Dr Kalokerinos has been proved correct time and again (Maggini S, Wenzlaff S, Hornig D, 2010).

Further, distinguished international researcher, Professor R K Chandra, has stated: "There is a complex three-way interaction between nutrition, immunity, and infection. Nutritional deficiency impairs immunity and increases the severity, duration, and perhaps the incidence of infection. Similarly infection itself can suppress the immune responses and worsen malnutrition" (Chandra R K, 1985, pp. 5-16).

Natural Therapists have always advised patients that a healthy diet is critical in protecting against infection and disease, advice that is now not only scientifically acceptable, but even more relevant with the huge increase in immune-deficiency diseases such as cancer, asthma, arthritis and allergies, as well as AIDS.

This section examines some general methods of protection against infectious diseases, concentrating on strengthening the entire immune response by raising the individual's dynamic vitality or, in homoeopathic terms, their *Vital Force.* Because diet represents a constant input to the system, it is one of the most important factors in immune response.

2.1.1 Nutrition and the immune system

The immune system is composed of many cell types that collectively provide protection from bacterial, viral, parasitic and fungal infections and from growth of abnormal cells. These include the lymph nodes, spleen, thymus, tonsils, adenoids, appendix, bone marrow, and gut associated lymphoid tissue which comprises around 70% of our entire immune system.

A varied, balanced diet of complex carbohydrates, proteins and good fat is essential for proper immune function and overall good health.

- Complex carbohydrates include grains, legumes, fruits, vegetables. These foods contain vitamins, minerals, antioxidants and other phytonutrients, plus provide an excellent source of fibre. There is a predominance of low GI (glycaemic index) foods. Refined carbohydrates are stripped of these essential nutrients. Avoid chemicals, preservatives and colouring.
- Protein foods include eggs, fish, chicken, lean meats, cheese, nuts and seeds. Adequate protein is essential for growth and repair of tissues and is required by the liver to assist with the body's removal of toxins.

- Beneficial fats - omega 3, omega 6 and monounsaturated - consumed at appropriate levels support healthy cells. These include fish/fish oils, flaxseeds, olive oil, nuts and seeds, and avocado.

Long term nutrient depletion and diets high in sugar, refined foods and saturated fats can adversely affect health as well as compromise the immune system.

As our gut is very important to our entire immune system, restoring and maintaining good gut flora with lactobacillus or chlorophyll rich foods/ supplements will enhance our immune response.

A qualified naturopathic practitioner can guide you in planning the most appropriate diet for your individual needs.

I highly recommend a relatively new book by Dr Jennifer Barham-Floreani, *Well Adjusted Babies* (Barham-Floreani J, 2009). It is full of useful advice in many areas, including nutritional guidance.

2.1.2 Nutritional deficiencies associated with immune deficiency

The vitamins and minerals listed below in Table 2-1 and Table 2-2 are generally considered to be the most important for regulating immune response. While a balanced diet is essential for overall good health, individual nutrients consumed in excess may still compromise immunity. Conversely, a deficiency in any nutrient (not just those listed) may adversely affect immune response. Consult a qualified practitioner for professional advice.

Table 2-1 Effects of Vitamin and Mineral Deficiencies on the Immune System

Vitamin	**Effects of Deficiency**
A	Reduces the number of white blood cells and the effectiveness of lymphocytes, significantly increasing frequency/severity of infections
B (Complex)	[Particularly B6 (Pyridoxine) and B9 (Folic Acid); also important are B1, B2, B5, and B12.] The body cannot produce antibodies (including antibodies to vaccines), and dramatically reduces the number of white blood cells; the Thymus and lymphatic organs begin to waste away.
C	Reduces production of antibodies and phagocytosis (destruction of foreign cells by white cells); reduces resistance to infection and increases severity of infection if acquired.
E	Increases susceptibility to infection, including reduction of antibody production; this vitamin works closely with other anti-oxidants and affects T-Cell-dependent antibody response.
Mineral	**Effects of Deficiency**
Copper	Decreased antibody-forming cell response of the B-cell system; reduces assimilation of Iron.
Iron	Reduces T-cell response to infection and phagocyte activity of lymphocytes.
Magnesium	Impairs antibody-forming cell response in the Spleen as well as white cell levels.
Selenium	Impairs T-cell dependent antibody responses, particularly when linked to Vitamin E deficiency.
Zinc	One of the most important minerals; significantly affects cell-mediated immune response.

2.1.3 Sources of nutrients for the immune system

Table 2.2 lists common food sources containing the nutrients identified above.

Table 2-2 Foods and Herbs Important in Supporting the Immune System

Nutrient	**F O O D S**	
	Animal Origin	**Vegetable Origin**
Vitamin A	Fish liver oils (cod, salmon, halibut), butter, egg yolk	Carrots, apricots, sweet potatoes, green leafy vegetables, mint, red peppers
Vitamin B9 (Folic Acid)	Organ meats, eggs	Brewers yeast, soy products, fresh nuts, wheatgerm/bran, oats, unpolished rice, green leafy vegetables, beans
Vitamin B6 (Pyridoxine)	Salmon, mackerel, tuna, chicken, egg yolk	Brewers yeast, wheatgerm/bran, kidney beans, sunflower seeds, walnuts, legumes, bananas, molasses, cabbage
Nutrient	**Animal Origin**	**Vegetable Origin**
Vitamin C		Citrus fruits, pineapple, blackcurrants, strawberries, tomatoes, peppers, raw cabbage, broccoli, carrots, parsley, lettuce, potatoes
Vitamin E	Beef, egg yolk, herring	Safflower and sunflower seeds, seed oil (esp. wheat germ oil), almonds, nuts, soy products, leafy green vegetables, corn
Copper	Oysters, crab, lamb	Brewers yeast, almonds, seeds, mushrooms, buckwheat, beans, dried legumes, prunes, molasses
Iron	Liver, red meats, oysters, clams, poultry, eggs	Molasses, wheatgerm, legumes, whole-grain cereals, dark green leafy vegetables, apricots, yeast, figs, dates
Magnesium	Seafood, eggs	Dates, almonds, walnuts, brazil nuts, cashews, brewers yeast, green leafy vegetables, parsnips, barley, soybeans, molasses
Selenium	Liver, eggs, mackerel, tuna	Brazil nuts, garlic, brewers yeast, wheat germ/bran, whole grains, brown rice, onions, broccoli, cabbage

Zinc	Oysters, herring, liver, beef, egg yolks	Sunflower and pumpkin seeds, whole grains, wheat germ/bran, peas, nuts, carrots, green leafy vegetables, yeast, mushrooms, ginger

Anti-oxidants no doubt play an important part in general health and resistance to disease. Those who subscribe to the anti-oxidant theory of long life and good health will note that Vitamins A, C, and E and Selenium all feature in the table above.

2.1.4 Other factors that can affect immune response

Apart from diet, there are other important factors are involved in stimulating general immune competence. The most significant of these are listed as follows:

- *Environmental:* We absorb many toxins from our environment such as chemicals and heavy metals. These may come from the foods we eat, the air we breathe, the water we drink, or what we are surrounded by. We need to be aware of this factor, to avoid excessive exposure and reduce the burden.
- *Physiological and emotional stress, and a lack of sleep, rest and relaxation:* They lower immune response in both adults and children. While we are constantly under some form of stress in our lives, it is important to have strategies to deal with these stresses to minimize the negative impact. Meditation, relaxation, spiritual interests, music, enjoyable hobbies, etc, can create a more a balanced lifestyle.
- *Natural Supplements:* Although it would be preferable to obtain the necessary micro-nutrients, vitamins, enzymes, amino acids, and so on from wholesome foods, this is not always possible. The nutritional value of food rapidly deteriorates through storage, heating, cooling, irradiation, chemical treatments, and other forms of processing. It may therefore be advisable to include some natural supplements in the diet to ensure that deficiencies of essential nutrients do not develop.
- *Constitutional Remedies:* Many homoeopaths believe that if children or adults are given appropriate constitutional remedies, **all** aspects of their health will improve, enabling them to cope more effectively with any viral or bacterial invasion of the body. They are convinced that such invasions are actually the **result** of prior susceptibility due

> to constitutional weakness, and not the **cause** of this weakness. This view is well supported in practice, so these practitioners believe that if a child becomes infected, homoeopathic treatment of the disease will very likely have good results, with the added advantage of the child's immune response being allowed to develop naturally.

However, even the healthiest of people may succumb to specific infectious diseases, which is why other homoeopaths (myself included) believe that specific protection for the more serious infectious diseases is desirable. Constitutional treatment should be undertaken, but should be supplemented with the necessary specific prophylactics. This debate is continued in Section 4.

A number of other modalities provide general toning for the system. While not as deep acting as homoeopathic constitutional high potencies, these can provide valuable support for the entire being. For example, massage, Reiki, Bach Wildflower remedies, and so on are of great value in many cases and will definitely improve immune strength. Chiropractic or osteopathic treatment may also be of value (Lovett L, 1990; Barham-Floreani J, 2009).

2.1.5 Conclusions for general immunity

The effort involved in adapting diet and lifestyle to maximise the vitality of the immune system is especially important for young children whose immune systems are still maturing. Breastfeeding mothers can benefit both themselves and their children by living wisely.

As shown in Section 1, vaccination cannot guarantee full protection against specific infectious diseases, and may in fact place additional strain on children when they are most vulnerable. Even if vaccination is used, one cannot assume that a child's health is automatically protected. Excellent diet and lifestyle are always necessary.

The late Dr Glen Dettman recommended that parents who decide to vaccinate their children must ensure they receive high doses of Vitamin C for at least one week before and after vaccines are administered. I suggest a minimum of 3000 mg daily, spread out in three doses through the day. If this dosage is excessive for the individual, diarrhoea will develop. If so, the dose can be reduced until the diarrhoea ceases.

If food intake is considered inadequate to provide needed nutrients, supplements may be indicated; however, it should be remembered that care is necessary in giving supplements to young children. Fresh, unprocessed foods and simple herbs are always the best alternative when available.

2.2 Specific methods to prevent infectious diseases

Anything which improves a child's (or an adult's) general health will improve their resistance to any infection. However, it is clear that taking specific action to target specific diseases will provide a greater level of protection – we know this because even extremely healthy people occasionally succumb to the common cold, or flu. Further, some diseases such as meningococcal disease have occurred in healthy young sportsmen and sportswomen who have shared drink bottles.

If the disease-specific methods of protection did not provide a more certain method of disease prevention, then the rates of vaccine and HP effectiveness would be 0% in very healthy children, since the immunisation would provide no further increase in immunity. Evidence shows this not to be the case.

In my doctoral studies completed in 2004, I showed that there are really only two forms of disease-specific prevention (immunisation) against infectious diseases; vaccination and homœoprophylaxis (HP). Most of what follows in Sections 3, 4 and 5 will be a comparison of these two methods.

2.3 General vs. Specific methods to prevent specific diseases

If our aim is to provide the greatest level of prevention possible against specific infectious diseases, then we need to use disease-specific prevention.

This in no way lessens the importance of general methods to improve immunity and health overall. These will always benefit the child by not only raising their ability to cope with infections when exposed, but also to resolve infections naturally if the disease develops.

My recommendation is always to do both – provide the best diet and lifestyle for your child, use constitutional support where possible, and support this with appropriate disease-specific prevention if you feel it is necessary to protect against specific infectious diseases.

PART 2: SPECIFIC METHODS OF DISEASE PREVENTION

3 QUESTION 3: What are the risks and benefits of the vaccination option?

It's pretty simple really – if a health professional tells you that vaccination is safe and effective, politely ask them to give you, in writing, their personal guarantee that if you vaccinate your child then they will be fully liable if your child either gets the targeted disease, or is adversely affected by the vaccine in any way.

If they won't give you their personal guarantee, then you know that you are fully justified in asking questions, and doing your own independent research, before making your reasoned decision regarding vaccination. You also know that they are in no position (morally or legally) to criticise your decision to make up your own mind.

All I ask of readers is that you make up your own mind based on the information that I present, plus whatever else you can get your hands on. If some of the information in this Section seems to over-represent the doubts about vaccination, this is simply because the information stressing the benefits is usually all one can obtain from health authorities. There needs to be a balance. When you have gathered a balanced cross-section of information, you are then in the best possible position to weight up the pros and cons not only of vaccination but also of the homoeopathic alternative.

It is worth remembering that promotional material from pharmaceutical companies, medical associations and (unfortunately) most health departments must be treated with great caution. Significant economic forces are at play. For example, "In 1995, an international high technology research firm, Frost & Sullivan, projected that the worldwide human vaccine market will increase from $2.9 billion to more than $7 billion by the year 2001" (Fisher BL, 2000).

More recent estimates show the extent to which the worldwide market has grown. In 2010, *Pharmaceutical Technology* concluded "The market for vaccines is increasing quickly, and major pharmaceutical companies such as Pfizer (New York) and

GlaxoSmithKline (London) are competing for a greater share of it. Two new market-research reports describe the market's recent growth and predict future market expansions.

The world market for preventative vaccines was worth $22.1 billion in 2009, compared with a value of $19 billion in 2008, according to market-research firm Kalorama Information. The firm's latest report, titled "Vaccines 2010: World Market Analysis, Key Players, and Critical Trends in a Fast-Changing Industry," predicts that the worldwide vaccine market will grow at a compound annual rate of 9.7% during the next five years. The growth will result from the introduction of new products and the expanding use of current products…

In its new report titled "Vaccines Review and Outlook 2010," Canon Data Products Group predicts that the vaccine market will grow at an estimated annual rate of 14% during the next five years, thus outpacing the growth in the oncology market. The global vaccine market will achieve $34 billion in sales by 2012, according to Canon's report."(Greb E. 2010).

Readers must draw their own conclusions as to how this type of economic pressure may influence the public statements of such bodies.

3.1 Basic arguments for routine vaccination

In simple terms: according to modern science, tiny living organisms known as *antigens* (i.e. viruses or bacteria) cause infectious diseases. When faced with an invasion of antigens, the body sends out *antibodies* to combine with and neutralise the antigens. It was found that by *attenuation* (chemically or biologically reducing the virulence of the antigen) and introducing this substance into humans through injection or ingestion (oral doses), antibodies would be produced. This increased pool of disease-specific antibodies would help to combat any subsequent invasion by a virulent strain of the antigen by quickly stimulating further antibody-based response to the antigen. Because the organism was partially deactivated, recipients would not get the disease. Thus, vaccination developed into one of the most common medical interventions currently practiced.

According to orthodox science, there are two broad types of immunological response:

(i) Humoral immunity, which is concerned with antibody and complement activities and is stimulated by antigen-specific groups (clones) of B-lymphocytes; and

(ii) Cellular immunity, which is dependent upon T-lymphocytes and designed to directly destroy or contain antigen cells.

Antibody-related immunity is due to those activated B-lymphocytes that do not become plasma cells, but continue to reside as 'memory' cells in lymphoid tissue. Even more recent study suggests that the principal first defence against viral attack is the production and release by virus-infected cells of a small protein called *interferon,* which acts on other cells to render them resistant to viral infection. Interferon may be related to the body's Vitamin C status.

So in simple terms, the following is a summary of the arguments supporting routine vaccination:

- When a person is exposed to an infectious disease (*antigens*), the body produces *antibodies* and other sensitised white blood cells to combat the infection.
- After the infection subsides, the person is left with a pool of 'memory' cells, and this 'immunologic memory' helps the person resist the infection should contact with the disease occur again.
- An 'immunologic memory' can be artificially generated by administering *attenuated* (partly or totally killed or inactivated) doses of the antigenic material. These doses will be mild enough to avoid infection, but strong enough to stimulate production of antibodies and memory cells.
- Antibody production is increased by artificially slowing down the release of attenuated toxins by using chemical *adjuvants* (such as Aluminium Phosphate).
- Thus, vaccination can provide a high level of protection against infectious disease without the disadvantage of suffering the distressing symptoms of the disease, and possible residual effects.

In addition to these simple arguments, which are understandably appealing to many people, supporters of routine vaccination can point to undisputed successes with some vaccination programs, whereby introduction of the program resulted in an immediate reduction in the incidence of the disease. Interestingly, the number of successful programs is not as high as supporters claim. This is demonstrated in Section 3.4.1 following, in which the actual disease trends before and after mass vaccination programs were introduced are presented.

Nevertheless, pharmaceutical companies and their agents use these results to claim that vaccination is broadly effective against most infectious diseases, and suggest that elimination of these diseases will be achieved if as many people as possible are vaccinated.

For example, in a typical enthusiastically pro-vaccination article, Bedford and Elliman state that "Immunisation against infectious disease has probably saved more lives than any other public health intervention, apart from the provision of clean water. Although other factors were important, it would not have been possible to eradicate smallpox without vaccination; the eradication of wild polio from the western hemisphere is largely due to immunisation; and the immense reductions in *Haemophilus influenzae* type b infections, diphtheria, whooping cough, and measles are also evidence of the value of immunization" (Bedford H and Elliman D, 2002, p. 240).

They go on to say that "Health professionals have a duty to provide accurate information to enable parents to make a truly informed decision about their child's vaccinations", but then make clearly incorrect overgeneralizations such as "The routine vaccines are safe" (p. 240), and make a totally inaccurate claim against homoeopathy (discussed in Section 8.6.4).

The pro-vaccination arguments sound very persuasive, and have obviously appealed to the majority of doctors, government officials and politicians to the extent that now vaccination is not only big business but is legally required in some countries.

This has translated into high vaccine coverage rates in most developed countries. For example, data provided by the Australian

Childhood Immunisation Register (which commenced operation on 1/1/1996) showed that at 30th June 2004, 91% of one year olds, 92% of two year olds and 84% of six year olds were fully vaccinated according to the NH&MRC standard vaccination schedule. A more recent study showed over 90% of children fully covered at 12 and 24 months of age, and around 75% at 72 months (Dept. Health and Ageing, 2008). Summaries of age group data are published by the Department of Health and Ageing (www.health.gov.au) Health Insurance Commission in the quarterly Communicable Diseases Intelligence bulletin.

3.2 Problems associated with routine vaccination - summary

There are three basic weaknesses in the theory and the practical implementation of vaccination:

- The primary cause of disease is not simply antigenic, since not all unvaccinated or previously unexposed people become infected when similarly exposed to an identical antigen. The disease *initially* results from sensitivity on a very subtle level of the organism, which causes an inability to cope with invading antigens. This raises the question regarding why some people have natural immunity while others do not. Many other factors are involved in immunity, including genetic characteristics, placental transfer, breastfeeding, as well as individual health, nutritional status, and emotional response to stress. Homoeopaths also believe that inherited chronic predisposing weaknesses called *miasms* are a significant factor (more of that in Section 4).
- Injection or ingestion of antigens does not necessarily produce the same results in all individuals. At best, these vaccines increase toxins in the body which may cause some of the many side effects associated with vaccination. These side effects are aggravated by the relatively massive doses of antigen administered compared to natural exposure, plus chemicals such as Aluminium Phosphate and Thimerosal used in the vaccines. Further, if injected, the antigenic and chemical material enters the bloodstream almost directly, bypassing the outer or primary immunological defences in the respiratory and the gastro-intestinal tracts. In addition, the protection given by injected antigens is usually temporary, whereas natural exposure to infectious diseases virus generally produces near-permanent immunity (but not 100%).

- Repeated injections of antigens tend to both sensitise the recipient to the disease and destroy the vitality of the immune system on a number of levels. This has been scientifically established, as noted in references to various medical practitioners and researchers in this Section and Section 9. Natural Therapists believe that damage also occurs on the inner, dynamic level from which an individual derives their entire physical and emotional health (Vithoulkas G, 1980).

The *best* position that advocates of routine vaccination can take is that the program offers a significant level of protection against targeted diseases, and that the known side-effects (and yet to be demonstrated side-effects) are less than the potential risks of the disease, and are worth the risk.

It will be shown below that perhaps the most important question to be asked concerning the long-term side-effects of routine vaccination has not been adequately considered. What is needed is a twenty year study of two groups of children from infancy, with one group to receive routine vaccinations and one group to remain unvaccinated. Their general health and a complete disease history should be compared at the end of the period. **Until such a study is carried out, no 'scientific' claims can be made about the long-term safety and efficacy of vaccines.**

This is even more apparent when one considers the current movement towards using combination vaccines. For many years the triple antigen vaccine (DPT) was the best known combination vaccine. Then the measles-mumps-rubella (MMR) vaccine appeared in the 1980's. These are called trivalent vaccines because they have three antigenic components. We are now being exposed to hexavalent vaccines (6 components) such as DTaP/HBV/IPV/Hib, and some researchers are proposing a combination vaccine containing all antigenic components.

The editors of the *British Medical Journal* made the following statement "The safety, efficacy, and immunogenicity of a combined vaccine may be affected by interactions, not only between antigens but also between these and other components such as adjuvants, stabilisers, and preservatives. Research on combination vaccines is more difficult than on single antigen vaccines because they are replacing widely used single vaccines, making trials with placebos unethical. The disease may no longer be common, so the production of antibodies or immunogenicity, rather than protection from the disease (clinical efficacy), has to be assessed. This may be satisfactory when antibody concentrations correlate closely with protection, but for some diseases (for example pertussis) this is not the case. Thus post-marketing surveillance is essential" (BMJ Editorial, 2003a).

In other words, we can "study" a new vaccine thoroughly, but we don't really know what will happen until after the vaccine is released. Very often we must wait years until a complete picture of possible adverse events becomes available, and years before the efficacy of the vaccine in a variety of practical situations can be established.

They go on to give an example of how the diphtheria vaccine is more effective when conjugated (combined) with an effective whole cell pertussis vaccine, but much less effective if combined with the less effective acellular pertussis vaccine. Similar results are found with the Hib vaccine. They continued; "However, there has been a rise in Hib cases in fully immunised children in the United Kingdom. This is probably in part due to the use of a combined DTaP/Hib preparation" (BMJ Editorial, 2003).

Despite assurances to the contrary, we are dealing with uncertainty.

Thus, it is clear that vaccination does not offer a perfect solution.

A reasonable person should therefore ask the question: "*Is there a genuine alternative to vaccination?*" As will be shown in Section 4, the answer is a definite *YES*.

As parents, the first line of protection you can give your child involves:

- Ensuring adequate ongoing nutrition for yourselves and your children with a balanced diet
- No more than a moderate alcohol intake, and no smoking
- Breastfeeding, where possible, to around nine to twelve months
- Providing an emotionally stable home environment for your children
- Ensuring safe and effective treatment if an infectious disease is contracted. Well known medical homoeopath Dr Dorothy Shepherd wrote that, during local outbreaks of disease, conventional

practitioners would complain that she always had the "easy" cases; her reply was that her method of treatment - homoeopathy - made her cases appear easy (Shepherd D, 1967).

- Constitutional treatment, which will elevate general vitality and immune competence.

Then to maximise the second line of protection against specific diseases, parents may support the above general measures with disease-specific preventatives against targeted infectious diseases. This is when the decision between vaccination and the homoeoprophylaxis needs to be made.

In this Section we shall examine vaccination, and in Section 4 following we shall examine the homoeopathic option, or *homœoprophylaxis*. In both Sections, my aim is to present balanced information. It is clear that the object of this book is to provide parents with choices, and this aim is not served by only presenting the negatives of vaccination, and the positives of homœoprophylaxis. Vaccination is a legitimate option, with both strengths and weaknesses.

We shall begin by looking at the historical use of mass vaccination in Australia, the timing of which is usually similar to that in other developed countries. Then we shall consider in turn the general effectiveness and the general safety of vaccines.

We shall examine the actual data showing deaths and notifications of targeted diseases, both before and after the introduction of mass vaccination, as well as a broad look at the type of evidence produced by the medical community supporting the effectiveness of vaccines.

The major problems with vaccination in general will be discussed. This will be followed by a look at individual vaccines (this information has now been placed in Appendix 9.2). The following material will support the conclusions summarised in Table 3-1.

Table 3-1 A Summary of Conclusions Concerning Vaccination

SUMMARY OF CONCLUSIONS

1. Vaccination does provide protection against many infectious diseases
   (a) The long-term success of vaccination programs has been overstated.
   (b) Most new vaccines are thoroughly trialled (but not always).
   (c) The effectiveness of most vaccines seems high, but field results are variable.

2. The safety of vaccines is not known with certainty.
   (a) Short-term testing is undertaken, but results are not consistently reliable.
   (b) Long-term testing of single health effects is incomplete.
   (c) Long-term testing of adverse events and of overall wellness has not been done.

3. Vaccination is a generally (but not completely) effective method of disease prevention. The short-term adverse events have been underestimated, and the true long-term health consequences have not been researched thoroughly.

It can be seen from these general conclusions that vaccination has some benefits and some risks. These will be compared in Section 5 with the benefits and the risks of homœoprophylaxis. Readers will then be better able to make an informed decision as to which method of disease-specific prevention they wish to use.

3.3 The historical use of vaccination

The historical use of vaccines in Australia from 1966-2000 was summarised by McIntyre and others, and is shown in Table 3.2 following (McIntyre et.al. 2002), with subsequent main new vaccines following.

Table 3-2 The Use of Mass Vaccination in Australia

Vaccine	Public sector		Private sector	
	Australia	**Exceptions**	**Australia**	**Exceptions**
OPV (oral polio vaccine)	1966		1994	Qld (? 1998) NSW 1966 Tas 1966
DTPw (whole cell P)	1953		1994	WA 1988
Rubella (adolescent girls)	1971			
MMR (infant dose)	1989		1994	NSW 1989 Qld 1989
MMR (adolescent dose)	1994	SA 1996	1994	WA 1993 SA 1996
ADT	1982		1994	WA 1988
CDT	1975		1994	WA 1988
Hib vaccines (infants born from Feb 1993)	1993 April		1993 April	
Hib vaccines (all infants aged <5 years)	1993 July	WA 1993 Jan NT 1993 April	1993 July	WA 1993 Jan NT 1994
DTPa boosters (infants aged 18 mths and 4-5 yrs)	1997 Sept	Tas 1997 Oct Qld 1997 Dec	1997 Sept	Tas 1997 Oct Qld 1997 Dec

Vaccine	Public sector		Private sector	
	Australia	Exceptions	Australia	Exceptions
DTPa (infants aged 2, 4 and 6 months)	1999 Feb	NT 1997 Aug SA 1997 Aug Tas 1999 Feb Qld 1999 April	1999 Feb	NT 1997 Aug SA 1997 Aug Tas 1999 Feb Qld 1999 April
Hep B (at-risk infants)	1987	NT 1988 Jan SA 1996	Not funded by the C'wealth	NSW 1987
Hep B (adolescent dose)	1998 Jan	Qld 1998 March Tas 1998 March NT 1998 April NSW 1999 SA 1999	?1998	Qld 1998 March Tas 1998 March NT 1998 April NSW 1999
Hep B (universal infant dose)	2000 May	NT 1990 Aug	2000 May	NT 1994
Vaccines on the current National Immunisation Program became free of charge in the public and private sector in all jurisdictions in 1999/2000. All scheduled childhood vaccines became free in the private sector in the Australian Capital Territory in 1993 (except for MMR vaccine which became free in the private sector in 1994) and in the Northern Territory in 1994. **2000-2007**				
Vaccine				
Pneumoccal conjugate 7-valent	2001	Non Aboriginal and Torres Straight Is.		
Varicella			2001	
Meningococcal C conjugate	2003		2002 Aug and Oct	

Vaccine	Public sector		Private sector	
	Australia	Exceptions	Australia	Exceptions
Pneumococcal conjugate 7-valent	2005 Jan	adults		
Pneumococcal conjugate 23-valent	2005 Jan	infants		
Inactivated Polio (IPV) replacing OPV	2005 Nov			
Varicella	2005 Nov			
Human papilloma virus	2007 Apr			
Rotavirus	2007 May	NT 2006 Oct		

Key to Vaccines for Tables 3-2 and 3-3:

(note that some of the technical names will be explained in Appendix 9.2 on individual vaccines, such as PRP-OMP for Hib vaccination)

OPV Oral polio vaccine (or, IPV – inactivated polio (combination) vaccine)

DTPw Diphtheria-tetanus-whole cell pertussis vaccine

DTPa Diphtheria-tetanus-acellular pertussis vaccine; infant/child formulation (or,

dTpa Aadult/adolescent formulation DTPa vaccine)

ADT Combined diphtheria-tetanus vaccine; adult formulation (or, dT)

CDT Combined diphtheria-tetanus vaccine; child formulation

Hib Haemophilis influenzae type b vaccine: Hib1 = PRP-T, HbOC (non-indigenous children); Hib2 = PRP-OMP (all children)

MMR Measles-mumps-rubella vaccine.

Hep B Hepatitis B vaccine: HepB1 = monovalent; HepB2 = monovalent or in combination with DPTa; HepB3 = in combination with Hib(PRP-OMP); HepB4 = for teenagers who have not received infant doses).

HPV Human papiloma virus vaccine.

MenCCV Meningococcal C conjugate vaccine.

7vPC 7-valent pneumococcal conjugate vaccine.

23vPPV 23-valent pneumococcal polysaccharide vaccine.

VZV Varicella (Chicken Pox), 1 = children with a negative history of varicella.

Pneum Pneumococcal vaccine: Pneum1 = 7-valent conjugate vaccine; Pneum2 =23-valent polysaccharide vaccine; Pneum3 = Pneum2 for indigenous Australians

Inf Influenza, annual vaccine: Infl = for indigenous Australians.

Rotavirus vaccine.

The standard Australian Vaccination Schedule in 2010 is shown in Table 3-3. It will be similar to schedules used in most developed countries, although some national differences will exist, such as the national indigenous vaccination program in Australia.

Table 3-3 Standard Australian Vaccination Schedule

	Option 1	Option 2
Birth	Hep B	
2 months	Combined DTPa-Hepatitis B HiB; Polio; Pneum (7vPCV); Rotavirus	Combined Hib (PRP-OMP) - Hepatitis B; DPTa; Polio; Pneum (7vPCV); Rotavirus
4 months	Combined DTPa-Hepatitis B HiB; Polio; Pneum (7vPCV); Rotavirus	Combined Hib (PRP-OMP) - Hepatitis B; DPTa; Polio; Pneum (7vPCV); Rotavirus
6 months	Combined DTPa-Hepatitis B HiB; Polio; Pneum (7vPCV); Rotavirus	DPTa; Polio; Pneum (7vPCV); Rotavirus
12 months	MMR; Meningococcal C; Hib	Combined Hib (PRP-OMP) - Hepatitis B; MMR; Meningococcal C;
18 months	Chicken pox	
4 years	DTPa; MMR; Polio	
12-13 years	HPV	
14 years	DTPa	
	Seasonal Influenza	
	Additional vaccines for Aboriginal and Torres Straight Islanders	

This information will be useful when examining disease trends in Section 3.4.1 following.

3.4 The general effectiveness of vaccines

The effectiveness of vaccines can be tested by directly examining clinical trials and other epidemiological testing of individual vaccines. It also can be tested by examining the historical trends in a disease both before and after mass vaccination was introduced.

We shall begin by looking at historical data, then consider vaccine testing in general, and finally look at some individual vaccines.

3.4.1 Actual disease trends - a diagrammatic summary

One of the most common claims made by advocates of routine vaccination is that the procedure is responsible for eliminating common infectious diseases from communities which have been well vaccinated.

This argument is *not* generally supported by historical data, and the trends in infectious diseases give some indication of the true impact of vaccines.

The diagrams for the following diseases have been prepared from figures kindly provided by the Department of Health and Human Services (USA), Department of Health and Social Security (UK), and the Commonwealth Department of Health (Australia):

- Whooping Cough
- Measles
- Poliomyelitis
- Tetanus
- Diphtheria

Where available, figures for both notifications and deaths are included for each disease, as well as the dates when vaccination programs were introduced on a community wide basis.

Detailed information on each of the following diseases is presented in Appendix 9.1, and further comments on individual vaccines are given in Appendix 9.2.

3.4.1.1 Whooping Cough

As shown in the diagrams which follow (refer Figures 3-1 to 3-4), deaths from whooping cough were virtually eliminated *before* vaccination programs were introduced; however, there was some reduction in notifications following vaccination. The whooping cough vaccination is generally recognised as one of the least effective routine vaccines and, as will be shown, has an uncertain safety record.

Figure 3-1 shows that whooping cough in the USA was clearly declining prior to the introduction of mass vaccination. The reader does not need scientific qualifications to understand this fact, just an ability to observe and an open mind.

Note: in all the following Figures, the arrows show when mass vaccination programs were introduced. When figures are scaled down, the ratio is shown as e.g., "/25".

Figure 3-1 Whooping Cough: USA

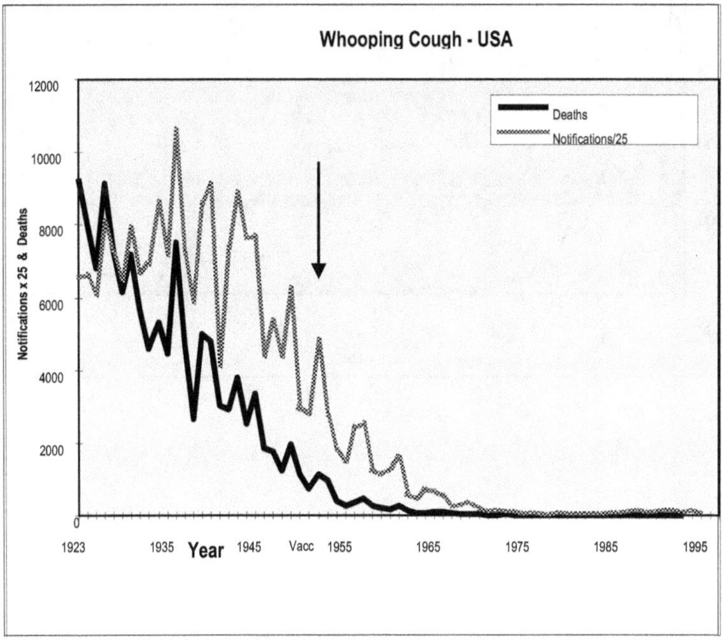
Whooping Cough - USA
Deaths
Notifications/25
Notifications x 25 & Deaths
12000
10000
8000
6000
4000
2000
0
1923
1935
Year
1945
Vacc
1955
1965
1975
1985
1995

The UK experience of the 1960's and late 1970's is regularly cited in defence of routine vaccination; many UK parents stopped vaccinating their children at these times due to stories of terrible damage resulting from the Triple Antigen vaccine. Claims of thousands of deaths due to the decline in vaccination rates are heavily exaggerated (see Figures 3-2 and 3-3). In fact, the figures clearly support suggestions by Professor Gordon Stewart, amongst others, that whooping cough attacks were grossly over-reported in 1978 and 1982 by doctors eager to prove to parents that vaccination is necessary (refer section 9.2.13). The ratio of deaths to notifications is also totally unbalanced (refer section 9.2.13, Table 9-4).

Figure 3-2 Whooping Cough: England & Wales

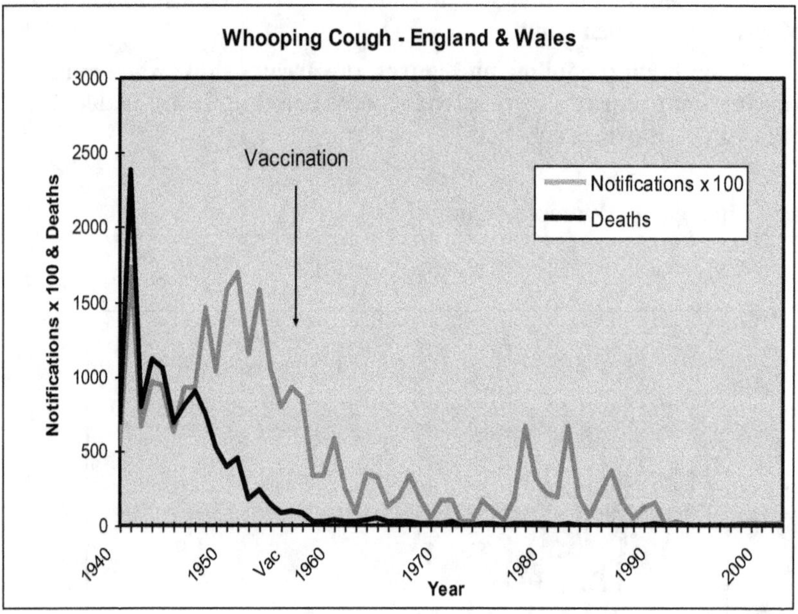
Whooping Cough - England & Wales
Notifications x 100 & Deaths
3000
2500
2000
1500
1000
500
0
Vaccination
Notifications x 100
Deaths
1940
1950
Vac
1960
1970
1980
1990
2000
Year

Figure 3-3 Whooping Cough: England & Wales 1965-1985 (Detail)

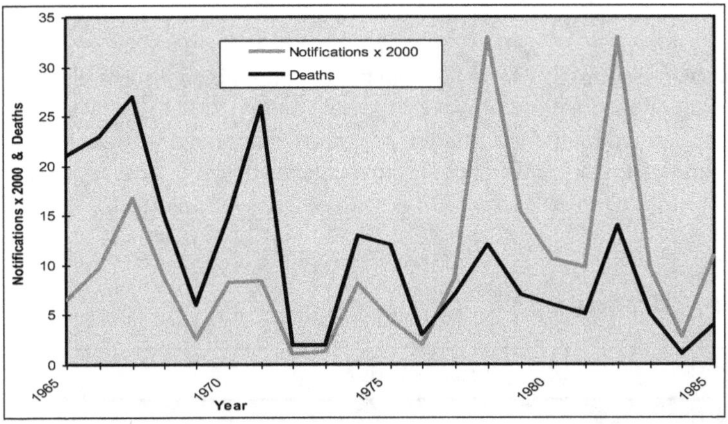
Notifications x 2000
Deaths
Notifications x 2000 & Deaths
35
30
25
20
15
10
5
0
1965
1970
1975
1980
1985
Year

I was not able to discover the full figures for notifications of whooping cough in Australia over the period of time examined. However the figure for deaths shown in Figure 3-4 indicates once again that the trend was already in decline well before the introduction of mass vaccination.

Figure 3-4 Whooping Cough: Australia

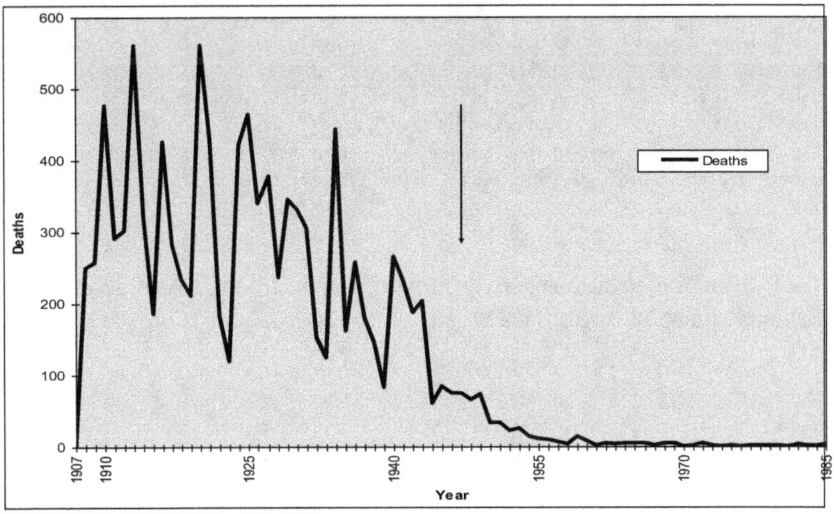
Deaths
Deaths
600
500
400
300
200
100
0
1907
1910
1925
1940
1955
1970
1985
Year

3.4.1.2 Measles

Deaths from measles were also practically eliminated prior to the introduction of vaccination; however, the decline in notifications was clearly accelerated by the vaccination programs, and credit must be given to vaccination for its clear impact on the incidence of the disease.

Figure 3-5 Measles: USA

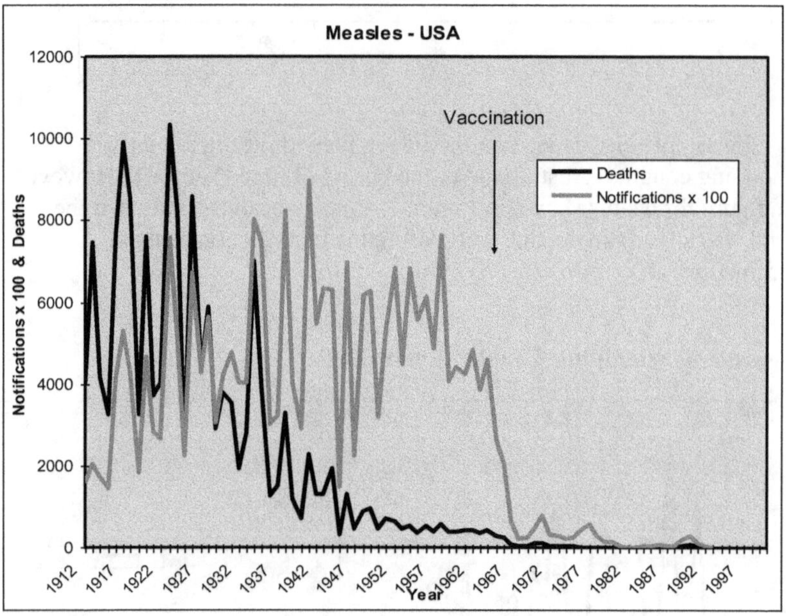
Measles - USA
Vaccination
Deaths
Notifications x 100
Notifications x 100 & Deaths
12000
10000
8000
6000
4000
2000
0
1912
1917
1922
1927
1932
1937
1942
1947
1952
1957
1962
1967
1972
1977
1982
1987
1992
1997
Year

Similar conclusions may be drawn from the UK and Australian figures in the following Tables.

Figure 3-6 Measles: England & Wales

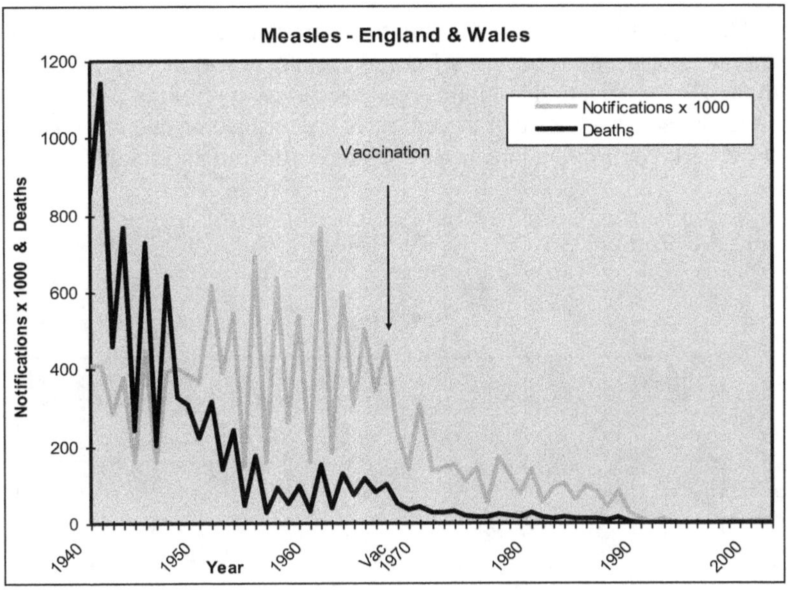
Measles - England & Wales
Notifications x 1000 & Deaths
1200
1000
800
600
400
200
0
Notifications x 1000
Deaths
Vaccination
1940
1950
Year
1960
Vac
1970
1980
1990
2000

Figure 3-7 Measles: Australia

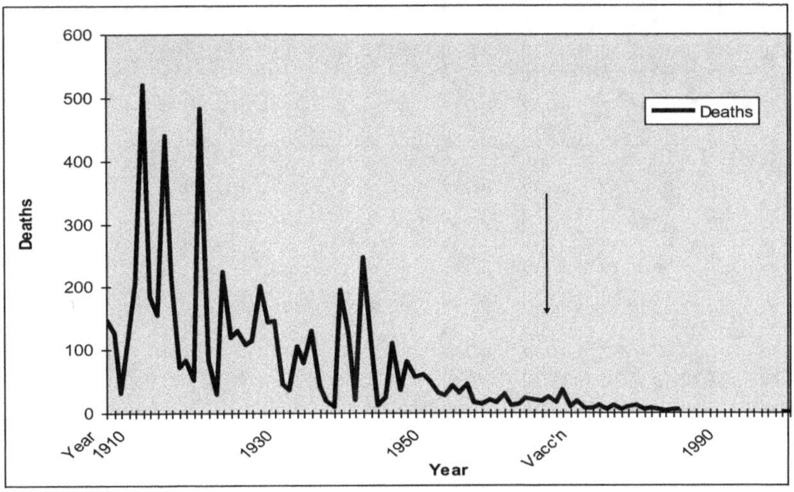
Deaths
600
500
400
300
200
100
0
Deaths
Year
1910
1930
1950
Vacc'n
1990
Year

3.4.1.3 Poliomyelitis

The figures for polio are difficult to interpret accurately. The peaks in deaths and notifications occurred *before* vaccination was introduced. Although the vaccination programs *appeared* to have reinforced the decline, there is evidence that these figures are misleading due to a change in the criteria for notifications from 1958 onwards (refer section 9.2.15).

Figure 3-8 Polio: USA

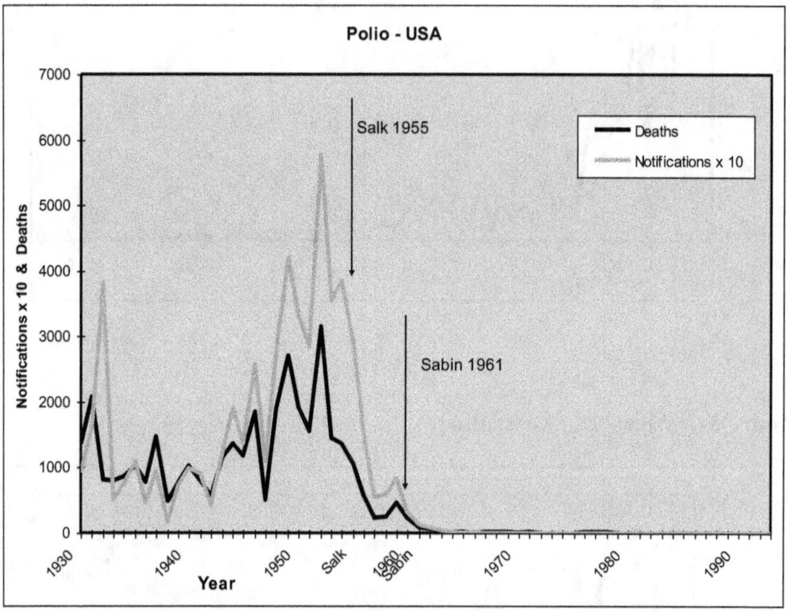
Polio - USA
Salk 1955
Sabin 1961
Deaths
Notifications x 10
Notifications x 10 & Deaths
7000
6000
5000
4000
3000
2000
1000
0
1930
1940
1950
Salk
1960
Sabin
1970
1980
1990
Year

Figure 3-9 Polio: England & Wales

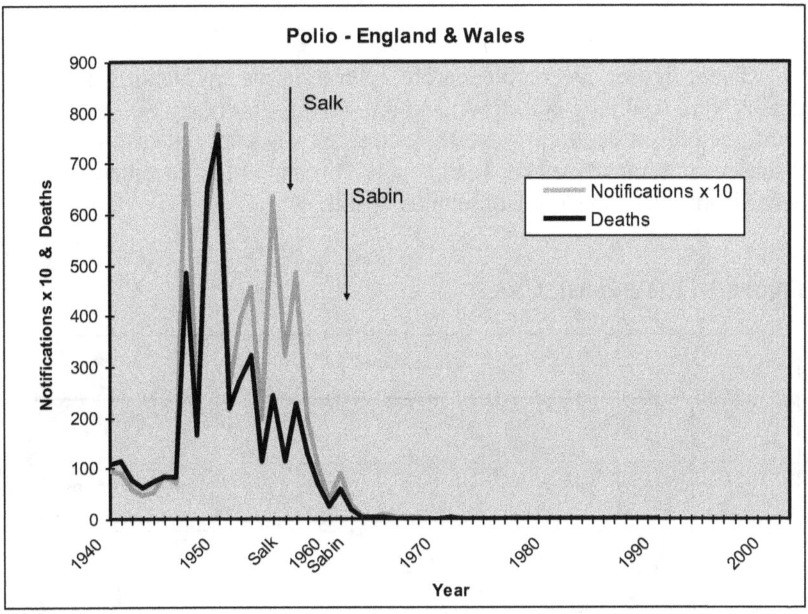
Polio - England & Wales
900
800
700
600
500
400
300
200
100
0
Notifications x 10 & Deaths
Salk
Sabin
Notifications x 10
Deaths
1940
1950
Salk
1960
Sabin
1970
1980
1990
2000
Year

Figure 3-10 Polio: Australia

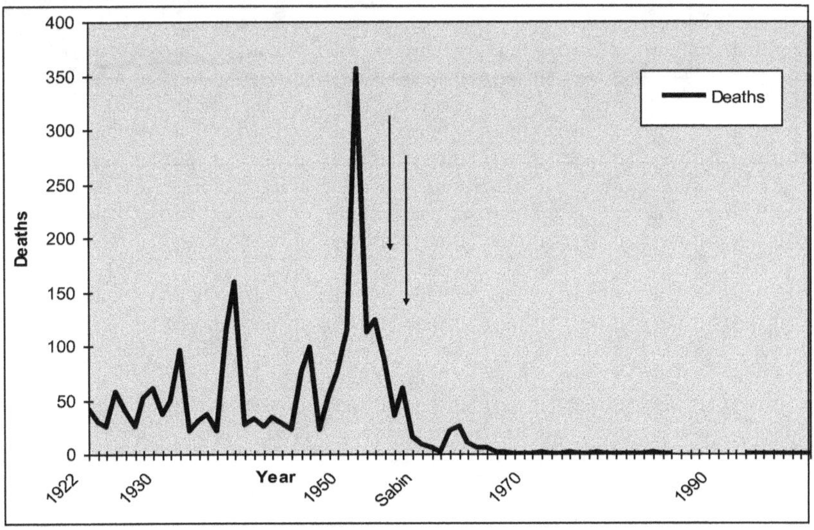
400
350
300
250
200
150
100
50
0
Deaths
Deaths
1922
1930
Year
1950
Sabin
1970
1990

3.4.1.4 Tetanus

These figures also require careful interpretation. While trends in deaths were declining before vaccination, the program may have reinforced this reduction. Nevertheless, tetanus is a special case since the disease is not transferred between people - no amount of vaccination can actually eradicate the 'pool' of tetanus in soil, etc.

Figure 3-11 Tetanus: USA

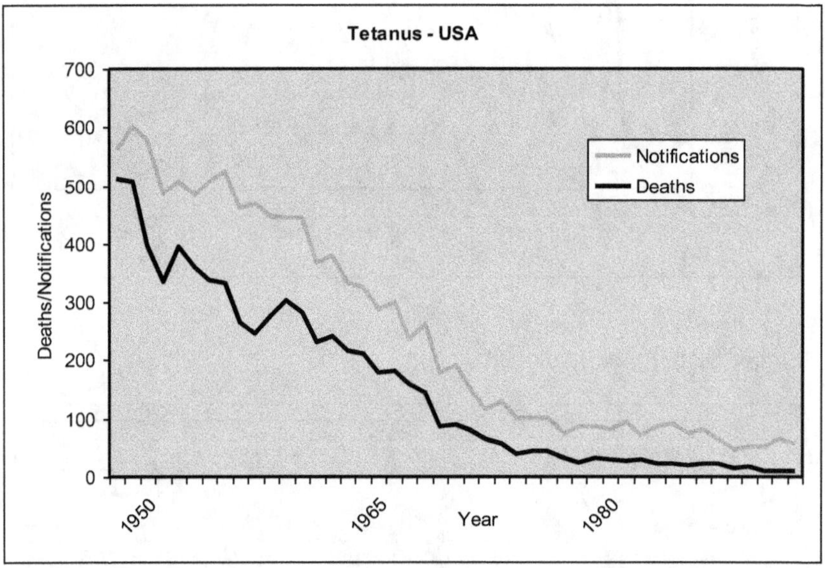
Tetanus - USA
700
600
500
400
300
200
100
0
Deaths/Notifications
Notifications
Deaths
1950
1965
Year
1980

Figure 3-12 Tetanus: England & Wales

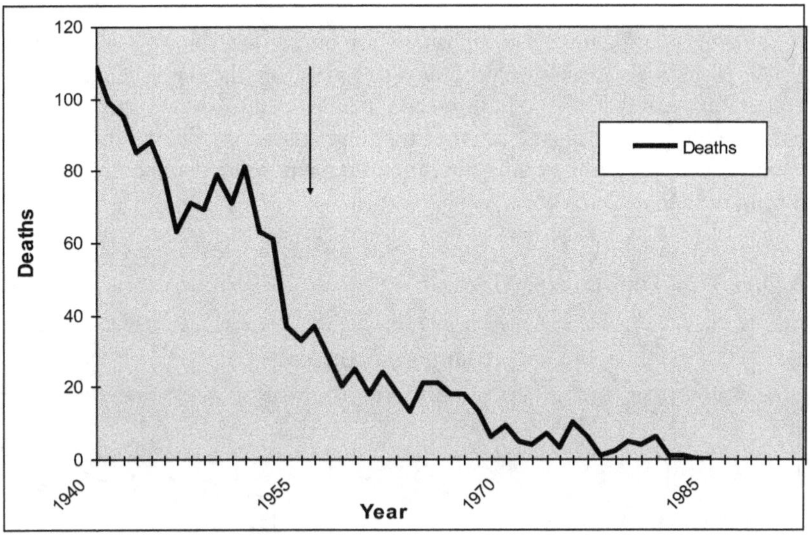
120
100
80
60
40
20
0
Deaths
Deaths
1940
1955
1970
1985
Year

Figure 3-13 Tetanus: Australia

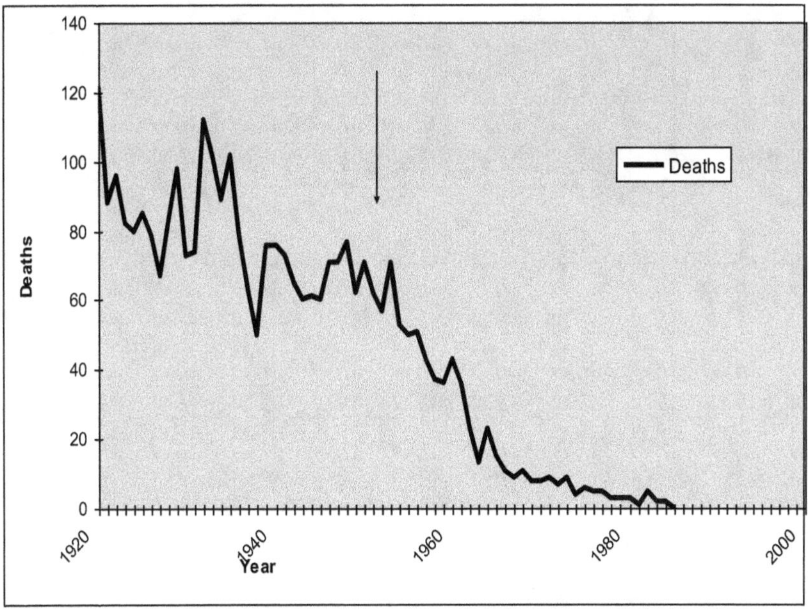
140
120
100
80
60
40
20
0
Deaths
Deaths
1920
1940
1960
1980
2000
Year

3.4.1.5 Diphtheria

Figures for deaths from diphtheria are only given for Australia and the USA. The USA vaccination programs began before the reported data collection started. Thus no definite conclusions can be drawn from Figure 3-14. However, it is clear from the Australian data that the diphtheria vaccination program had only a minimal impact on the decline in deaths during the 1900's.

Figure 3-14 Diphtheria: USA

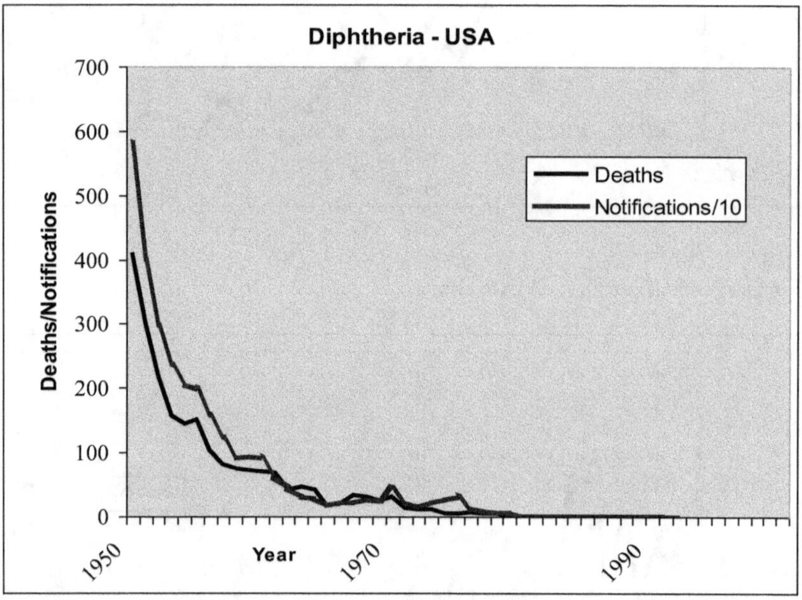
Diphtheria - USA
700
600
500
400
300
200
100
0
Deaths/Notifications
Deaths
Notifications/10
1950
Year
1970
1990

Figure 3-15 Diphtheria: Australia

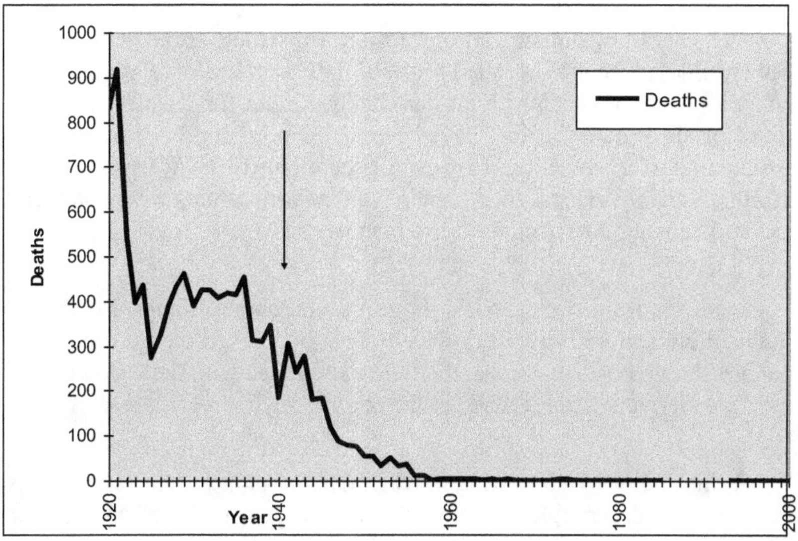
Deaths
1000
900
800
700
600
500
400
300
200
100
0
Year
1920
1940
1960
1980
2000

Conclusions regarding historical impact of vaccination

As the figures clearly indicate, vaccination programs have had mixed successes in lowering deaths and/or notifications for these infectious diseases. Although some programs clearly lowered the incidence (notification) of a particular disease, others obviously did not. Most programs had only a marginal impact on death rates for each of the diseases.

Certainly, **it cannot be generally claimed that vaccination has been responsible for the elimination of infectious diseases**, the credit for which must be largely attributed to improved sanitation and waste disposal, personal hygiene and nursing care, and the reduction of severe nutritional deficiencies in the countries considered. These improvements are what are still needed in third world counties, rather than vaccines which can and do produce terrible side effects in malnourished children (Kalokerinos A, 1974).

3.4.2 Clinical trials and other measures of vaccine effectiveness

The scientific gold-standard for testing substances is the randomised, double-blind, placebo-controlled trial. Initially there were relatively few such tests made of vaccines. This has changed in recent decades, and clinical trials of new vaccines have become the normal procedure prior to introduction of the vaccines. However, exceptions do exist; for example, no clinical trials of Hepatitis B vaccine in newborn infants were conducted prior to licensing the vaccine for use in newborns.

Evidence from clinical trials shows us a number of things. Firstly, the results of clinical trials can vary widely. Secondly, even though a clinical trial has shown positive results, the field experience with the vaccine can be very different when it is used in the community (see Table 3-4).

A third point worth making in general about pharmaceutical products is that even with scrupulous testing, the true long-term side effects of drugs and vaccines can only be revealed with hindsight, and often only decades after the drug or vaccine was released. This point is seen every year when drugs that have previously passed through double-blind clinical trials are removed from use due to unexpected side effects.

We see it also with vaccines; for example, in the replacement of whole cell vaccines with "safer" a-cellular vaccines and the withdrawal of the Rotavirus vaccine in 1999 (see Section 3.5.4). I am certainly not suggesting that a continuing search for improvements should not be made, but the point is that the orthodox community used to state that the whole cell vaccines were safe to use, and that the Rotavirus vaccine was safe. Now they are saying something else is much safer, thus confirming that the previous products were relatively unsafe.

Some examples of the issue of inconsistency of results are shown below in Table 3-4, for whooping cough (pertussis), measles and mumps. The NH&MRC figures will be given first, as they typically present the most optimistic figure for efficacy. Other trials will then be shown, to make the point that there is inconsistency with results.

A fourth point relates to the extent to which the integrity of researchers influences the results of clinical trials. This has repeatedly been shown in the orthodox literature to be of great concern, due often to the corrupting influence of pharmaceutical sponsors (McGauran N, 2010).

In the interests of accuracy, it is certainly possible to find many examples of vaccine failures in the medical literature (Lancet, 1988), but they at times are due to a batch of vaccines being incorrectly manufactured, or stored, or administered. These one-off examples do not prove that vaccines in general are ineffective. In fact it is clear from an objective look at research that vaccines do offer a level of protection against targeted infectious diseases. It is also clear that Health Department literature presents the best possible figures for efficacy. The real-life experience may be very different.

In summary, it is reasonable to conclude that current vaccines are generally tested in clinical trials, and most provide a significant level of protection against targeted diseases in the trial settings. However, the real efficacy of vaccines in practice may be much less than the best estimate given by authorities. Further, claims that vaccines were the reason why many infectious diseases have nearly disappeared are overstated.

Table 3-4 The Variability of Clinical Trials of Vaccine Efficacy

Pertussis
(1) NH&MRC (2003) *The Australian Immunisation Handbook*, 8th Edition, p. 207. States that pertussis vaccine is more than **80%** effective through to six years of age, following three doses at 2, 4 and 6 months of age.
(2) Gustafsson L, et al, (1996) A Controlled Trial of a Two-Component Acellular, a Five-Component Acellular, and a Whole-Cell Pertussis Vaccine. *NEJM* Vol 334:349-356 Feb. 8, 1996, No. 6
Two-component, acellular, DPT [efficacy **58.9%** (95% C.I. 50.0-65-9)]
Five-component, acellular, DPT [efficacy **85.2%** (95% C.I. 80.6-88.8)]
Whole-cell DPT [higher rates of crying, cyanosis, fever, local reactions than other 3 – efficacy **48.3%** (95% C.I. 37.0-57.6)]. Note: C.I. = confidence intervals
DT (as a control)
Vaccines given at 2, 4, 6 months of age, children were followed for signs of pertussis for an additional 2 years.

Measles

(1) NH&MRC (2008) *The Australian Immunisation Handbook*, 9th Edition, p. 203. States that measles vaccine is **95%** effective after one dose, and **99%** effective after two doses.

(2) Puri A., et.al. (2002) Measles Vaccine Efficacy Evaluated by Case Reference Technique. *Indian Paediatrics*. 39: pp. 556-560.

The relative risk was calculated to be 2.6, indicating that an unvaccinated child is 2.6 times more prone to develop measles as compared to a vaccinated child. Vaccine efficacy by case-reference method was **62%.** This and similar findings show that efficacy is significantly affected by the general health of the recipient.

Mumps

(1) NH&MRC (2008) *The Australian Immunisation Handbook*, 9th Edition, page 224. States that mumps vaccine has a **95%** seroconversion, but effectiveness between 60 and 90%.

(2) Schlegel M, et al, (1999) Comparative efficacy of three mumps vaccines during disease outbreak in eastern Switzerland: cohort study. *BMJ*; 319: p. 352 (7 August)

Attack rate in unvaccinated people 63% (a common result)

Rubini strain – 67%; Jeryl-Lynn strain – 14%; Urabe strain – 8%

Best efficacy – **84%** - (C.I. 64 – 94%)

This latter study shows that efficacy is heavily dependant on which strain of mumps the person is exposed to, and it can be significantly less than 95%.

3.5 General safety of vaccines

3.5.1 Routine vaccination - a summary of risks

In this section we examine the risks associated with the general practice of routine vaccination, and include relevant material extracted from the considerable but fragmented body of information on the dangers of this practice. The purpose of this summary is to provide factual information on which to base your own decision concerning vaccination, as well as to provide material which can be shown to health professionals willing to consider all the facts involved in this difficult issue.

As well, this section demonstrates that *any* person who says vaccination is a **totally** safe and effective procedure is either a fool or a liar - and probably both. This is not to say that the risks from vaccination are greater or less than the risks involved in the diseases themselves; that issue is considered throughout the book.

Note: One reviewer commented that medical professionals do not claim vaccination to be totally safe and effective. While this may be so officially (and responsible GP's don't make this claim), many parents say that they have never been informed of the possible risks, and that they have been told vaccination is safe and effective. **If it is officially recognised that vaccination has limitations, why do health officials refuse to even investigate an alternative (homoeopathy), which has no toxic side effects, has a written clinical record of effectiveness over 200 years, and now has considerable data to support effectiveness and safety?** - The corrupting influence of pharmaceutical lobby groups?

3.5.2 The general risks of routine vaccination

One of the first major works by an orthodox practitioner detailing the risks of routine vaccination was written in 1966 by Sir Graham Wilson (Wilson G, 1967). At the time, Sir Graham was Honorary Lecturer in the Department of Bacteriology at the London School of Hygiene and Tropical Medicine. Formerly Director of the Public Health Laboratory Service, England and Wales, he was clearly neither a radical, nor unqualified to discuss this topic.

In his conclusions, Sir Graham stated, "I want to make it abundantly clear that I am not an anti-vaccinationist . . . Vaccines, of one sort or another, have conferred immense benefit on mankind but . . . they have their dangers"(Wilson G, 1967, p.289).

While clearly a supporter of the general principle of vaccination, Sir Graham was also acutely aware of the possible dangers. He did not unquestioningly accept that every vaccine was worth using simply because it had been developed; neither did he believe in the indiscriminate use of vaccines. His work principally examined the short to medium term observable risks of vaccination, and although written 40 years ago, his findings, which are summarised in Table 3-5, are still valid today, since some of the vaccines are still in use, and the principles of the method remain largely unchanged.

Table 3-5 Wilson's Summary of Direct Adverse Reactions to Vaccination

Type of Reaction	Vaccine Involved
1 Severe Systemic (involving entire system)	1 Measles
2 Specific Homologous disease, e.g. Polio	2 Polio
3 Specific Heterologous (different in origin) disease, e.g., Tetanus	3 Diphtheria, Tetanus, Pertussis
4 Intoxication, e.g., with Tetanus Toxin	4 Diphtheria, Tetanus
5 Provocation Disease, e.g., Polio	5 Comb. Tetanus/Pertussis, Polio
6 Suppuration	6 Diphtheria toxoid
7 Neuritis (nerve inflammation)	7 Tetanus antiserum
8 Encephalomyelitis (inflammation of brain, spinal cord)	8 Pertussis, Tetanus
9 Anaphylaxis (allergic reaction to vaccine)	9 Egg based vaccines, Tetanus
10 Damage to foetus	10 Vaccinia

Sir Graham's work represents only the first step in this review of the risks of vaccination, and although there are major factors he did not consider, his research clearly shows that vaccination is *not* a risk-free procedure that can be used without question or careful patient evaluation.

In his own words, "The inherent danger of all vaccination procedures should be a deterrent to their unnecessary or unjustifiable use"(Wilson G, 1967, p.282).

Another respected medical writer and general supporter of vaccination was George Dick, Professor of Pathology at London University, who also held responsible Public Health positions. Professor Dick stated that, "Every vaccine carries certain hazards and can produce untoward reactions in some people . . . in general, there are more vaccine complications than is generally appreciated."(Dick G, 1978, p. 15). While he believed that, in the case of some diseases, the benefits of vaccination outweighed the risks, he also spoke out against indiscriminate vaccination.

Medical journals such as the *Lancet*, the *British Medical Journal*, and *JAMA*, all contain many references to the possible dangers of vaccination. In addition to these references, a number of distinguished medical authors in Britain, the United States, and Australia have strongly argued against indiscriminate vaccination. For example, one of the best known of these medical authors in Britain, Professor Gordon Stewart, conducted a very public campaign against the pertussis (whooping cough) vaccine some decades ago, supporting his arguments with facts and figures.

Some will also be familiar with the writings on this subject of the late Professor Robert Mendelsohn, and Dr Harold Buttram, both from the United States. Medical Homoeopath, Dr Richard Moskowitz, has also made valuable contributions to the debate.

In Australia, Dr Archie Kalokerinos pioneered work which identified the risks of vaccination in malnourished children (Kalokerinos A, 1974). He was later joined in this and other research by the late Dr Glen Dettman.

Internationally, many concerned doctors contributed to *The International Vaccination Newsletter*, which was started in 1993 by Belgium MD, Dr Kris Gaublomme.

Dr H L Coulter and B L Fisher have thoroughly and accurately researched and documented the risks of the Triple Antigen vaccine (Coulter H L and Fisher B L, 1985). Every concerned parent should purchase this 470 page paperback, which gives access to medical literature without the need for struggling with difficult and obscure references; it also contains disturbing information concerning 'behind the scenes' actions of pharmaceutical companies. This book led to vaccine damage compensation being introduced into the USA – a remarkable accomplishment.

Coulter and Fisher list fourteen significant short-term side effects of the DPT vaccine, which can also apply to other vaccines. These are listed in Table 3-6 below.

Table 3-6 Coulter & Fisher's Short-Term Side Effects of the DPT Vaccine

	Type of Reaction
1	Skin reactions
2	Fever
3	Vomiting and diarrhoea
4	Cough, runny nose, ear infection
5	High pitched screaming, persistent crying
6	Collapse or shock-like episodes
7	Excessive sleepiness
8	Seizure disorders - convulsions, Epilepsy
9	Infantile spasms
10	Loss of muscle control
11	Inflammation of the brain
12	Blood disorders Thrombocyteopenia, Haemolytic Anaemia
13	Diabetes and Hypoglycaemia
14	Death and Sudden Infant Death Syndrome (SIDS)

Many parents can attest to the accuracy of this list first hand. Indirectly, pharmaceutical companies also acknowledge its accuracy, as indicated by the warnings to health personnel printed on vaccine instruction leaflets. Their findings are also supported by medical research; for example, that conducted by Cody, Baraff, and others (Cody CL et al, 1981).

In addition to these short term side effects, Coulter and Fisher list three major areas of possible long term damage, shown in Table 3-7.

Table 3-7 Coulter & Fisher's Long-Term Side Effects of the DPT Vaccine

Type of Effect
1. severe neurological damage
2. brain damage, learning disabilities, and hyperactivity
3. allergy and hypersensitivity

Possibly the most disturbing aspect of their book, however, is the number of reported case histories where doctors administering vaccines completely ignored patients' previous reactions to vaccination, in some cases resulting in death. Such cases give parents undeniable evidence that they are ultimately responsible for their children's health, a responsibility which cannot be passed on to others.

This conclusion was reinforced by a survey of doctors in Australia, which showed that "54% would give DPT when it is clearly contra-indicated." (MacIntyre C R, Nolan T, 1994). Subsequent surveys have shown that little has changed in the last 10 years.

In Section 3.5.9, a pre-vaccination checklist is presented as an Appendix. It would be interesting to know how many parents of vaccinated children have actually been shown the list prior to vaccination. My guess is – not many. In Section 3.5.9, a list of adverse events following vaccination that are required to be reported is given as an Appendix. **Many parents tell stories of how a doctor has refused to acknowledge that an event, which the parents know was caused by vaccination, is actually vaccine-related.** In other words, many events go unreported. Further examples of non-compliance problems will be given in this Section.

Coulter and Fisher's work was effectively verified by the medical community itself. In 1991, the US Government's principal advisory body on health, The Institute of Medicine, released a report titled the *Adverse Effects of Pertussis and Rubella Vaccines* (Institute of Medicine, 1991). Their findings are summarised in Table 3.8 following.

Table 3-8 Summary of the Institute of Medicine's Conclusions by Adverse Event for DPT and RA 27/3 Rubella Vaccine

Conclusion	DPT VACCINE	RA 27/3 RUBELLA VACCINE
No evidence bearing on a causal relation (i.e., cannot tell yes or no from evidence)	Autism	
Evidence insufficient to indicate a causal relation (i.e., cannot tell yes or no from evidence)	Aseptic Meningitis, Chronic Neurologic Damage, Erythema Multiforme or other rash, Guillain- Barré Syndrome, Haemolytic Anaemia, Juvenile Diabetes, Learning Disabilities and Attention Deficit Disorder	Radiculoneur-itis and other neuropathies Thrombo-cytopenic Purpura
Evidence does not indicate a causal relation (probable no)	Infantile Spasms, Hypsarrythmia, Reye Syndrome, Sudden Infant Death Syndrome	
Evidence is consistent with causal relation (possible yes)	Acute Encephalopathy Shock and 'unusual shock-like state'	Chronic Arthritis
Evidence indicates a causal relation (probable yes)	Anaphylaxis and protracted, inconsolable crying	Acute Arthritis

Although the work of Coulter and Fisher is very thorough, there are other aspects to consider. Perhaps the most serious potential consequences of routine vaccination relate to subtle damage to a child's immune system and the possible creation of genetic abnormalities. Some of these effects are outlined below.

* Dr Moskowitz, who has written extensively about vaccination, has shown that, just as 'slow viruses' (e.g. Subacute Sclerosing Panencephalitis - SSPE) can occasionally occur in nature as a result of a badly managed viral infection, the unnatural process of vaccination can lead to slow viruses developing in the body, giving rise to the "far less curable chronic diseases of the present, with their amortisable suffering and disability" (Moskowitz R, 1985).
* In 1982, Drs Buttram and Hoffman warned of "the probability of

widespread and unrecognised vaccine-induced immune system malfunction, and the need for scientific investigation of these effects". They identified "the lowering of the body's resistance resulting from vaccinations. Since this effect is often delayed, indirect, and masked, its true nature is seldom recognised."(Buttram H and Hoffman J C, 1982).

* Dr Buttram also expressed concern that a 'Jumping Gene' phenomenon may arise because vaccines are often prepared in animal embryos or serum. This may cause the vaccines to become "carriers, incorporating their genetic material into the invaded cells . . . permanently weakening the immune system of the individual" (Buttram H, 1987).

The IOM went further. In September 1993 they released a report entitled *Adverse Events Associate with Childhood Vaccines: Evidence Bearing on Causality*. Their report was summarised in a Special Communication in the *JAMA*, which in part stated that "The committee found that the evidence favoured acceptance of a causal relation between diphtheria and tetanus toxoids and Guillain-Barré syndrome and brachial neuritis, between measles vaccine and anaphylaxis, between oral polio vaccine and Guillain-Barré syndrome, and between unconjugated Hib vaccine and susceptibility to Hib disease. The committee found that the evidence established causality between diphtheria and tetanus toxoids and anaphylaxis, between measles vaccine and death from measles vaccine-strain infection, between measles-mumps-rubella vaccine and thrombocytopenia and anaphylaxis, between oral polio vaccine and poliomyelitis and death from polio vaccine-strain viral infection, and between hepatitis B vaccine and anaphylaxis" (JAMA special communication, 1994)

The community-wide incidence of these events is very very low (it is of course 100% if your child is one of those affected), but they happen, and this proves that **no vaccine is completely safe**.

The NH&MRC have listed the potential ill effects of vaccines (NH&MRC, 2008, back cover). As we saw when examining the NH&MRC figures for vaccine efficacy, their summary presents vaccination in the best possible light. Readers should not accept that the NH&MRC material is a complete list of possible adverse events, but as a starting point only. A comprehensive study of long-term damage has never been undertaken, or at least, has never been published

Table 3-9 presents an example of common adverse events following vaccination publicly released by the South Australian Government. It is similar to the NH&MRC list, and in fact the latest SA site (2010) defaults to the NH&MRC website. Other examples of further complications will be presented in Section 3.6.

http://www.health.sa.gov.au/immunisationcalculator/immcalc-about-imm.htm.

Table 3-9 Adverse Events Following Vaccination

Vaccine	Side effects of vaccination
DTPa Diphtheria Tetanus Pertussis (acellular)	DTPa vaccine (Serious adverse events are less common than with DTPw) □Irritable, crying, unsettled and generally unhappy □Drowsiness or tiredness □Localized pain, redness & swelling at injection site □Occasionally injection site nodule . may last many weeks (no treatment needed) □Low grade temperature (fever)
Hepatitis B	□Localized pain, redness & swelling at injection site □Occasionally injection site nodule . may last many weeks (no treatment needed) □Low grade temperature (fever)
Hib	□Localized pain, redness & swelling at injection site □Occasionally injection site nodule . may last many weeks (no treatment needed) □Low grade temperature (fever)
Influenza	□Drowsiness or tiredness □Muscle aches □Localized pain, redness & swelling at injection site □Occasionally injection site nodule . may last many weeks (no treatment needed) □Low grade temperature (fever)

Vaccine	Side effects of vaccination
MMR Measles Mumps Rubella	Occasionally injection site nodule . may last many weeks (no treatment needed) Seen 7 to 10 days after vaccination: Low grade temperature (fever) lasting 2-3 days, faint red rash (not infectious), head cold and/or runny nose, cough and/or puffy eyes Drowsiness or tiredness Swelling of salivary glands
Meningococcal type C	Irritable, crying, unsettled and generally unhappy Loss of appetite Headache (usually observed in adolescent/adults) Localized pain, redness & swelling at injection site Occasionally injection site nodule . may last many weeks (no treatment needed) Low grade temperature (fever)
Pneumococcal (7vPCV) (23vPPV)	Conjugate vaccine (7vPCV) Localized pain, redness & swelling at injection site Occasionally injection site nodule . may last many weeks (no treatment needed) Low grade temperature (fever) Polysaccharide vaccine (23vPPV) Localized pain, redness & swelling at injection site Occasionally injection site nodule . may last many weeks (no treatment needed) Low grade temperature (fever)
Polio	OPV: (Oral Polio Vaccine) Occasional diarrhoea (no treatment usually needed but parent or carer must wash hands carefully after changing nappies) IPV: (Inactivated Polio Vaccine – injected) Muscle aches Localized pain, redness & swelling at injection site Occasionally injection site nodule . may last many weeks (no treatment needed)

Vaccine	Side effects of vaccination
	Low grade temperature (fever)
Rubella	Bruising or bleeding Local inflammation and discomfort Swollen glands Localized pain, stiff neck, joint pains Rash Low grade temperature (fever)
Varicella (chickenpox)	Localized pain, redness & swelling at injection site Occasionally injection site nodule . may last many weeks (no treatment needed) Low grade temperature (fever) Seen 5-26 days after vaccination: Pustular rash (2-5 lesions) usually at injection site which occasional covers other parts of the body

Some other general points are:

- Other writers have produced evidence that the contamination of animal sera (blood) used in vaccine production with various animal retro-viruses is an ongoing problem (Rappenport J, 1988).
- A 1994 study of 446 children and adolescents demonstrated that children who received the pertussis vaccine were 5.43 times more likely to develop asthma in later years, over twice as likely to have ear infections, and significantly more likely to spend longer periods in hospital than those who had not receive the vaccine (Odent M. et al, 1994c). Thus, clear evidence is emerging of a long term weakening of the immune system due to vaccination.
- Dr Robert Gallo, the US expert who first identified the AIDS virus, raised the possibility of a relationship between the spread of AIDS in Central Africa and the World Health Organisation's (WHO) Smallpox vaccination campaign (Gallo R, 1987).
- WHO figures show that the greatest spread of the HIV infection coincides with the areas receiving the most intense vaccination programs. This may also explain why the disease in Africa is more evenly spread between males and females than it is in the West.

- Dr Eva Snead noted that, since 1953, the polio vaccine has been cultured in cells from the African Green Monkey. At times, these cells have been shown to be contaminated with the SV-40 virus, which is closely related to the AIDS virus. Dr Snead speculated that contaminated polio vaccine may be responsible for the current epidemics of leukemia, childhood cancer, and birth defects as well as immune deficiency diseases (Snead E L, 1987).

In addition to these physical consequences, practising homoeopaths have stated for over 150 years that vaccination causes changes on the dynamic plane. These dynamic changes may produce a range of physical complications, as well as insidious complications over time, that is, chronic 'miasmic' diseases. (*Note:* In homoeopathy, a *miasm* is a diathesis or predisposition to a group of symptoms).

Table 3-10 below gives my summary of possible long-term side-effects; this list is by no means complete. Some of the side effects listed have been demonstrated by research, while others are still to be proved. These effects are *not* intended to be mutually exclusive, and the frequency of these side effects occurring in practice is certainly in dispute; miasmic damage, for example, is believed by homoeopaths to be a common reaction.

Table 3-10 A Summary of Some of the Long-Term Side-Effects of Vaccination

	Type of Reaction
1	Severe neurological damage
2	Brain damage affecting learning and behaviour
3	Allergy and hypersensitivity
4	General damage to the immune system
5	Slow viruses
6	Genetic abnormalities - Jumping Gene phenomenon
7	Viral transference
8	Trigger mechanism for immune system diseases
9	Dynamic (miasmic) damage.

This information, most of which reports the concerns of scientifically trained people, should be sufficient to make all but the most biased reader hesitate before imposing mass vaccination on future generations of our children. At the very least, it shows that in general terms, **mass vaccination is not a risk free procedure**. Parents deserve to be told the truth when they are forced to make decisions regarding their children. The "never you mind, doctor knows best" approach employed by many in orthodox medicine is condescending, and as unacceptable today as it should have been in years gone by.

3.5.3 Vaccination and Sudden Infant Death Syndrome (SIDs)

At the end of this Section, a special report on the link between vaccination and some cases of cot death (SIDs) is presented (see Section 3.5.8). It is not suggested that vaccination is the only cause of SIDs, but the material provides clear, objective evidence that it is a contributing factor in some cases.

Some commentators have stated that the conclusion regarding SIDs is meaningless because this is the age at which SIDs occur anyway, so they will always occur near one of the 2, 4 or 6 months vaccines. Two points need to be made here.

1. It is entirely plausible that one reason why early infancy is the prime time for SIDs is the fact that the infant's immune system is stressed by vaccines at birth, as well as at 2, 4 and 6 months of age.

2. The material presented in Section 3.5.8 does not rely on opinion, it relies on objective observations. And the observations point to one of the causes of SIDs being vaccination.

I repeat, I am not in any way suggesting that vaccination is the only cause of SIDs – it clearly is not (unvaccinated children die from SIDs). I certainly believe that vaccination is a contributing factor in some cases of SIDs.

3.5.4 Why vaccines cause damage

Having examined some of the damaging effects of vaccination, this section briefly considers the causes.

Sir Graham Wilson listed six major causes for the adverse reactions he had identified (Wilson G, 1967). These causes are summarised in table 3-11 below.

Table 3-11 Summary of Direct Causes of Vaccine Damage

	Type of Direct Cause
1	Normal toxicity
2	Faulty production
3	Faulty administration
4	Allergy
5	Other causes: abnormal sensitivity of patients
6	Indirect effects: damage to foetus, provocation disease

Point 1 acknowledges that vaccines contain potentially toxic material. Examples of these toxins will be given when we examine each individual vaccine in Section 9.2 below. Sometimes however, the researchers and the regulators just get it wrong – either by underestimating the potential problems with a particular vaccine, or simply by not following their own rules. A classic example of this relates to the withdrawal of the Rotavirus vaccine in October 1999 following its release earlier in the year. The following material was presented by Michael Belkin concerning the actions of Dr John Modlin, the then Chairman of the ACIP (Advisory Committee on Immunisation Practices), the body providing immunisation recommendation in the USA. He stated:

"..at the February 1999 ACIP meeting Chairman Modlin lobbied for the ACIP to recommend the Rotavirus vaccine for premature infants, although no safety studies had been done, much less peer reviewed or published … As a member of the Vaccines and Related Biological Products Advisory Committee (VRBPAC) and Chairman of the Rotavirus working group, Modlin had data showing a risk of intussusception (life threatening bowel obstructions) in clinical trials of Rotavirus before that February 1999 meeting. The Rotavirus vaccine was withdrawn from the market in October 1999 after 113 cases of intussusception. One premature baby died after getting rotavirus vaccine in a vaccine cocktail and another five-month-old died after developing intussusception five days after the receipt of the vaccine" (Belkin M, 2000).

Point 2 suggests that at times batches of vaccines are even more dangerous than usual. For example, "A toxic batch of pertussis vaccine caused gross brain damage to a baby vaccinated 23 years ago, the Irish Supreme Court has ruled. Three judges unanimously held that the Wellcome Foundation, the vaccine's manufacturers, liable for the plight of Kenneth Best, now 23, but with a mental age of around 12 months". It had been found that "Wellcome's tests had been inadequate and that the company had been negligent in releasing the batch, which had failed the mouse weight gain test and exceeded recommended potency and toxicity levels" (BMJ report, 1992).

While Sir Graham focused on problems related to the vaccine itself (points 1 to 2), problems with the administration of the vaccine (point 3), and problems with recipients (points 4 to 6), there is another class of reasons why the procedure of vaccination can lead both to significant acute and chronic problems. These causes are listed in Table 3-12 following.

The six procedural causes listed create what I call a *perverted response syndrome* (PRS). In other words, the natural mechanisms of immunity are perverted by the process of vaccination. The acute fevers, diarrhoea, and rashes arising during a natural infection show that the body is fighting the antigen and driving it from the body.

Since vaccines rarely invoke the full immune response (despite adverse reactions), the modified antigen may linger in the body. In fact, the chemical adjuncts are designed to cause this. The *slow viruses* referred to by Dr Moskowitz may arise as a consequence of this perverted response.

A note should be made here regarding the mercury-based preservative thimerosal. This chemical has recently been withdrawn from use in most (not all) infant vaccines, although it is still used in vaccines for adults. The orthodox position is something along the lines of – *thimerosal levels are so low that they pose no risk, however in order to protect very low birth weight infants, and just to reduce the total levels of mercury exposure which have been increased because of food and general environmental chemical, we will remove the chemical from infant vaccines.*

Table 3-12 Summary of Procedural Causes of Vaccine Damage

Type of procedural cause
1 *Administration* The procedure of injection by-passes the normal pathways of infection which our immune system is designed to protect.
2 *Adjuvants* The use of chemicals such as aluminium phosphate both pervert the natural immune response and insert neuro-toxins directly into the system.
3 *Preservation* Chemical preservatives are used to stabilise vaccines. One of the most common is thimerosal, which is a mercury-based compound. Mercury is also neuro-toxic*.
4 *Attenuation* The procedure of altering the antigen with chemicals, heat, etc., leads to an unnatural response and possible toxicity.
5 *Preparation* The procedure of preparing some vaccines in animal (and human) tissues leads to possible genetic abnormalities and disease transference.
6 *Quantity* The quantities of the modified antigen injected are massive in relation to the quantities involved in a natural infection.

Assurances that there is such a thing as a "safe" level of mercury reminds one of assurances given years ago about "safe" levels of lead in petrol, and then the reversal of this position saying that there is no such thing as a safe level of lead. The other issue here is the long-term safety of the new chemicals being used in place of thimerosal – we just won't know until the chemicals have been injected into our children for many years. Constantly in this debate we come back to the question – why take the risk of potential damage when a non-toxic alternative is available?

NOTE: - a startling new report on the link between thiomersal and autism was released in June 2005. I have included extracts from this report as Appendix 4 to Section 3.5.

So, *even if* vaccines were produced without impurities and correctly administered only to people who show no obvious sensitivity, the PRS itself would still represent significant cause for concern.

3.5.5 The link between vaccination and chronic diseases

As part of my research at Swinburne University from 2000 to 2004, I studied the link between different methods of immunisation, including vaccination and homœoprophylaxis, and the long-term incidence of asthma, eczema, ear problems, allergies and behavioural problems. The aim was to use these conditions as markers of overall health. This is the type of research that should be undertaken by orthodox researchers.

The findings have been published in part in *Homœoprophylaxis – A Fifteen Year Clinical Study*, and the following material is taken from that book (Golden I, 2004).

The relationship between vaccination and the five conditions studied is shown in Table 3-13. For those who need a brief introduction to the statistical measures used, a brief introduction is given in Table 3-16.

In summary, the figures in Table 3-13 show that there is a positive relationship between vaccination and all but one of the conditions studied; the Odds Ratios are greater than 1 for every condition except behavioural problems. However, not all the measures are statistically significant (P less than 0.05). **The findings which are statistically significant (confidence greater than 95%) are shown in bold type**. In particular, the figures show a clear and certain link between vaccination and asthma, using orthodox statistical measures of linkage and confidence.

The findings would have been stronger if the numbers surveyed were greater than the 781 children surveyed. Such research is easy to do with adequate funding. The question to be asked of orthodox authorities is - **why has this type of research examining the link between vaccination and long-term diseases not been carried out systematically over the last few decades?**

Surely a procedure which is imposed on the majority of citizens of a country should be tested beyond immediate short-term reactions, and occasional long-term investigations of individual effects. If orthodox authorities are so sure of the long-term safety of vaccination, let them test it objectively, and publish the results. The fact that the results of such testing have not been published leaves open to question the motives of the supporters of vaccination; **if the long-term testing hasn't been done – why not? If the testing has been done – why are the results not published?**

Table 3-13 Long-term Health Effects of Vaccination

Conditions Studied	**Measurement**	**Vaccination** All diagnoses	**Vaccination** GP diagnoses
Asthma	Odds Ratio	**1.75**	**1.89**
	Chi Test P	**0.0025**	**0.0007**
Eczema	Odds Ratio	1.315	**1.76**
	Chi Test P	0.121	**0.006**
Ear/Hearing	Odds Ratio	1.149	**1.517**
	Chi Test P	0.459	**0.04**
Allergies	Odds Ratio	1.220	1.518
	Chi Test P	0.239	0.061
Behaviour	Odds Ratio	0.869	0.784
	Chi Test P	0.593	0.613

I am not alone in these concerns. Some orthodox medical researchers have expressed similar concerns. For example, well known researchers into the link between diabetes and vaccination, Classen and Classen, stated in the *British Medical Journal* that "We believe that the public should be fully informed that vaccines, though effective in preventing infections, may have long-term adverse events". They questioned the value of many safety trials that only recorded reactions shortly following vaccination and thus could not detect long-term autoimmune dysfunctions. "An educated public will probably increasingly demand proper safety studies before widespread immunisation. We believe that the outcome of this decision will be the development of safer vaccine technology" (Classen J B & Classen D C, 1999, p. 193).

One does not need to engage in conspiracy theories to be left with doubts. **But when it comes to the health and safety of our children, there should be no doubts!**

3.5.6 New research into vaccine damaged children

One way to gain an understanding of the damage that vaccination can cause is to examine the symptoms of children who have been treated with homoeopathic potencies of the vaccines which were suspected of causing damage. For example, if case taking reveals that a child has experienced a change in his or her personality ever since receiving the triple antigen vaccine, then one possible treatment strategy is to give to the child potencies of the triple antigen vaccine, along with constitutional and/or symptomatic treatment when appropriate.

If we observe that certain symptoms are removed only by using potencies of a particular vaccine, then we can assume that the vaccine caused the symptoms – simply because there is really no other reason (outside of extreme co-incidence) why the symptoms would be cured.

When we examine a significant number of cases involving various vaccines, we gain some understanding of the range of possible symptoms that vaccinations can cause. We are in effect discovering long-term vaccine damage symptoms in reverse – by finding out what symptoms the homoeopathic treatment for vaccine damage can remove.

Because of my interest in this area for over 25 years I do get regular referrals for patients where vaccine damage is suspected. Some years ago one of my senior students and I analysed a group of my cases where a homoeopathic potency of a vaccine caused a significant removal of disease symptoms. The symptoms were tabulated, and compared to a list prepared totally independently by South African medical homoeopath the late Dr Tinus Smits, who is also experienced in the treatment of vaccine damaged children (web site: http://www.tinussmits.com/english/). The two lists show a remarkable similarity, as shown in Table 3-14.

Table 3-14 Conditions Responding to Treatment for Vaccine Damage

	I. Golden (26)			T. Smits (26)			Combined (52)		
	#	Σ	%	#	Σ	%	#	Σ	%
Behavioural problems	6			4			10		
Speech/learning problems	3			7			10		
Autism	1			0			1		
Epilepsy	3			2			5		
Tourette's syndrome	1	14	28.6%	0	13	25.5%	1	27	27.0%
Listlessness	0			4			4		
Allergies	2			1			3		
Sleep disturbance	2	4	8.2%	0	5	9.8%	2	9	9.0%
Upper respiratory tract problems	8			8			16		
Ears/hearing problems	6			3			9		
Asthma	5			0			5		
Lower respiratory tract problems	1	20	40.8%	7	18	35.3%	8	38	38.0%
Skin problems		6	12.2%		8	15.7%		14	14.0%
Gastrointestinal problems		2	4.1%		7	13.7%		9	9.0%
Raynaud's	1			0			1		
Arthritis	1			0			1		
Migraines	1	3	6.1%	0	0	0.0%	1	3	3.0%
TOTALS		**49**	**100.0%**		**51**	**100.0%**		**100**	**100.0%**

The figures show the count by conditions, which is why there are about twice as many symptoms as there are patients. We clearly see that the top three areas where symptoms have been removed are (1) respiratory tract, (2) brain and (3) skin. To an experienced practitioner, this list makes perfect sense when we consider the types of condition that present for treatment following vaccination – eczema, asthma, and behavioural/learning difficulties.

This work was expanded in 2008 with the publication of my book *Vaccine Damaged Children – Treatment, Prevention, Reasons* (Golden I. 2008), and again in 2010 when additional data was added to the analysis. The latest findings are shown in Table 3-15.

It is important to remember that this book is based on real-world experiences – it is not a theoretical work. Children are vaccinated. Vaccine damage does occur. Vaccine damage is usually treatable, subject to individual strengths and weaknesses and the extent of the initial damage. We **do** have choices and options in both the treatment and prevention of both acute and chronic disease. These are realities we must deal with based on credible information.

If the unthinking advocates of vaccination could see the profound effects of vaccine damage which practitioners face every day in their clinics, they may be more reasonable in their comments. They also may be more considerate towards parents who choose not to vaccinate based on extensive research into potential short and long term effects of vaccination.

People who have chosen not to vaccinate after careful research, are often bitterly criticised by others who are typically ignorant and uninformed about the real issues. This includes some orthodox medical people who have never done any individual research, but who parrot the pronouncements of pharmaceutical funded studies which have found their way into the official policies of Health Departments in this and other countries.

I have the utmost respect and regard for parents who have and are making this difficult journey. They do it knowing that they are actually the most responsible of all participants in this debate, and are placing the wellbeing of their children above their own personal comfort and social acceptance.

Table 3-15: Summary of Results 2001,2008

	2001			2008	
Result	**No**	**%**		**No**	**%**
1 = Strong improvement	9	14.1%		29	11.4%
2 = Improvement	17	26.6%		71	27.8%
3 = No improvement	5	7.8%		12	4.7%
4 = Patient worse	4	6.3%		6	2.4%
5 = Result unclear	13	20.3%		64	25.1%
6 = No follow up	16	25.0%		66	25.9%
7 = Reaction, no follow up	0	0.0%		7	2.7%
Total	**64**	**100.0%**		**255**	**100.0%**
Results excluding no follow ups					
Result	**No**	**%**		**No**	**%**
1 = Strong improvement	9	18.8%		29	15.9%
2 = Improvement	17	35.4%		71	39.0%
3 = No improvement	5	10.4%		12	6.6%
4 = Patient worse	4	8.3%		6	3.3%
5 = Result unclear	13	27.1%		64	35.2%
Total	**48**	**100.0%**		**183**	**100.0%**

The data from my research has enabled symptom profiles of different vaccines to be constructed, two of which are shown below for the DPT and MMR vaccines. They throw light onto the long-term adverse effects of vaccines which the orthodox authorities ignore, which they avoid committing research funds to uncover, and which they pretend are not significant. **Long-term vaccine damage is highly significant, and imposes a huge cost financially and emotionally to the entire community. It is avoidable, it benefits only pharmaceutical multinationals, and history will judge it to be the greatest failure of orthodox medicine in the 20th and 21st centuries.**

Figure 3-16: Symptom profile of the DPT vaccine

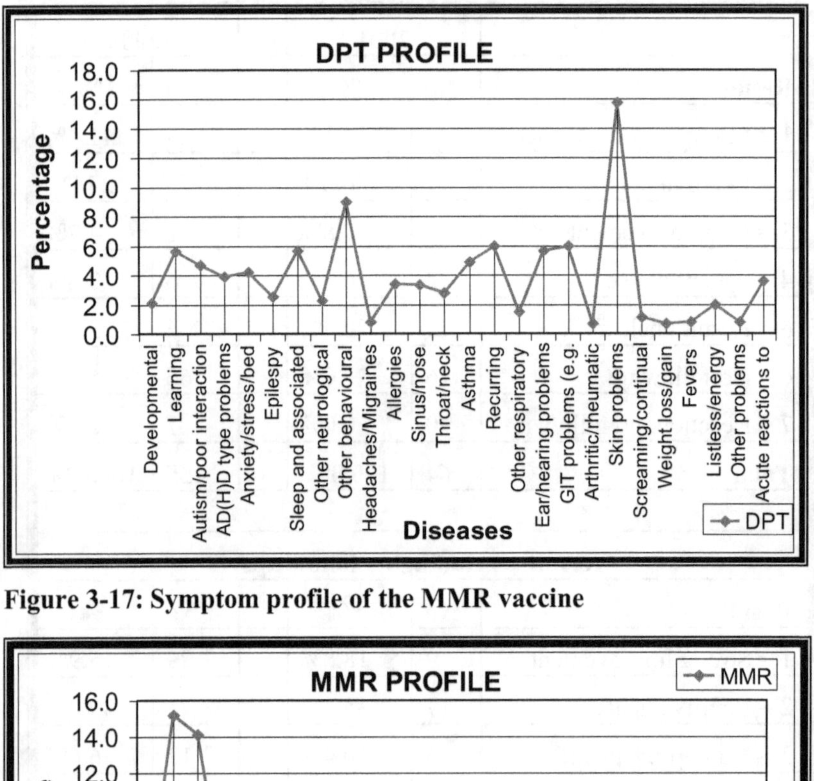
DPT PROFILE
Percentage
18.0
16.0
14.0
12.0
10.0
8.0
6.0
4.0
2.0
0.0
Developmental
Learning
Autism/poor interaction
AD(H)D type problems
Anxiety/stress/bed
Epilespy
Sleep and associated
Other neurological
Other behavioural
Headaches/Migraines
Allergies
Sinus/nose
Throat/neck
Asthma
Recurring
Other respiratory
Ear/hearing problems
GIT problems (e.g.
Arthritic/rheumatic
Skin problems
Screaming/continual
Weight loss/gain
Fevers
Listless/energy
Other problems
Acute reactions to
Diseases
DPT

Figure 3-17: Symptom profile of the MMR vaccine

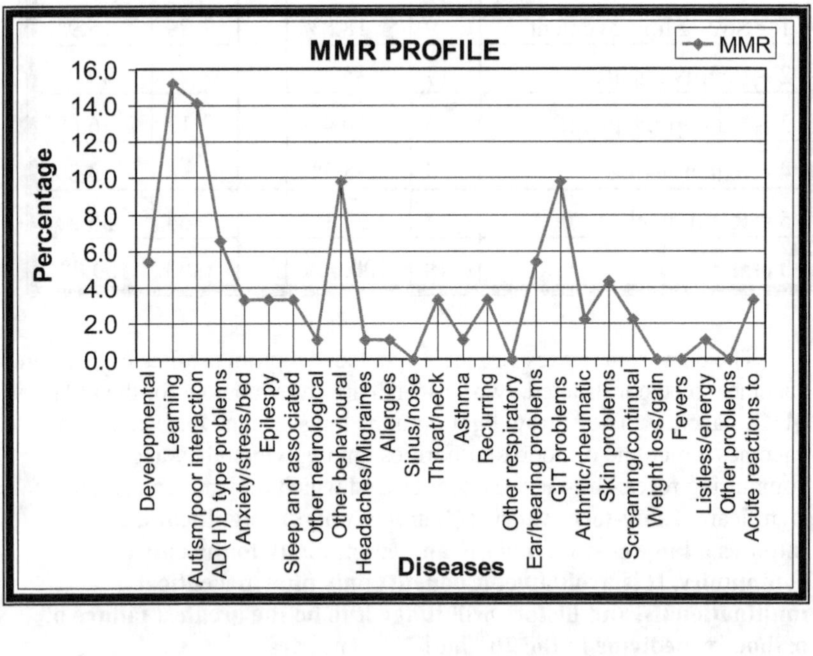
MMR PROFILE
MMR
Percentage
16.0
14.0
12.0
10.0
8.0
6.0
4.0
2.0
0.0
Developmental
Learning
Autism/poor interaction
AD(H)D type problems
Anxiety/stress/bed
Epilespy
Sleep and associated
Other neurological
Other behavioural
Headaches/Migraines
Allergies
Sinus/nose
Throat/neck
Asthma
Recurring
Other respiratory
Ear/hearing problems
GIT problems
Arthritic/rheumatic
Skin problems
Screaming/continual
Weight loss/gain
Fevers
Listless/energy
Other problems
Acute reactions to
Diseases

A final point to note here is that potencies of vaccines are appropriate to use in treating vaccine damage – NOT for use in the prevention of infectious diseases. Whilst they may have some protective effects, the Nosodes of the targeted diseases are much more appropriate for prevention purposes.

3.5.7 Conclusions to Section 3.5

The above material, and the information provided in the following three Appendices, demonstrates that **vaccination is *not* a totally safe procedure**; although the safety of some vaccines has been improved, it appears that unquestioning acceptance of routine vaccination is unjustified. It certainly shows that **parents should *not* leave the decision to vaccinate their children to others with a vested interest in the procedure.**

Many parents struggle with the question of whether the risk of vaccine-induced damage is greater or less than the risk of damage due to the infectious diseases that vaccines are designed to prevent. **Until appropriate long-term studies are carried out, the question of long-term safety will remain unresolved**.

Since there is sufficient evidence to raise genuine doubts concerning the value of routine vaccination, the examination of the other method of disease-specific protection against infectious diseases in Section 4 becomes even more appropriate. It is indeed a shame that orthodox authorities are not prepared to examine the following material with an open and "scientific" mind. As mentioned in Section 3.5.10 below – 'Secrecy is the antithesis of the true scientific method'.

An open and honest examination of all issues, on both sides of the debate, is what is most needed to restore confidence that our children are subjected only to safe and effective procedures.

A NOTE FOR PARENTS WHEN READING THE LITERATURE: This is not an easy topic to research. The language used is often difficult to access without scientific training. Further, when an article questioning vaccines is published with a plain English summary, it is attacked using technical terms which make the attack sound "scientific".

My experience is that the more intentionally complex a response is, the less it can be trusted. Truth does not need to be hidden behind complexity. Just remember that for every argument for, there is an equally convincing argument against any finding. And ask, if you can, who is funding the author.

Table 3-16 A Simple Explanation of Basic Statistical Measures

SOME SIMPLE STATISTICS – measuring the relationship between a condition (such as asthma), and possible causes (the type of immunisation used)

The **Odds Ratio** (OR) is a measure of the relationship between a condition (asthma), and a variable (the method of immunisation). When OR>1 (i.e., when the Odds Ratio is greater than 1), we can say there is a positive link between asthma and the method of immunisation. When OR<1, we can say there is a reduced likelihood of asthma if the particular method of immunisation is used.

The **Chi Squared Probability** (P) gives us a statistical measure of how definite the relationship shown by the OR really is. The lower the figure for P, the less the likelihood of the relationship being one of chance or co-incidence, and thus the greater the likelihood that the relationship is NOT one of chance, i.e., the more confidence we can have that the OR figure does accurately reflect the relationship between the condition and the variable.

Statisticians regard a measure as being statistically significant if P<0.05 (i.e., P is less than 0.05). This is when they talk about the 95% confidence level being achieved.

So IF the figures show that OR<1, and close to OR=0, with a P<0.05, THEN we can say with high statistical certainty that the method of immunization used is actually associated with a reduction in the incidence of asthma.

IF the figures show that OR>1, with a P<0.05, THEN we can say with high statistical certainty that the method of immunization used is actually associated with an increase in the incidence of asthma.

* * * * * * *

3.5.8 Appendix 1 to Section 3.5: Vaccination and Breathing Apnoea

Objective, scientific evidence shows a further area of possible damage relating to vaccination.

In a special scientific paper prepared for the Association for Prevention of Cot Death, Dr Viera Scheibner analysed the findings of computer printouts from babies monitored by COTWATCH (a true breathing monitor, as opposed to a motion monitor) designed by the late Leif Karlsson. These figures are presented with the kind permission of Dr Scheibner.

A number of the printouts recorded episodes of apnoea (cessation of breathing) and hypopnoea (shallow or low volume breathing) before and after DPT vaccination was given. (*Note:* The longer the duration of apnoea or hypopnoea, the greater the risk of Cot Death). Remember, this data is derived from computer monitoring; it is not personally influenced by subjective assessments of the operators or observers. This is objective, scientific evidence.

The data clearly shows that vaccination caused a dramatic increase in episodes where breathing either ceased altogether or nearly ceased. However, the most disturbing aspect of this data is the fact that these episodes continued periodically for months following vaccination. A similar breathing pattern occurred in tests conducted with other children.

Dramatic support for her conclusions appeared in the journal, Australian Doctor, under the heading, "Immunisation implicated in infants' apnoea". Dr P Sanchez, Assistant Professor of Paediatrics at the University of Texas, found that nineteen percent (19%) of infants in his study group "developed either new or increased episodes of apnoea in the 24-48 hours after they were given DPT and Hib conjugate vaccines" (Sanchez P, 1993).

This is precisely what Dr Scheibner has found through the use of Cotwatch!

Dr Scheibner's clear conclusions lend further support to the concerns expressed by other researchers: "The effect of vaccinating babies has never been systematically studied, recorded or analysed. Vaccination is the single most prevalent and most preventable cause of infant deaths. In the face of mounting evidence about the ineffectiveness of vaccination in preventing infectious diseases and the great number of serious short and long term adverse effects of vaccines, the call for suspension of vaccination is now inevitable" (Scheibner V, 1990).

In an extensive recent contribution, Dr Scheibner stated that "Cotwatch computer printouts demonstrate increased stress level in breathing more than 6 weeks after vaccination" (Scheibner V, 2004, p. 12). She also demonstrated how some cases of "shaken baby syndrome" that occurred weeks or months after vaccination were actually consistent with vaccine damage. This is a major contribution, as orthodox researchers typically only look for adverse events that follow relatively soon after vaccination. This clearly results in many cases of vaccine damage being misdiagnosed as being unrelated to vaccination.

EXPLANATORY NOTES: Special Scientific Paper of the Association for Prevention of Cot Death.

- *Figure 3-18* - Computer printout of a three-week record of breathing of an eight month child before and after receiving the third DPT shot.

  Each vertical line represents a histogram of events within one hour. The full length of each vertical line represents 60 events. The horizontal lines show events from 6 to 20 seconds. The events are apneas (6-15 seconds) and hypopneas (more than 15 seconds). The figures on the left-hand side are integrals of the weighted apnea-hypopnea density (WAHD). Non-stressed breathing is characterised by WAHD values in hundreds and (occasionally) not exceeding 2500. The stress-induced breathing pattern is characterised by values over 2500, but is also indicated by persistent values from 1000 to 3000.

- *Figure -19* - The first printout is a summary of Figure 3-18 [18 days less three days of the initial part of Figure 3-18].

  Each vertical column represents a summary of events for 24 hours. An arrow indicates the day when the DPT vaccine was administered. Within 24 hours of the injection, the WAHD values went from 758 to 3437.

  The 48 hour reaction (13,247) was almost four times that of the 24 hour reaction. This was followed by 48 hours of lowered stress reaction (WAHD values of 1084 and 686).

Days 5 and 6 were again characterised by acute stress-induced breathing patterns (WAHD values of almost 12,000), followed by lower, yet still elevated WAHD values for several days.

The acute stress-induced breathing on day 16 is of special interest.

Twenty-seven days after the shot, the child was still experiencing elevated WAHD values (around 2000) for several days, with one major incident on the 27th day.

Two months after the DPT injection, the child experienced elevated WAHD values for another two weeks, with one acute pattern on the 59th day.

Figure 3-18 Computer Printout of Three-Week Record

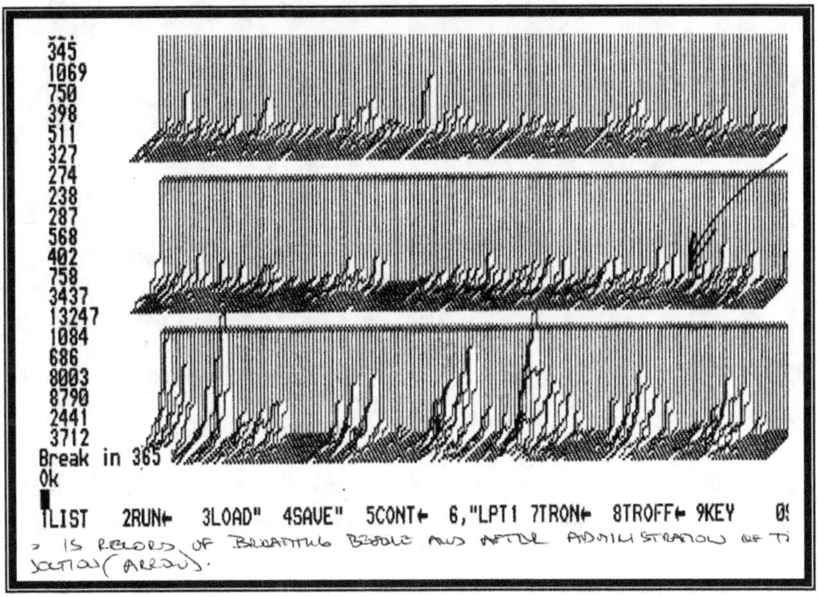
345
1069
750
398
511
327
274
238
287
568
402
758
3437
13247
1084
686
8003
8790
2441
3712
Break in 365
Ok
1LIST 2RUN← 3LOAD" 4SAVE" 5CONT← 6,"LPT1 7TRON← 8TROFF← 9KEY

Figure 3-19 Computer Printouts Summarising Breathing Patterns Over Two Months

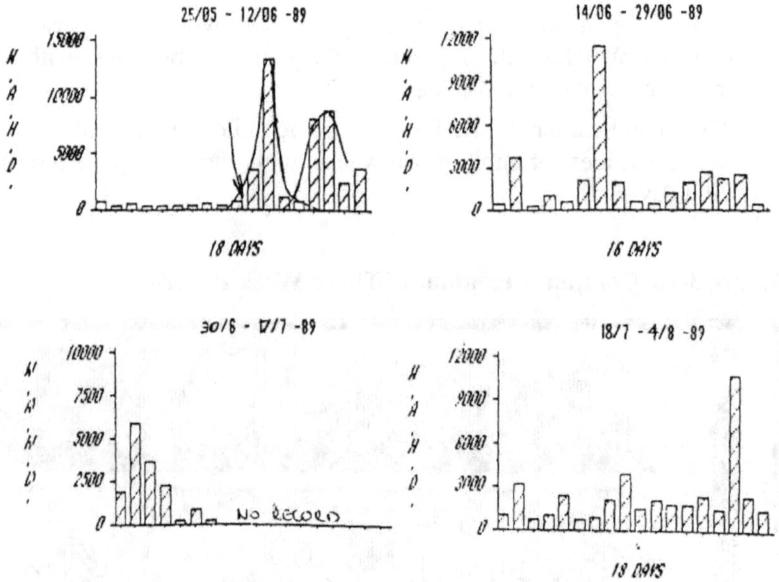
14/06 - 29/06 -89
18/7 - 4/8 -89
No record

(All figures copyright Leif Karlsson, 1989).

3.5.9 Appendix 2 to Section 3.5: Pre-vaccination checklist

The *Australian Immunisation Handbook*, 2008, gives a pre-vaccination checklist, and a pre-vaccination assessment of conditions that may preclude vaccination (NH&MRC, 2008, pp. 9-24, especially p.16).

Parents are asked to advise if any of the following conditions apply (Table 1.3.1 in the *Handbook*):

> The person to be vaccinated is currently unwell; has a disease which compromises immunity (eg. leukaemia, cancer, HIV/AIDS) or is having treatment which lowers immunity (eg. oral steroid medicines such as cortisone and prednisone, radiotherapy, chemotherapy); has had a severe reaction following any vaccine; has any severe allergies, especially to vaccine contents; has been vaccinated in the past month; has had an injection of

immunoglobulin, or received any blood products or a whole blood transfusion within the past year; is pregnant; has a past history of Guillain-Barré syndrome; was a preterm infant; has a chronic illness; has a bleeding disorder.

Another Table is then provided with strategies to deal with these situations.

Then the vaccination provider should ask the parents:

- Did you understand the information provided to you about immunisation?
- Do you need more information to decide whether to proceed?
- Did you bring your/your child's vaccination record card with you?

Anecdotal evidence suggests that many parents would acknowledge that the 3rd question was asked (have you got your vaccination record card). Many would say that the checklist was not provided to them, and they were not asked if more information was needed. No doubt compliance will improve as the threat of legal action grows.

The pre-vaccination assessment makes it clear that if a child has a temperature above 38.5°C, they should not be vaccinated. If they have diarrhoea or vomiting they should not be given the oral Polio vaccine. If they have allergies to any of the following then certain vaccines should not be given (specified in the NH&MRC Table 1.3.2) – streptomycin; neomycin; polymyxin; gentamicin; yeast protein; egg protein; gelatin; thiomersal; phenoxyethanol. Finally, if they have had "previous severe local and/or systemic adverse event" when previously vaccinated, then no vaccines should be given without reference (particularly anaphylaxis).

It is acknowledged that live vaccines should not be given to individuals with impaired immunity. This includes MMR, MMRV, VV, Rubella, Yellow Fever, BCG, oral rotavirus, and oral typhoid vaccines.

The *Handbook* also lists what it terms "false contraindications" to vaccination (NH&MRC Table 1.3.4) which includes the following conditions: a mild illness without fever (T <38.5°C); family history of any adverse events following immunization; past history of convulsions; treatment with antibiotics; treatment with locally acting (inhaled or low-dose topical) steroids; replacement corticosteroids; asthma, eczema, atopy, hay fever or 'snuffles'; previous diseases similar to the vaccination targets; a premature infant; history of neonatal jaundice; low weight in an otherwise healthy child; any neurological conditions including cerebral palsy and Down syndrome; contact with an infectious disease; child's mother is pregnant; child to be vaccinated is being breastfed; woman to be vaccinated is breastfeeding; recent or imminent surgery; poorly documented vaccination history.

So the NH&MRC recommends that unless there is a history of anaphylaxis or a compromised immune system with a live vaccine, then vaccination should proceed. This would appear to contradict in places the more cautious advice in some vaccine information pamphlets.

3.5.10 Appendix 3 to Section 3.5: Reporting of adverse events following vaccination

The *Australian Immunisation Handbook*, 2008, gives comprehensive guidance to vaccine providers as to what type of adverse events following vaccination should be reported (NH&MRC, 2008, pp. 58-66, and 360-363). They encourage the reporting of any serious or unexpected event, and list contact details for notification of AEFIs (adverse events following immunisation) in each state (NH&MRC Table 1.5.3 p.66)

If all vaccine providers followed the official guidelines, and listened to parents openly and objectively without feeling the need to defend their system, then many parental concerns would be satisfied. Further, we as a community would have a much better idea of the true safety of vaccines. Unfortunately, many parents attest to a failure in this area. Because there is a current reluctance to openly acknowledge possible adverse events, many parents are concerned that the orthodox system has "something to hide".

In fact the *Handbook* lists on page 61 a series of events where they claim there is no causal link with vaccination, including: sudden infant death syndrome (SIDS); autism and MMR vaccine; multiple sclerosis and hepatitis B vaccine; inflammatory bowel disease and MMR vaccine; diabetes and Hib vaccine; asthma and any vaccine.

This is clearly a defensive list, because as shown elsewhere in this book there are a significant variety of references which would attest to vaccination causing these conditions in SOME recipients (certainly not in every vaccinated person). Once again, parents are left with a sense that there is "something to hide".

Secrecy is the anthesis of the true scientific method. The scientists should never forget this.

The NSW Health Department has advised that the following adverse events should be reported (last updated 13/9/2004, see http://www.health.nsw.gov.au/factsheets/guideline/adverse.html)
"A person with any condition that is serious or unexpected that occurs any time after he or she received a vaccination and is considered by the doctor to be possibly related to that vaccination. Such conditions may including:
• Abscess; • Acute flaccid paralysis; • Allergic reaction; • Anaphylaxis; • Arthralgia; • Arthritis; • Brachial neuritis; • Death; • Disseminated BCG; • Encephalopathy; • Encephalitis; • Extensive limb swelling; • Fever - over 40.5°C; • Guillain-Barré Syndrome (GBS); • Hypotonic - hyporesponsive episode (shock, collapse); • Local reaction (severe); • Lymphadenitis (includes suppurative lymphadenitis); • Meningitis - diagnosis must be made by physician; • Nodule; • Orchitis; • Osteitis; • Osteomyelitis; • Parotitis; • Rash (severe or unusual); • Screaming (persistent); • Seizure; • Sepsis; • Subacute sclerosing panencephalitis; • Thrombocytopenia; • Toxic-shock syndrome; • Vaccine associated paralytic poliomyelitis; • Other severe or unusual events"

Quite a list, some of which would rarely occur. However, the question becomes – if there is a viable alternative to these unlikely but possible risks, then why take the risk at all?

The government publishes the rates of adverse events. Two examples are shown in Tables 3-17 and 3-18.

Table 3-17 Reporting Rates of Adverse Events Following Immunisation (AEFI) Per 100,000 Vaccine Doses,* Children Aged Less Than Seven Years, ADRAC Database, January to June 2004

Suspected vaccine or AEFI category	AEFI records (n)	Vaccine doses* (n)	Reporting rate per 100,000 doses	Difference
Diphtheria-tetanus-pertussis	122	255,758	47.7	-16.6
Diphtheria-tetanus-pertussis-hepatitis B	32	226,240	14.1	-4.8
Haemophilus influenzae type b	44	227,364	19.4	-2.4
Haemophilus influenzae type b-hepatitis B	8	127,501	6.3	-5.0
Poliovirus (oral or inactivated)	50	478,488	10.4	-4.4
Measles-mumps-rubella	78	239,256	32.6	+1.4
Meningococcal C conjugate	51	179,379	28.4	-10.3
Total	**205**	**1,749,075**	**11.7**	**-8.1**
'Certain' or 'probable' causality rating	73	1,749,075	4.2	-5.8
'Serious' outcome	17	1,749,075	1.0	-0.2

* Number of vaccine doses recorded on the Australian Childhood Immunisation Register (ACIR) and administered between 1 January and 30 June 2004.

Table 3-18 Reporting rates of adverse events following immunisation (AEFI) per 100,000 vaccine doses,* children aged less than 7 years, ADRS database, 2007

	AEFI records (n)	**Vaccine doses* (n)**	**Report. rate per 100,000 doses**
Vaccine			
DTPa-containing vaccines	334	1,064,713	31.4
DTPa-IPV	287	669,451	42.9
Pentavalent (DTPa-IPV-HepB)	8	17,862	44.8
Hexavalent (DTPa-IPV-HepB-Hib)	39	377,400	10.3
Haemophilus influenzae type b	17	111,389	15.3
Haemophilus influenzae type b-hepatitis B	118	422,838	27.9
Measles-mumps-rubella	118	527,082	22.4
Meningococcal C conjugate	30	282,527	10.6
Pneumococcal conjugate	158	825,018	19.2
Rotavirus vaccine¶	72	219,791	33.2
Varicella	28	251,766	11.1
AEFI Category			
Total People	**470**	**3,702,124**	**12.7**
'Certain' or 'probable' causality rating	150	3,702,124	4.1
'Serious' outcome	53	3,702,124	1.48

Available from:
http://www.health.gov.au/internet/main/publishing.nsf/Content/cda-cdi3204a.htm

This web site contains detailed information regarding the nature of the adverse events reported. If GPs did report all reactions, this would be a most valuable site. But we know they do not, and so this is a glimpse only.

The Australian Vaccination Network (AVN) has begun collecting information concerning AEFI (adverse events following immunisation), and they can be lodged at the following web site: http://www.avn.org.au/

3.5.11 Appendix 4 to Section 3.5: Thiomersal and autism

On June 16, 2005, a report by Robert F Kennedy Jnr, an environmental lawyer in the USA, was published online by Salon.com and by Rolling Stone magazine. Kennedy reported on the official cover-up of the link between thiomersal (the mercury based preservative used in many vaccines) and autism. I recommend all of you who need evidence as to why we must take responsibility for our own health decisions to read this report. The online publication references are:

http://www.salon.com/news/feature/2005/06/16/thimerosal/index_np.html

Kennedy reported on a meeting in June 2000 of a group of top government scientists, health officials, and representatives from every major vaccine manufacturer, at the isolated Simpsonwood conference centre. The participants were warned that "There would be no making photocopies of documents, no taking papers with them when they left"

The meeting discussed a study by a CDC (Centre for Disease Control) epidemiologist named Tom Verstraeten, who had analysed the agency's database containing the medical records of 100,000 children, that thiomersal appeared to be directly linked to a dramatic increase in the incidence of autism and many other child neurological disorders - "Since 1991, when the CDC and the FDA had recommended that three additional vaccines laced with the preservative be given to extremely young infants -- in one case, within hours of birth -- the estimated number of cases of autism had increased fifteenfold, from one in every 2,500 children to one in 166 children". Kennedy reported how the epidemic of autism spread, for no other apparent reason, to those developing countries who have introduced thiomersal-based vaccines – China, India, Argentina and Nicaragua.

Kennedy continued – "But instead of taking immediate steps to alert the public and rid the vaccine supply of thimerosal, the officials and executives at Simpsonwood spent most of the next two days discussing how to cover up the damaging data". He then goes on to outline the extent of the cover-up, how vaccine manufacturers paid off certain influential politicians to protect them, how the CDC pressured the IOM to release a neutral report on thiomersal, how scientific studies have been buried, and how the public has been mislead.

Read this report and draw your own conclusions!

As I said elsewhere, people who are capable of independent research have found that health officials and vaccine manufacturers have not been completely open and honest when it comes to describing the safety and effectiveness of vaccination. Kennedy's report provides yet another example of this recurring pattern of deceit and cover-up. The average GP just repeats what they are told, and what they are told is unreliable.

This is why many people have doubts. This is why many people question official pronouncements. **Those who complain about the anti-vaccination lobby would do better to deal honestly with the public, and then there would be no need to doubt**.

3.6 Specific vaccines examined

It is appropriate to examine the vaccines currently used in Australia to prevent some of the diseases described in Section 1. Whilst there are differences between developed countries, the information now shown in Appendix 9.2 will be applicable to most readers. The list also includes vaccines for what may be described as "overseas travel" conditions. Of course, these diseases may be currently active in countries where some readers live. A range of material will be presented relating to the vaccines considered.

Much of the technical information about the vaccines currently in use in Australia is available from *The Australian Immunisation Handbook*, 9th ed. 2008 (which, as said before, I am unable to quote directly). This information is generally applicable to other countries that tend to use similar vaccination schedules. The information is also publicly available on a variety of web sites and in various official publications. An example of a web site showing current vaccines used are:

http://www.mydr.com.au/default.asp?Article=3271 check ref

The vaccines examined in Appendix 9.2 include the following:

9.2.1	Chicken Pox
9.2.2	Cholera
9.2.3	Diphtheria
9.2.4	Haemophilis influenzae type b (Hib)
9.2.5	Hepatitis A
9.2.6	Hepatitis B
9.2.7	Hepatitis C
9.2.8	Influenza
9.2.9	Japanese encephalitis
9.2.10	Measles
9.2.11	Meningococcal infections
9.2.12	Mumps
9.2.13	Pertussis (Whooping Cough)
9.2.14	Pneumococcal infections9.2.15 Poliomyelitis

Index of Vaccine Manufacturers (with abbreviations used below)

AP	Aventis Pasteur
BH	Baxter Healthcare
Ch	Chiron
CSL	Commonwealth Serum Laboratories
DC	Delpharm Consultants
EHS	Ebos Health & Science
GSK	GlaxoSmithKline
Md	Medeva
MSD	Merck Sharp & Dohme
Nov	Novartis
Oct	Octapharma
SPPL	Sanofi PasteurPty Ltd
Stat	Statens Serum Institut
SyP	Solvay Pharmaceuticals
W	Wyeth

Reminder: Appendix 9.2 now contains the analysis of the vaccines above.

3.7 Some last minute findings

One of the problems associated with preparing the new edition of a book is lack of time to incorporate every reference accumulated in the years since the previous edition. I have many hundreds of electronic files and paper reports, all of which I would like to have studied carefully and incorporated into the 7th edition. Some I have, some I haven't, and some I have just made brief notes about which I will now show. Remember, the purpose of all this information is to make a case that **VACCINES ARE NOT COMPLETELY EFFECTIVE, NOR COMPLETELY SAFE, AND THE LEVEL OF SAFETY IS UNPROVEN.**

Once this is established, it follows logically that it is worthwhile examining options, and in particular the homoeopathic option which is the only other disease-specific immunisation option to vaccination.

European Inquiry Suggests Swine Flu Pandemic Driven by Big Pharma for Profit

American Chronicle. **29/9/2010.**

Makers of the Swine Flu vaccine had a very profitable year in 2009. By last June, CSL Limited's annual profits had reportedly risen 63 percent over 2008, GlaxoSmithKline's 2009 earnings spiked 30 percent in the third quarter alone, to $2.19 billion and Roche made 12 times more in the second quarter of 2009 than of 2008, all because of a Swine Flu pandemic that, according to a Parliamentary Assembly of the Council of Europe (PACE) investigation, was driven by collusion between the World Health Organization (WHO) and Big Pharma.

****

Australians snub free swine flu vaccine

Big Pond News. **10/9/2010** » 07:18am

The Australian Institute of Health and Welfare (AIHW) has put the total number of vaccinated Australians at the end of February at about 3.9 million, or 18 per cent of the population.

****

Four children die after routine vaccination

Times of India , **Aug 23, 2010**, 03.43am IST

LUCKNOW: A day after four children died in villages of Mohanlalganj tehsil here during a routine immunisation drive.

****

UK's £1bn swine flu blunder left 20m vaccines unused

London Evening Standard. **1/7/2010**

British taxpayers footed a £1.2 billion bill to fight a swine flu pandemic that never matched the dire predictions, an official report revealed today.

Britain spent £654 million preparing for a possible flu pandemic, and £587 million responding to the H1N1 outbreak — a total of £1.24 billion. That includes £1.01 billion on drugs, among them antivirals, doses of vaccine and antibiotics.

The investigation reveals that drug company GSK did not sign a "get-out" clause in its contract with the Government, which left the country with unwanted vaccines. Last year GSK made revenues of £883 million from sales of the vaccine.

****

Government 'too cosy with flu vaccine maker'

By Brigid Andersen – ABC News Online Investigative Unit. **28/4/2010.**

Jodi Hahn says the Government needs to set up a national reporting body to report cases of adverse reactions to vaccines among children. The Federal Government has been accused of making flawed decisions because of its overly "cosy" relationship with flu vaccine manufacturer CSL.

Health officials are investigating the death of a two-year-old Brisbane girl and more than 250 reports of adverse reactions among children who have received the seasonal flu vaccine, and Australia's chief medical officer has issued a warning to doctors to stop using the CSL shots on the under-fives.

Now the vaccine manufacturer is facing claims it has undue influence over the Federal Government and that this "close relationship" has blocked the rollout and funding of more advanced flu vaccines on the Australian market.

****

FURY AT VACCINE SCANDAL

Express.co.uk Sunday **January 10,2010**

By Lucy Johnston

HUNDREDS of public sector workers who claim their lives have been wrecked by vaccines say the Government has abandoned them.

Up to 200 doctors, nurses, firefighters, prison officers, police officers, forensic scientists and binmen say they have developed serious physical and mental health problems after injections essential for their work over the past 10 years. All have given up their jobs and some are now 60 per cent disabled.

****

21 Deaths in Japan After H1N1 Vaccine

japantimes.co.jp. **November 22, 2009**

The frequency of cases of severe side effects detected in the administration of H1N1 vaccines in Japan has been higher than for seasonal flu vaccines said the Japanese Health Ministry.

68 cases of serious side effects were recorded according to a health ministry survey. Eight more deaths were reported outside the survey, bringing the death toll after vaccination to 21

****

12 Babies die during vaccine trials in Argentina

EFE via COMTEX . Thursday, **July 10, 2008**; Posted: 05:23 PM

Buenos Aires,- At least 12 babies who were part of a clinical study to test the effectiveness of a vaccine against pneumonia have died over the past year in Argentina, the local press reported Thursday.

The study was sponsored by global drug giant GlaxoSmithKline and uses children from poor families, who are "pressured and forced into signing consent forms," the Argentine Federation of Health Professionals, or Fesprosa, said.

"This occurs without any type of state control" and "does not comply with minimum ethical requirements," Fesprosa said.

The vaccine trial is still ongoing despite the denunciations, and those in charge of the study were cited by the Critica newspaper as saying that the procedures are being carried out in a lawful manner.

****

French judges probe firms over vaccinations source

Reuters. PARIS | Fri Feb 1, 2008 3:32am EST

French authorities have opened a formal investigation into two managers from drugs groups GlaxoSmithKline (GSK.L) and Sanofi Pasteur over a vaccination campaign in the 1990s, a judicial source said late on Thursday.

Judge Marie-Odile Bertella-Geffroy also opened an investigation for manslaughter against Sanofi Pasteur MSD, a joint venture between Sanofi Aventis (SASY.PA) and Merck (MRK.N), the same source said.

The investigations follow allegations that the companies failed to fully disclose side effects from an anti-hepatitis B drug used in a vaccination campaign between 1994 and 1998.

There was no immediate comment from the companies or the two managers involved.

From 1994 to 1998, almost two thirds of the French population and almost all newborn babies were vaccinated against hepatitis B, but the campaign was suspended after concerns arose about possible secondary effects from the treatments.

Some 30 plaintiffs have launched a civil action in the case, including the families of five people who died after vaccination.

****

Risk of Vaccine Induced Diabetes in Children with a Family History of Type 1 Diabetes

Newly published data in the *Open Pediatric Medicine Journal* , 2008, 2, 7-10, reveals siblings of diabetics have an extremely high risk of developing vaccine induced type 1, insulin dependent diabetes. The hemophilus vaccine for example may cause over 2% of these children to develop type 1, insulin dependent, diabetes. Other vaccines have an effect of similar magnitude.

1874-3099/08 2008 Bentham Science Publishers Ltd. John Barthelow Classen*

****

Vaccine Damage: Parents receive $2bn compensation pay-outs
WDDTY. **04 October 2007**

Vaccine manufacturers have paid out nearly $2bn in damages to parents in America whose children were harmed by one of the childhood jabs such as the MMR (measles-mumps-rubella) or DPT (diphtheria-pertussis-tetanus). In all, around 2,000 families have received compensation payments that have averaged $850,000 each. There are a further 700 claims that are going through the pipeline. None of the claims is for autism as medical researchers say they have failed to find a link between the disease and the MMR vaccine, despite the initial findings made by Dr Andrew Wakefield.

****

3.8 A summary of the risks and benefits of vaccination

In Table 3-1, it was suggested that the following conclusions would be supported by the analysis in this Section:

1. Vaccination does provide protection against many infectious diseases

   (a) The long-term success of vaccination programs has been overstated

   (b) Most new vaccines are thoroughly trialled (but not always)

   (c) The effectiveness of most vaccines seems high, but field results are variable

2. The safety of vaccines is not known with certainty

   (a) Short-term testing is undertaken, but results are not consistently reliable

   (b) Long-term testing of single health effects is incomplete

   (c) Long-term testing of overall wellness has not been done

3. Vaccination is a generally (but not completely) effective method of disease prevention. The short-term adverse effects have been underestimated, and the true long-term health consequences have not been researched thoroughly.

It is up to the readers to decide for themselves how well these statements have been proved. As I said at the beginning of this Section – if some of the information in this Section seems to over-represent the doubts about vaccination, this is simply because the information stressing the benefits is usually all one can obtain from health authorities. At times this information is just over-enthusiastic. At other times it is deliberately selective, misleading, and simply incorrect.

Whatever decision you come to about the material presented above, I believe that one conclusion cannot be disputed, based as it is on published material from vaccine manufacturers, medical researchers and health authorities. That is:

Vaccination is neither completely effective nor completely safe.

This conclusion makes the consideration of an alternative not only sensible, but obligatory. Section 4 following examines the only other disease-specific alternative to vaccination – homœoprophylaxis. Once both options have been carefully examined, then an informed and objective decision can be made about which is the best option for one's child.

The most disappointing aspect of this whole debate is that many so-called scientists refuse to consider all available information and alternatives, and make pronouncements such as "homoeopathy is ineffective" based on speculation, not facts. Such an approach is not scientific. It is also tragic that scientists deliberately withhold information from the public, as with the SV40 cover-up. This explains why a growing number of independently minded people no longer accept without question statements by health authorities.

The refusal to accept official pronouncements without question clearly irritates many in authority, but in fact it is the authorities' refusal to be totally honest with the public that is the real reason why many anti-vaccination groups have been established around the world, and why conspiracy theories have multiplied.

Truth makes speculation redundant.

However, even if the scientists refuse to follow the basic principles of science, that is no reason for parents not to base their own decisions on an objective analysis of available information.

The fact that you are prepared to go through this process of research and decision-making leaves you better informed than most, if not all, of those people who may criticise your questioning of the orthodox approach.

Never forget this fact, and be proud of your willingness to face tough choices out of love and concern for the wellbeing of your children. **Whatever decision you finally make, you can do no more than this.**

4 QUESTION 4: What are the risks and benefits of the homœoprophylaxis option?

We shall examine the homoeopathic method of immunisation, or homœoprophylaxis (HP), in the following way:

Firstly, we shall give a general explanation and introduction to homœoprophylaxis (Section 4.1).

- A brief history of homoeopathy
- Historical references to homœoprophylaxis
- How homœoprophylaxis works
- Some relevant facts concerning homœoprophylaxis
- Questions commonly asked about homœoprophylaxis

Then we shall examine the HP program that I am using, and the research that supports it (Section 4.2).

- Available research into homœoprophylaxis
- My basic homœoprophylaxis program (2004)
- The general effectiveness of homœoprophylaxis
- Cuban data
- The general safety of homœoprophylaxis
  - Short-term safety
  - Long-term safety

Next we shall look at some special topics relating to homœoprophylaxis.

- A comparison of different homœoprophylaxis programs (4.3).
- The use of homœoprophylaxis by Australian homoeopaths (4.4).
- Suggested homœoprophylaxis for overseas travel (4.5).
- A response to the homoeopathic sceptics (4.6).

Finally, we shall draw general conclusions about homœoprophylaxis based on the material examined (Section 4.7).

A word of warning to readers who are not used to reading statistics – some of the information presented in the Sections outlining my research on HP may get a little difficult to read in places. Unfortunately there is not much I can do about this, as a table of data is a table of data! I am sure that you will be able to get the general idea from the comments I have attached, even if the figures don't mean a lot. It is necessary, however, that the main results are presented here to show the fact that there is a considerable body of evidence available to support the use of homœoprophylaxis.

4.1 A history and explanation of homœoprophylaxis.

4.1.1 A brief history of homoeopathy

Homoeopathy was founded in the late 1700's by a brilliant German physician, Samuel Hahnemann. He determined that most disease (as opposed to accidents and injuries) initially occurred on a deeper, inner level, with physical symptoms arising as a result of the subsequent disturbance to the person's *vital force,* or their inherited, inner, self-healing capacity or energy. He concluded that since disease arose on this level, prevention or cure would need to take place on the same level.

Hahnemann was the first practitioner to make full practical application of the natural law that *like cures like*, or the *Law of Similars.* This Law was known to Hippocrates and Paracelsus. He prepared remedies by *potentising* substances until all that remained of the particular substance was the dynamic (healing) energy. He treated patients using potentised doses of substances which, if taken in their crude form, would cause *similar* (disease) symptoms in healthy individuals. For each patient, the specific remedy was selected on the basis of this principle. The most similar of all remedies was called the *similimum.*

So, for example, in orthodox medicine Ipecac syrup is given to some people who may have swallowed toxic substances because Ipecac causes nausea and vomiting, and will cause the contents of the stomach to be expelled. In homoeopathic treatment, if we have a patient with persistent nausea and vomiting, Ipecac in potency is one of the remedies we consider (among many hundreds of possible remedies) to treat the patient. If the patient has a clean, moist tongue despite their gastrointestinal problems, then Ipecac is the remedy chosen, as it also has this characteristic and somewhat unusual symptom as part of its total symptom picture (usually the tongue is coated in GIT problems).

> *Note:* Potentisation is achieved by repeated dilutions and *succussions* (vigorous shaking of diluted material against a firm support). Using the centesimal scale of potentisation, one drop of the 'mother tincture' of the medicinal material is added to 99 drops of a neutral medium and shaken vigorously; this is the first, or '1c', potency. One drop of this solution is added to 99 drops of neutral medium and shaken to create the second, or 2c potency. These steps are repeated to create potencies as high as 100,000c. One drop of 3c potency, for example, contains only 1/1,000,000 of the original material; however, practical results have proven that the potentisation process releases the dynamic healing energy of the medicinal substance concerned. **Dilution alone without the succussions will not produce a medicinally active substance**.

Homoeopathy rapidly gained popular acceptance when it proved successful in treating the infectious diseases sweeping through Europe at that time. For example, historical records show that:

- In 1813, Hahnemann achieved a success rate of 100% in treating 183 Typhus patients; at that time Typhus was considered incurable.
- Scarlet Fever was effectively both treated and prevented by Hahnemann using the remedy Belladonna.
- During the European Cholera epidemics of the mid-1800's, the death rate was between 54% and 90%, while the death rate amongst persons who received homoeopathic treatment was between 5% and 16%.
- During the 1918-1920 Influenza (Spanish Flu) epidemics in the United States, the mortality rate was around 30%; the mortality rate among individuals treated homoeopathically was less than 1%.

Although support for homoeopathy declined in the early 1900's due to the spectacular advances of modern science, it is still widely used throughout Europe; for example, over 40% of French medical practitioners use Homoeopathic medicine. In England, the late Queen Mother was Patron of the British Homoeopathic Association, and the Queen never travels without her black box of homoeopathic remedies. UK has five homoeopathic hospitals in the National Health scheme. In India, the majority of medical practitioners use homoeopathic remedies, and they are also used in South America, South Africa and, to a lesser extent, in the United States. Homoeopathy is widely used in the prvious Eastern bloc countries. The WHO estimated that in 2007 over 500,000,000 were using homoeopathy around the world. It is one of the most used forms of complementary medicine on the planet.

The body of orthodox scientific research into homoeopathy is growing. For example, Dr Chauvanon showed that Diphtherinum (8M) produced a negative Schick test for a period of 10 years (Sankaran P, 1960). French Homoeopath, Dr O A Julian, described a mechanism of cure when using Homoeopathy (Julian OA, 1980). More recently, a number of major Meta analyses of the many scientific trials of homoeopathic treatment have been published in major scientific journals (Cucherat M, et al., 2000; Linde K, et al., 1997; Kleijnen J, et al., 1991).

In the mid 1980's, Professor J Beneviste and colleagues demonstrated the ability of potentised material to produce pathological changes (Beneviste J. et al, 1988). This latter research caused uproar in the orthodox scientific community. It also led to Beneviste being hounded out of his academic position in a series of cowardly and quite "unscientific" personal attacks on him. The orthodox establishment could not allow a respected scientist to question the principles upon which their entire system was based. If any readers want an example of the desperate way in which the orthodox scientific establishment fights to maintain their authority, then the Beneviste affair is compelling reading. It has been repeated more recently with the attacks on Dr Andrew Wakefield.

Despite the growing body of orthodox scientific evidence supporting the effectiveness of homoeopathic treatment, the homoeopathic paradigm is still irreconcilably different to that of the orthodox paradigm (given the present state of "scientific" understanding). This difference, plus the difficulty of applying orthodox research methods to homoeopathy, means that practical evidence must be used to support the validity of the homoeopathic method.

Considerable practical evidence does exist which shows not only that homoeopathic medicine offers an effective and safe means of treating disease, but that it also stimulates the body's immunological defence systems (both specifically and generally), thus giving prophylactic protection comparable with that of routine vaccination, without the potential side-effects. Examples of the historical use of homœoprophylaxis are given in Appendix 9.3.1 at the end of the book.

4.1.2 Historical references to homœoprophylaxis

The purpose of this section is to provide readers with some evidence of the frequent references to homoeopathic disease prevention (HP) in our literature over the entire life of homoeopathy. It is by no means a complete review. The references are listed in chronological order to give some feeling for the development of HP. This section is taken from *Homœoprophylaxis - A Practical and Philosophical Review, 3rd ed.*, (Golden I, 2001).

Note that this historical material has been moved to Appendix 9.3.1. Please review as required towards the end of the book. You will find that HP was first used by the founder of homoeopathy Dr Samuel Hahnemann, and by many homoeopathic "masters" since then.

4.1.3 How homœoprophylaxis works

Homoeopathy is a system of medicine which was developed by applying inductive logic to careful and extensive observations of healing methods and results. Philosophically, it is centred on a natural law referred to as *the Law of Similars*.

When referring to the treatment of patients, the Law of Similars (Treatment) states that a substance which is capable of producing a group of symptoms in a healthy person is capable of removing a group of SIMILAR symptoms in an unwell person.

The example of Ipecac was given above, showing that a substance which can cause nausea and vomiting in healthy people can, when used in potency, treat symptoms of nausea and vomiting in patients whose have other symptoms that are similar to the characteristic symptoms of Ipecac.

However, Dr Hahnemann also noted, and practically used, another aspect of the Law of Similars as it related to the prevention of disease. This may be stated in one of two ways:

(a) A substance which is capable of producing symptoms in a healthy person SIMILAR to the characteristic symptoms of an infectious disease, is capable of preventing these characteristic symptoms in a previously unprotected person (for example, the remedy China is one of the preventatives for malaria, and Nosodes are another example); or

(b) A substance which is capable of removing the characteristic symptoms of an infectious disease in an infected person, is capable of preventing the characteristic symptoms of the disease in a previously unprotected person (for example, Belladonna and scarlet fever, and Pulsatilla and measles).

There is some uncertainty as to whether the disease is actually prevented when using HP, or whether the characteristic symptoms are substantially lessened so that the person does not appear to have the disease. This idea was first suggested to me many years ago by Mr Alan Jones, one of Australia's most experienced homoeopaths. In many ways it doesn't really matter - the potential for damage from the disease is eliminated in a way that causes no harm. However, IF it can be shown that HP renders diseases sub-clinical, THEN it will have the added benefit of not only preventing distressing disease symptoms, but also of invoking a full antibody response, meaning that the length of protection offered by the method will be as great as if the person contracted the disease with all its typical clinical symptoms. Research is needed to resolve this potentially important point.

To give a practical example of both the treatment and prevention aspects of the Law of Similars we can begin with Dr Hahnemann's own first experience with the Law of Similars. While translating Cullen's *Materia Media* (a book of remedies) from English into German, he disagreed with the description of the overdose effects of Cinchona bark, which is used in the treatment of malarial fevers (Quinine). Having the inquiring mind of a true scientist, Dr Hahnemann took a dose of the bark, which produced fever-like symptoms. Soon after the fever subsided ,he took another dose, and the fever-like symptoms returned and then again subsided. From his medical training he knew that the symptoms which the bark produced were *similar* to the fever symptoms of malaria, the disease which the bark was used to treat. Dr Hahnemann realised that this was a practical example of the Law of Similars (for treatment).

Later, when treating patients with scarlet fever, Dr Hahnemann successfully used potencies of Belladonna, chosen on the basis of the Law of Similars. He also found that potencies of Belladonna would prevent scarlet fever, once again chosen on the basis of the Law of Similars (Hahnemann S, 1801).

We know that homoeopathy is relatively effective in practice, and that it is a logical and systematic method of medicine derived from fixed Laws of Nature. However, it is not readily explainable in terms of orthodox medicine, because science is not yet able to easily measure the energy profiles of different substances and the intensity of energy stimulae. Further, orthodox medicine is based totally on the need to explain all events in terms of molecular reactions, something which apparently makes it incompatible with the homoeopathic model.

It is most important to acknowledge that just because orthodox science cannot explain homoeopathy, it cannot be concluded that homoeopathy does not work; it can only be said that orthodox science has not yet developed the techniques required to adequately test (in ways they understand) homoeopathically prepared (potentised) substances .

This means that we must examine other areas of knowledge for an explanation. While the following may not satisfy some readers, it should be noted that since we are considering a practical discipline of disease prevention; what is most important is demonstrating whether it works, and *not* whether it can be easily explained in conventional terms.

Every major religion on the planet accepts that there is more to "us" than just bones and flesh. There are also many examples of how non-material influences can change our physical bodies. For example, the shock of hearing the news that a loved one has died may result in a person's hair turning white overnight. The physical change was a result of a non-physical (or energy) disturbance to the non-physical body. There are references available to healing on this energetic level (Golden I, 2002b).

It is also known that different people have inherited and/or acquired different degrees of sensitivity or susceptibility to different external influences. For example, a few people are highly sensitive to the Rhus tree; if such people walk near a Rhus tree they develop typical allergic symptoms (itching and watering eyes and nose, itching blotchy skin eruptions). When given appropriate doses of potentised Rhus Tox, their sensitivity decreases and, in many cases, is eliminated.

In a similar way, we can desensitise people to the influence of the measles virus by using appropriate remedies; they may then be exposed to the Measles virus without developing the symptoms associated with measles.

The homoeopathic method works on the first line of defence - the initial predisposition to be sensitive to a substance - rather than the last line of defence - the antibody-antigen reaction. It works on something which homoeopaths call *idiosyncrasy* – or the particular and peculiar sensitivities which each individual has to substances in their environment.

So the most easily understood explanation of how homœoprophylaxis works is by analogy, such as the Rhus Tox example above. I have discussed more technical explanations of the mechanism of action elsewhere, and am currently working on a new energetic model of homœoprophylaxis (Golden I, 1987, 1989a). The debate will continue!

4.1.4 Some relevant facts concerning homœoprophylaxis

Note: The abbreviation HP is used (depending on the context) to mean either:

(i) Homoeopathic prophylaxis (homœoprophylaxis), or

(ii) Homoeopathic prophylactics (the actual remedies used in a preventative program).

1. The use of HP began with Hahnemann, and has subsequently been used by some of the greatest homoeopathic prescribers, such as: Dr H C Allen, Dr C M F Von Boenninghausen, Dr J C Burnett, Dr J H Clarke, Dr A H Grimmer, Dr J T Kent, Dr S R Phatak, Dr P Schmidt, Dr D Shepherd, and Dr M L Tyler, to name only a few. Although this endorsement would be sufficient reassurance for many readers, there are other reasons for supporting the use of HP.

2. The method *does* work. The fact that potentised substances, selected using the Law of Similars, will reduce the likelihood of a patient developing the characteristic symptoms of an infectious disease has been established clinically over a period of 200 years, and is well reported in homoeopathic literature.

3. Protection against targeted diseases is not certain, as is the case with both conventional vaccination and even with immunity acquired through contracting the diseases themselves. Examples of the protection offered by HP over the years are given in Table 4-1 below. The consistency of results at around 90% is what makes the list impressive.

4. The question regarding the duration of protection is less certain. While Dr Chauvanon estimated that the efficacy of Diphtherinum (8M) was at least ten years, as measured by the Schick test, the dilemma is the same as for conventional vaccines, where length of protection is also uncertain (Sankaran P. 1972).

5. In comparing side-effects of potentised substances with those from conventional vaccines, it can be confidently stated that there is a zero possibility of a crude toxic reaction, except in patients with *extreme* sensitivity to the diluting medium of the remedy (e.g. milk sugar, maize starch, alcohol and water, etc). My research shows a level of (presumably dynamic) reactions to doses of the remedies at less than 2% (including some beneficial reactions); in all cases, these reactions were mild and temporary, with no evidence of ongoing adverse reactions or lessening in overall vitality (the reverse is actually reported to be the case). Experience suggests that these reactions were 'clearing' inherited or acquired damage caused by previous vaccines, or 'layers' left by poorly managed diseases.

- By comparison, Sir Graham Wilson's pioneering work revealed that there is overwhelming evidence of toxic side effects from conventional vaccines (Wilson G. 1967). More recent work by Dr Harris Coulter adds further weight to these findings (Coulter H. 1990). Many other references in the orthodox literature have been cited in Section 3 and Appendix 9.2.
- Many distinguished homoeopathic authors have warned of the potential for vaccinations to cause dynamic (Miasmic) damage (Burnett JC, 1884). Experienced homoeopathic practitioners also know this from their own clinical practices.

6. Some homoeopaths argue that we do not fully know the dynamic (Miasmic) long term consequences of potentised prophylactics (my latest research presented below has now partly answered this concern with data that demonstrates the long-term safety of HP). They conclude that is it desirable to allow a child to contract a disease and treat the disease according to the Law of Similars.

   This argument is appealing in theory, and can be sustained where both parents and practitioners wish to follow this approach. However, there are complications in practice:

   (a) Some diseases can be tragically severe in tiny infants, even with reasonable treatment. In the case of whooping cough, for example, I would rather prevent this disease in a three month old infant than have to treat it. I would certainly see prevention of meningococcal disease as a far better option than treatment, as the disease can be rapidly fatal.

   Without doubting the effectiveness of homoeopathic treatment, such treatment presumes that an accurate prescriber is locally available, and somewhat ignores the suffering for both child and parents while treatment occurs.

   (b) Many parents are not impressed with the argument that a child should be allowed to contract every disease and, if no alternative method of protection is offered, they will resort to conventional vaccination.

   Although it may be appropriate to express one's views concerning the value of treatment rather than protection, hopefully very few practitioners would refuse to offer assistance to parents who disagreed with what those parents might see as a theoretical or unrealistic option.

I would strongly argue that if parents prefer to vaccinate their children rather than provide no specific protection, we as practitioners are professionally obliged to make them aware of the homoeopathic alternative. It is then up to the parents concerned to choose between the two options for protection, based on the information available to them.

7. Some homoeopaths argue that disease-specific protection can be stimulated by using constitutional remedies. Even though this method undoubtedly works to an extent, there are many examples of individuals with a high vital force contracting specific infectious diseases. Disease-specific prophylaxis is more effective in producing the highest level of disease-specific immunity. I wish to stress that I totally support classical constitutional treatment. If chronic health issues are manifesting, then such treatment should take precedence over an HP program, which can be delayed. The bottom line is that there is no reason why both cannot be used if required, with the relevant remedies appropriately spaced apart under the direction of an experienced homoeopathic practitioner.

4.1.5 Questions commonly asked about homœoprophylaxis

This section covers some of the most frequently asked questions about homoeoprophylaxis. Suggestions for further inclusions in this section are welcomed and may be sent to the author, c/- Aurum Healing Centre, PO Box 695, Gisborne, Vic 3437 (please include a stamped, self-addressed envelope if a reply is required), or email brief inquiries to admin@homstudy.net.

1 *Do homoeopathic remedies produce antibodies?*

To date, not enough research has been done to settle this point, although the task would be by no means difficult to undertake. Whilst there have been reports of antibody production as a result of administering homoeopathic medicines, there are also reports to the contrary. However, unlike conventional vaccines, **the homoeopathic alternative does not rely on antibody formation**. The issue of antibody production is therefore a non-essential distraction.

2 *How do the homoeopathic remedies give protection?*

This question is not simple to answer, especially in terms consistent with orthodox biochemical mechanisms. See Section 4.1.3 above. Basically, the homoeopathic remedies reduce the patient's sensitivity to the dynamic stimulus of the virus or bacteria, thus lessening the patient's predisposition to being overcome by this stimulus.

If a person is known to be sensitive to a particular substance, then appropriate potencies of the substance can reduce or remove the sensitivity. The example used in Section 4.1.3 was of an individual who develops an itching, blotchy rash from contact with a Rhus tree. Homoeopaths know from considerable clinical experience that administration of a high potency of Rhus Tox can desensitise the patient to being affected by the Rhus tree.

Similarly, we can desensitise a patient to being affected by pertussis, diphtheria, etc by administering high potencies of a substance which is 'similar' to pertussis or diphtheria, etc. This is why the Nosodes are frequently used, but it is also the reason why other remedies may be just as effective: Dr Hahnemann first used potentised Belladonna to protect against scarlet fever. We do not know in advance whether or not an individual will be sensitive to exposure of different organisms, although experience tells us that many milder infectious diseases have high attack rates (e.g., measles, rubella), and some others with low attack rates have severe consequences (e.g., meningococcal disease). This is one reason for desensitising (immunising) people prior to exposure.

3 *Can the effect of the homoeopathic remedies be measured?*

Effectiveness cannot be readily measured using conventional biochemical testing. The effectiveness of homoeopathic remedies is measured by results. However, this is no different to the method often used to measure the effectiveness of conventional vaccines (i.e., by epidemiological studies). More sensitive measuring techniques will undoubtedly be developed as scientific knowledge increases; such techniques will eventually convince the sceptics that homoeopathy's 200 years of practical experience should be given the attention it deserves. In the meantime, the results of substantial long-term statistical analysis of HP are presented below.

4 *Can a change of diet affect a child's immunity when using homoeopathic remedies?*

As discussed in Section 2.1 earlier, diet and lifestyle can have a significant impact on the general health of a child, and an indirect effect on the child's general immunity.

The most important factor when administering homoeopathic remedies is to ensure that remedies are not given close to mealtimes, and preferably away from any intake of food or drink. Coffee (which children don't normally drink) is a known possible antidote; highly spiced foods and some of the more powerful herbs can also act as antidotes. Also worth noting is the capacity of strong odours, such as camphor or liniment, to antidote remedies if the remedy bottle is opened near the source of the odour. If parents are careful and sensible, however, the medicines should not be adversely affected.

5 *How long does the protective effect last?*

As with vaccines, the length of protection is uncertain. Dr Chavanon's work (referred to in Section 4.1.4) clearly demonstrates that low potencies (30C) have a brief action over a few weeks, and that high potencies (8M) have the potential to last up to ten years.

6 *If I have a break in the program, does this lesson the effectiveness?*

Generally, no. However, if only one dose has been taken, protection is less certain than if a number of doses have been given. In my programs since 1991, once the first triple dose of a particular remedy is given, a significant level of protection is believed to be established.

7 *Is the level of protection offered the same for all diseases?*

I have presented data for individual diseases in *Homœoprophylaxis - A Fifteen Year Clinical Study* (Golden 2004a). This shows the following levels of efficacy for 3 diseases; whooping cough – 88.3%; measles – 91.0%; mumps – 94.1%. As can be seen, the levels of effectiveness are reasonably close. We expect protection levels to be similar for different diseases.

8 *Is HP "homoeopathic vaccination"?*

No. We do not have homoeopathic vaccines. The only time potencies of vaccines should be used is to assist in the treatment of the symptoms of vaccine damage. These remedies are not the most appropriate medicines for preventative purposes. Those people who suggest that the principles of vaccination and homœoprophylaxis are very similar are incorrect. They work very differently, and are based on completely different principles.

4.2 An outline of available research into homœoprophylaxis.

As was shown above, HP has been used successfully for over 200 years. There has been considerable clinical evidence showing its safety and effectiveness, but little formal statistical research.

The findings of my literature review of published formal research into HP in humans is summarised in Table 4-1.

Most of the studies are relatively short-term, where the remedy was selected to prevent a single disease. My studies were long-term, and the remedies covered a number of diseases.

Table 4-2 shows the chronological development of my research from 1986 to 2004. More details of this research will be given below. It should be noted that this research has produced the following:

(a) The largest study of long-term HP ever undertaken in the world, showing the effectiveness and the safety of the method.

(b) A comparison of the effectiveness and safety of vaccination, HP, constitutional prevention, and no preventative method at all.

(c) A comparison of the effectiveness and safety of different HP programs.

(d) A survey of the attitudes to and the use of HP by Australian homoeopaths.

We shall look in turn at three areas of interest in my research findings:

(1) Section 4.2.1: the homoeoprophylactic programs I have used from 1986 to 2005.

(2) Section 4.2.2: the overall effectiveness of my programs, and of HP programs in general.

(3) Section 4.2.5: the overall safety of my program, and of HP programs in general.

Table 4-1 Some Measures of the Effectiveness of Homœoprophylaxis

Year	Researcher	Numbers of Participants	Length of Survey	Ages	Effectiveness %
1907	Eaton	2,806	< 1 year		97.5
1950	Taylor -Smith	82 (12 definately exposed)	< 1 year	all ages	100.0
1963	Gutman	385	< 1 year	adults	86.0
1974	Castro & Nogeira	HP 18,000 Other 6,340	3 months	Less than 15 years old	86.1
1987	English	694	2 years	children	87.0 - 91.5
1987	Fox	61	5 years	children	82.0 - 95.0
1998	Mroninski et al	HP 65,826 Other 23,539	6 months 12 months	0 – 20 years	95.0 91.0
1997	Golden	593 children 1,305 quest'res	10 years	1-5 years	88.8
2004	Golden	1,159 children 2,342 quest'res	15 years	1 - 5 years	90.4
2004	Golden	HP 159 Other 622	2 years	4 - 12 years	79.2

Table 4-2 Chronological Development of Isaac Golden's Research

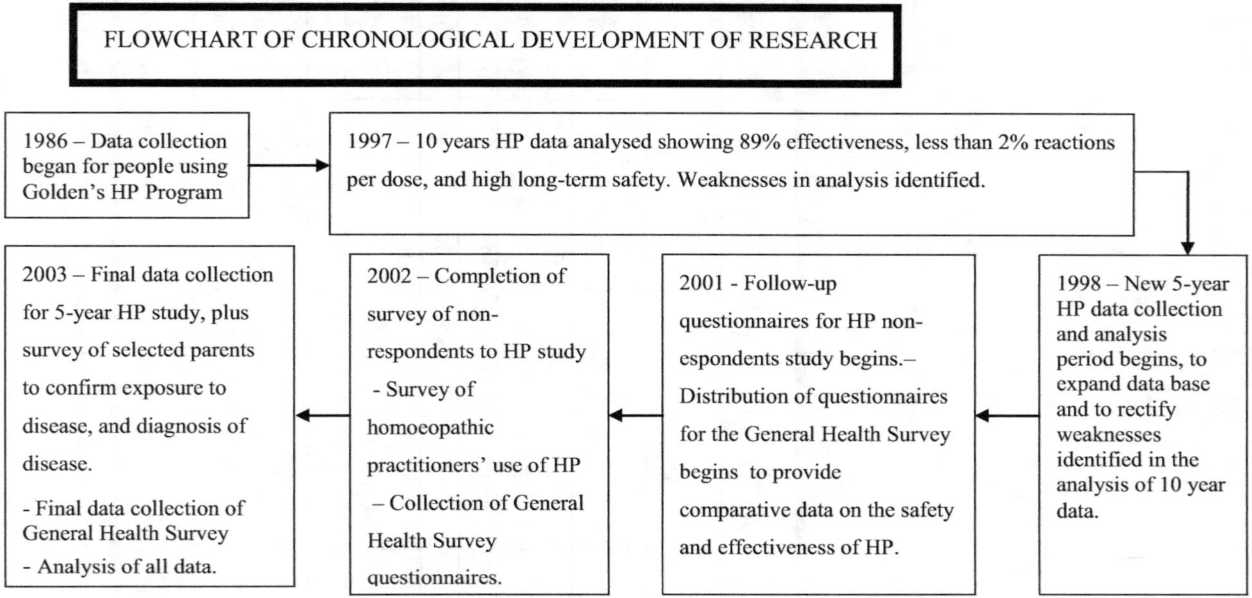
FLOWCHART OF CHRONOLOGICAL DEVELOPMENT OF RESEARCH
1986 – Data collection began for people using Golden's HP Program
1997 – 10 years HP data analysed showing 89% effectiveness, less than 2% reactions per dose, and high long-term safety. Weaknesses in analysis identified.
1998 – New 5-year HP data collection and analysis period begins, to expand data base and to rectify weaknesses identified in the analysis of 10 year data.
2001 - Follow-up questionnaires for HP non-espondents study begins.– Distribution of questionnaires for the General Health Survey begins to provide comparative data on the safety and effectiveness of HP.
2002 – Completion of survey of non-respondents to HP study - Survey of homoeopathic practitioners' use of HP – Collection of General Health Survey questionnaires.
2003 – Final data collection for 5-year HP study, plus survey of selected parents to confirm exposure to disease, and diagnosis of disease.
- Final data collection of General Health Survey
- Analysis of all data.

4.2.1 A specific homoeopathic preventative program

Homoeopathic preventative remedies have been used by practitioners with great effectiveness and reliability for over two centuries. Different practitioners have used a variety of remedies and potencies in a variety of situations.

This section examines the programs which I have developed since 1986. Following this, the statistical surveys conducted to assess the safety and effectiveness of these programs will be presented. As stressed previously, ***no* immunisation program, pharmaceutical or homoeopathic, can be guaranteed 100% effective**, but it is essential that we establish a reliable guide to the relative effectiveness and safety of vaccination and homœoprophylaxis. This guide should be based on evidence, not conjecture.

4.2.1.1 My basic homœoprophylaxis program (2004)

In Australia, routine vaccination is generally recommended for whooping cough, diphtheria, tetanus, poliomyelitis, measles, mumps, rubella, and Haemophilis meningitis (Hib). In addition, coverage against hepatitis B and meningococcal disease is recommended, and vaccines against pneumococcal disease, influenza, rotavirus and chicken pox all have been recommended for inclusion in routine vaccination programs. The list will grow as new vaccines are developed.

My current (2010) homœoprophylaxis program covers the following diseases; **whooping cough, tetanus, poliomyelitis, meningococcal disease, pneumococcal disease, and Haemophilis meningitis (Hib).** Optional remedies for measles, influenza and hepatitis B are provided, as well as a remedy for tetanus wounds. The program is designed to be used from one month of age, although it may be started at any age. An option for remedy substitution is described in Appendix 3.3(a).

The HP programs I have used over the years were developed initially following extensive research in the homoeopathic literature, and were modified as a consequence of subsequent personal clinical experience as well as formal research.

My first homœoprophylaxis program was released in 1986. It was substantially modified in 1991. In 1993, the program was slightly modified to include the Hib preventative. These programs are shown in the Tables in Appendix 9.3. The current program was first released in October 2004. The reasons for the changes made were published in the homoeopathic literature (Golden I, 2004). The main reasons related to a consideration of three factors; (i) identifying which diseases were potentially most serious, (ii) identifying which diseases were active in the community, and (iii) identifying which diseases were most discussed by and of concern to parents.

For example, coverage for meningococcal and pneumococcal diseases were included because of their potential seriousness. Coverage for diphtheria was removed because it is hardly present in the Australian community. Coverage for mumps was removed (as was rubella in 1991) because it is a mild disease in healthy children, and easily treated homoeopathically.

If some parents have a particular concern about any of these diseases which are no longer covered, they can be added back into the current program wherever the parents feel is most appropriate.

The current program is shown in Table 4-3 below. You will note that in many months it uses triple doses of the same remedy - marked with *. A triple dose is three doses of the remedy over 24 hours, e.g. a dose in the morning, a second in the evening, and a third the following morning. A triple dose is seen as providing a stronger, deeper acting dose of the remedy.

The disease-remedy relationship (including possible substitutions if Nosodes are not acceptable) is as follows:

. Whooping Cough -	*Pertussin*	Cuprum Metallicum
. Diphtheria -	*Diphtherinum*	Gelsemium
. Measles -	*Morbillinum*	Pulsatilla
. Poliomyelitis -	*Lathyrus Sativus*	Lathyrus Sativus
. Tetanus -	*Tetanus Toxin*	Hypericum
. Meningococcal -	*Meningococcinum*	Belladonna
. Pneumococcal -	*Pneumococcinum*	Belladonna
. Hib -	*Haemophilis*	Arsenicum Album

Table 4-3 The 2004 Long-Term Homœoprophylaxis Program

Code	Remedy Name	Disease	Months Given
The Main Program			
A1	Pertussin 200	Whooping Cough	1, 2*
A3	Pertussin 10M		14*, 26*, (52*)
G1	Pneumococcal 200	Pneumococcal Disease	3, 4*
G3	Pneumococcal 10M		16*, 30*, (58*)
C1	Lathyrus Sativus 200	Polio	5, 6*
C3	Lathyrus Sativus 10M		18*, 36*, (64*)
H1	Haemophilis 200	Haemophilis	7, 8*
H3	Haemophilis 10M	Influenzae type B	20*, 40*, (70*)
I1	Meningococcal 200	Meningococcal Disease	9, 10*
I3	Meningococcal 10M		22*, 44*, (76*)
B1	Tetanus Tox 200	Tetanus	11, 12*
B3	Tetanus Tox 10M		24*, 48*, (84*)
Additional Remedies Supplied			
E2	Morbillinum M	Measles	If required – use where preferred
J2	Hepatitis B M	Hepatitis B	If required – use where preferred
O	Oscillococcinum 200	Influenza	In flu season – monthly, or as treatment
M	Ledum 30	Tetanus wounds	If a wound – 3 times daily for 3 days

* - indicates the use of a triple dose, i.e. three doses in 24 hours.

( ) - indicates optional final booster if required.

The Supplementary Program

As with earlier programs, remedies may be used to give additional protection if exposure is likely during a localised outbreak. The remedies used are: A1, G1, C1, H1, I1, E2, J2, O, M. **If** exposure has already occurred, use expected treatment remedies (e.g., Pulsatilla 200 twice weekly following exposure to measles).

The status sheet accompanying the instructions for using the program is shown in Table 4-4. This is the record form which parents complete when they administer remedies to their child. It also shows the main program in a different, sequential layout.

The Supplementary program is shown in Table 4-5. This program is to be used IF the child is likely to be exposed to infection, e.g., visiting relatives with whooping cough, measles at kinder, meningococcal outbreak in the town. The reason for this is that no method of protection is 100% perfect, thus the supplementary remedies are like “extra insurance”, to minimise the likelihood of infection.

Most of the homoeopathic medicines listed in these tables are called *Nosodes*. These are potentised preparations of diseased substances; for example, the nosode Pertussin is the potentised expectoration from a patient with whooping cough. It must be stressed that no molecules of the organism are contained in the remedy. However, because HP is based on the Law of Similars, it is not essential to use Nosodes, and possible remedy substitutions have been shown above.

As discussed previously, when a person acquires immunity through natural exposure to a virus, the actual quantity of virus is minute, yet the change is effected on a dynamic level, and subsequently on the physical level. In homoeopathy, the effect is similar in that changes initially occur on a dynamic level. The homoeopathic remedy, Pertussin, is the virus potentised to a purely dynamic and non-material degree. Unlike vaccines, therefore, homoeopathic preparations copy the processes of Nature, with similar results in practice. Further, it must be stressed that vaccination is *not* a type of homoeopathy (as has been suggested by some).

Attacks on the homoeopathic option have criticised the use of Nosodes (Dwyer J, 1993). As has been demonstrated above, it is not necessary to use Nosodes, since significant clinical experience with the use of other remedies exists. Further, the issue may be seen in its true light when it is remembered that if *all* the remedies mentioned above were taken to a conventional laboratory, the scientists would be unable to distinguish one remedy from any other. We are using medicines of energy, not crude substances like those used in vaccines. The remedies are selected using the Law of Similars referred to earlier.

Table 4-4 Status Sheet for the 2004 Program

Age Rec. /Given	Remedy	Potency	Remedy Label	Date of Admin	Admin. By
1 month	Pertussin	200	A1		
2 months	Pertussin	200, 200, 200	A1		
3 months	Pneumococcinum	200	G1		
4 months	Pneumococcinum	200, 200, 200	G1		
5 months	Lathyrus Sativus	200	C1		
6 months	Lathyrus Sativus	200, 200, 200	C1		
7 months	Haemophilis	200	H1		
8 months	Haemophilis	200, 200, 200	H1		
9 months	Meningococcinum	200	I1		
10 months	Meningococcinum	200, 200, 200	I1		
11 months	Tetanus Tox	200	B1		
12 months	Tetanus Tox	200, 200, 200	B1		
14 months	Pertussin	10M, 10M, 10M	A3		
16 months	Pneumococcinum	10M, 10M, 10M	G3		
18 months	Lathyrus Sativus	10M, 10M, 10M	C3		
20 months	Haemophilis	10M, 10M, 10M	H3		
22 months	Meningococcinum	10M, 10M, 10M	I3		
24 months	Tetanus Tox	10M, 10M, 10M	B3		
26 months	Pertussin	10M, 10M, 10M	A3		
30 months	Pneumococcinum	10M, 10M, 10M	G3		
36 months	Lathyrus Sativus	10M, 10M, 10M	C3		
40 months	Haemophilis	10M, 10M, 10M	H3		
44 months	Meningococcinum	10M, 10M, 10M	I3		
48 months	Tetanus Tox	10M, 10M, 10M	B3		
52 months	Pertussin	10M, 10M, 10M	A3		
58 months	Pneumococcinum	10M, 10M, 10M	G3		
64 months	Lathyrus Sativus	10M, 10M, 10M	C3		
70 months	Haemophilis	10M, 10M, 10M	H3		
76 months	Meningococcinum	10M, 10M, 10M	I3		
84 months	Tetanus Tox	10M, 10M, 10M	B3		

Table 4-5 The Current Supplementary Program

Code	Medicine	Current Epidemic Exposed To
A1	Pertussin 200	Whooping Cough - take twice weekly for 2 weeks during outbreak
M	Ledum Palustre 30	Tetanus - take x3 daily for 3 days after breakage of the skin
C1	Lathyrus Sativus 200	Polio - take one dose every week during an outbreak.
G1	Pneumococcinum 200	Pneumococcal Disease - take every 2 weeks, for 6 weeks during an outbreak.
E2	Morbillinum 200	Measles - take weekly for 4 weeks during an outbreak.
I1	Meningococcinum 200	Meningococcal Disease - take weekly for 4 weeks during an outbreak.
H1	Haemophilis 200	Haemophilis Influenzae (HIB Meningitis) - take weekly for 4 weeks during an outbreak.
O	Oscillococcinum 200	Influenza - take weekly for 4 weeks during an outbreak.

The ignorance of such attacks is made more obvious considering that homoeopathic medicine is first dismissed because 'nothing is there', and then criticised as being 'toxic'. Logical and scientific criticism indeed!

Important Note: The second program was introduced in 1991 [refer Appendix 9.3] as a result of an additional two years of research, and information obtained from homoeopaths overseas. It was upgraded in 1993 to include a remedy for Hib meningitis. The original 1986 program [refer Appendix 9.3], as well as the following two programs *are* effective if used correctly; however, parents may upgrade if desired, and insert additional remedies into their program. It must also be stressed that, *if a disease has developed, use of these remedies may be contraindicated.* If your child contracts a disease, an experienced homoeopathic practitioner should be consulted since the appropriate remedy needs to be selected on the basis of careful evaluation of existing symptoms. In the case of an established disease, excellent results can be obtained with specific and accurately prescribed homoeopathic remedies. Remedies should only be obtained through a practitioner, or established homoeopathic Chemists such as Martin & Pleasance in Melbourne, Brauer Biotherapies in Tanunda, Gould's Pharmacy in Hobart, and Newtons Pharmacy in Sydney.

Explanatory Notes:

- One dose consists of two tablets or pilules of the medicine indicated. The pilules may be dissolved in a little water if preferred. Each dose must be administered at least 45 minutes before or after eating or drinking.
- The 1991 program is a direct result of research which clearly suggested the need for triple doses, not because single doses are ineffective, but to lessen the chance of a single dose being accidentally antidoted. It must be stressed that the original program is effective if used properly; however, any program may be improved as new information becomes available. Dr Hahnemann offered the clearest example of how intellectual evolution can lead to practical change.
- The program was generally available throughout Australia from me until 13 January 1993. My distribution of the program has since been restricted by the Government under TGA regulations (refer Section 8.6.3), and I cannot post it directly interstate or overseas. **However, homoeopaths around the country are legally able to provide the program to their patients, and these details are available from me.** So all that has happened is that the TGA restrictions have limited the amount of material available for my research, without lessening the availability of the program – an unproductive result!
- Instructions and a questionnaire are included with each program. Information from questionnaires is kept completely confidential and forms the basis of continuing research into the effectiveness of the program.

4.2.2 The general effectiveness of homœoprophylaxis.

A summary of published research showing the effectiveness of HP is shown in Table 4-1 above. The type of remedy used in these studies was either a *genus epidemicus* (GE) remedy, specific to a particular outbreak, or a Nosode prepared from diseased material. The figures show great consistency irrespective of the type of remedy used, and irrespective of whether long-term or short-term protection was used.

The figures include the two major research studies which I have published (Golden I, 1997; Golden I, 2004), which demonstrated an effectiveness of long-term HP of 88.8% and 90.4% respectively.

Table 4-6 Responses Received - 15 Year Clinical Study - 1988 to 2003

	Year and Survey							
	Sur.1	Sur.2a	Sur.2b	Sur.3	Sur.4	Sur.5	Sur.6	Sur.7
Series	1988	1989	1990	1991	1992	1993	1994	1995
1	50	40	23	19	11	11	9	6
2		39	13	8	11	10	4	6
3			48	25	18	15	7	10
4			2	60	47	33	26	18
5					55	30	24	20
6						135	77	65
7						3	64	25
8								48
9								3
10								
11								
12								
13								
14								
15								
Total	**50**	**79**	**86**	**112**	**142**	**237**	**211**	**201**

In order to gather statistics regarding the effectiveness of the different HP programs used since 1986, a questionnaire was sent each year to parents using my program. The results of the first survey (1988) were reported in the first edition of this book. The second survey, covering two periods - 1989 and 1990 - were included in the second edition. The third edition covered the 1991 survey, and the fourth edition included results from the fourth survey conducted during 1992 and the fifth survey in 1993, as well as a summary of the results accumulated since the program commenced. The fifth edition reported the 1994 (sixth) survey. In 1997, the combined results of eight surveys were reported with over 1,300 questionnaire responses.

Table 4-6 shows the questionnaire responses collected from 1986 to 2004 with 2,342 responses, which form the basis of the results studied in my doctoral thesis, and the results presented here.

Year and Survey							
(Cont.)	Sur.8a	Sur.8b	Sur.9	Sur.9	Sur.9	Sur.9	Sur.9
Series	1996	1997	1998	1999	2000	2001	2002/3
1	0	0	0	0	0	0	0
2	0	0	0	0	0	0	0
3	1	1	0	0	0	0	0
4	0	1	3	3	0	0	0
5	1	0	0	0	0	0	0
6	34	32	1	0	0	0	0
7	13	13	0	0	0	0	0
8	20	22	14	12	10	6	4
9	43	14	11	12	10	7	5
10		42	19	18	17	16	2
11			72	41	21	17	29
12				78	47	36	30
13					97	61	57
14						90	54
15							87
Total	**112**	**125**	**120**	**164**	**202**	**233**	**268**
708	Group A: Total Responses Series 1-5						
817	Group B: Total Responses Series 6-10						
817	Group C: Total Responses Series 11-15						
2342	**Total Groups: TOTAL RESPONSES**						

Table 4-7 summarises the results, divided into three series of 5 years each. The single figure measure of the effectiveness of HP over the entire survey period is 90.4%. These results have been analysed in considerable detail in *Homœoprophylaxis – A Fifteen Year Clinical Study* for those who enjoy statistics (Golden, 2004). It is available from P.O. Box 695, Gisborne, 3437 for $32.00 (including postage and packing for Victorian state addresses).

Table 4-7 Summary of Results - Long-Term Homœoprophylaxis

Measures of Reactions & Efficacy	Data Series			
Data After Follow-Up Surveys	Series 1-5	Series 6-10	Series 11-15	Totals
Total Responses	**708**	**817**	**817**	**2342**
1. Previously vaccinated	73	102	110	285
	10.3%	**12.5%**	**13.5%**	**12.2%**
2. Definite reactions to remedies	51	81	81	213
Reactions per person	**7.2%**	**9.9%**	**9.9%**	**9.1%**
Reactions per dose (est.)	**1.2%**	**1.7%**	**1.7%**	**1.5%**
3. Definitely suffered from diseases covered by main program (a measure of failure)	18	11	11	40
	2.5%	**1.3%**	**1.4%**	**1.7%**
4. Definitely exposed to diseases covered by main program	177	127	113	417
	25.0%	**15.5%**	**13.8%**	**17.8%**
5. Definitely suffering diseases, after definite exposure and after taking the appropriate remedy (a measure of failure)	18/177	11/127	11/113	40/417
	10.2%	**8.7%**	**9.7%**	**9.6%**
6. Definitely not suffering diseases, after definite exposure and after taking appropriate remedy (a measure of success)	159/177	116/127	102/113	377/417
	89.8%	**91.3%**	**90.3%**	**90.4%**

4.2.2.1 Comments on the combined survey results

The following are brief comments on the major statistics in Table 4-7 using the same numbering system shown in the table.

* *Measure 2 - Definite reactions to remedies in the homoeopathic program*

Because the remedies contain no material doses of toxic material, the possibility of toxic reactions is zero. The resulting adverse reactions are, therefore, of interest, and may be divided into three types:

(i) acute hypersensitivity to the neutral base of the homoeopathic pilules which carry the potency; this type of sensitivity is extremely rare.

(ii) proving – where the effect of the remedy imposes symptoms onto the child.

(iii) clearing reactions, where a temporary healing response occurs as the potencies eliminate inherited or acquired damage; an excellent example of this was given in a response contained in the 1991 survey -

> (4102) She had Diphtherinum at 7 months; this was followed by a very bad cold and a drop in weight gain. At the time I thought it coincidence. Later when I mentioned which remedy had preceded the cold to Emily's father, he became very excited and told me that he "had nearly died of Diphtheria" when he was 6 years old.

* *Measure 3 - First measure of failure of the homoeopathic option*

This figure measures how many children suffered from a disease after taking the disease-specific remedy in the program. An average failure rate of less than 2% is found.

The weakness of this measure is that not every child in the program has been exposed to an infectious disease, while some children may have had multiple exposures. However, the imputed success rate of 98% is taken to be a maximum measure of efficacy.

* *Measure 5 - Second measure of failure of the homoeopathic option*

This figure measures how many children suffered from a disease after exposure, and after taking the appropriate remedy It is a more reliable measure. It is interesting to note how mild the disease symptoms were in the majority of cases, indicating that the homoeopathic remedy stimulated the child's ability to deal effectively with the disease. A failure rate of 10% compares very favourably with that of conventional vaccines.

* *Measure 6 - First measure of success of the homoeopathic option*

This measures how many children were exposed, but did *not* acquire the disease. Once again, the figure for efficacy of 90.4% compares favourably with the conventional option.

While these figures may be criticised on the basis that they are derived from parents' observations, this is the only feasible method of obtaining data while funds for more extensive research remain unavailable. As part of my doctoral research, I performed a number of checks on the last 5 years data to validate it. Table 4-8 below shows these checks.

STATISTICAL NOTE TO TABLE 4-8: *Sensitivity* is the proportion of respondents who have experienced a disease or exposure, and are correctly classified as having had the experience. *Specificity* is the proportion of respondents who have not experienced a disease or exposure, and are correctly classified as not having had that experience.

These tests have confirmed the reliability of the Series 11-15 data. Since these results were consistent with the Series 1-10 results, it is reasonable to conclude that the entire series of results (Series 1-15) are reliable.

Table 4-8 Tests to Validate the Results Reporting the Efficacy of Long-Term HP

No.	Test	Result
1	The accountability rate (the % of those surveyed who responded) of the final 5-years' data was calculated to ensure a significant level of accountability (>70%) and thus greater reliability of results.	>70% accountability of first year responses was achieved
2	Non-respondents were surveyed to ensure that the questionnaires that were received gave responses that were reflective of the entire population.	Responses from non-respondents were consistent with respondent replies.
3	Respondents who reported acquisition of a disease were surveyed to verify the accuracy of their initial report.	High level of accuracy of initial reports.
4	Respondents who reported exposure to a disease were surveyed to verify the accuracy of their initial report.	High level of accuracy of initial reports.
5	A more detailed statistical analysis of the data was undertaken to determine confidence limits for the figure for the efficacy of HP.	Confidence limits were: CI = 87.6% - 93.2% (P=0.05)
6	The accuracy of the measurements of efficacy based on notifications of and exposure to diseases was tested by calculating the *sensitivity* and *specificity* of the data.	High levels of *sensitivity* (disease = 90.9%, exposure = 95.6%), and *specificity* (disease = 98.1%, exposure = 99.2%).
7	A comparison with national disease attack rates was undertaken to provide an effective control group against which to compare results.	Weighted average national disease attack rate = 79%; HP associated with reduction in disease, P <0.01.

4.2.2.2 A second measure of effectiveness based on attack rates

One remaining statistical criticism of my long-term research is that no control groups were used. That is, there was no comparable group of children who **did not** use my HP program against which to compare findings from children who **did** use my program.

The reason why such comparisons are important is that if, for example, I found a level of effectiveness of 90% for immunisation, after exposure, against a disease that would normally only infect 10% of exposed persons, this would indicate very little protection, compared to an effectiveness of 90% against a disease that normally infected 95% of exposed persons who had not been immunised.

This leads to the difference between the *effectiveness* of a method of immunisation, and its *efficacy*.

Any review of orthodox literature reveals a range of estimates of vaccine *efficacy*, varying between diseases, and between different vaccines for similar diseases. In broad terms, the best estimates of efficacy range from 80% - 99%, where vaccine efficacy (VE) is commonly defined as

$$VE = \frac{ARU - ARV}{ARU} \times 100$$

where

ARU = Disease Attack Rate in unvaccinated children

ARV = Disease Attack Rate in vaccinated children

Now a similar comparison can be made for HP using known disease attack rates, which show the probability of an unimmunised person acquiring a disease following exposure. These rates can be used as a default control group for my study.

Table 4-9 summarises material from my doctoral thesis showing national attack rates for three diseases, and from *Homœoprophylaxis – A Fifteen Year Clinical Study* showing attack rates for HP for those diseases

(Golden I, 2004a, 2005). The efficacy of HP is thus able to be calculated for those three diseases, and once again shows a level comparable to that of vaccination. This also introduces the use of a default control group of unimmunised children against which the experience of children using HP may be compared. It is true that this is not a perfect control group, as the conditions of children using my program may be different from those of children studied nationally. However, such differences are likely to be small, and the published figures for national attack rates are relatively consistent.

Table 4-9 National Attack Rates and the Efficacy of HP

Disease	Attack Rate, Unimmunised %	Attack Rate, HP %	Efficacy of HP %
Whooping Cough	85.0	11.7	86.2
Measles	90.0	9.0	90.0
Mumps	70.0	5.9	91.6

4.2.2.3 A summary of findings of the combined surveys

No statistical study is ever perfect. There are always factors that can possibly affect the reliability of the findings. The orthodox community holds up the double-blind, randomised, controlled clinical trial to be the "gold standard" of testing. However, we know that every year drugs (and occasionally vaccines) that have been tested using this gold standard are withdrawn from use due to side-effects or failures in efficacy that were not identified during the testing process.

The gold standard is not perfect either!

The material I have presented above tells us the following:

1. HP has been used for over 200 years, with clinical reports showing a high level of effectiveness.

2. My research over nearly 20 years shows both the effectiveness and the efficacy of my long-term HP program of around 90%.

3. Substantial data verification procedures were applied to the last 5 years of my data. The results, after applying these checks, were consistent with the first 10 years of data. This supports the view that the 15 years of figures are reliable, without being perfect.

Now I have no doubt that an orthodox analyst with a case to make against HP will point out the remaining weaknesses in my data, and say that it proves nothing. However, the test that I am looking for is whether a reasonable person, with an open mind, believes that the historical experience with HP, supported by my data, shows that HP does offer a genuine option of a reasonably effective method of infectious disease prevention.

I believe that the material presented above does show that a genuine option exists. However, it is for you, the reader, to make your own judgement.

We shall now add to the strength of the above evidence the largest body of research supporting the effectiveness of HP that the world has seen. This has been generated from HP interventions in Cuban where they have immunised millions of people in 2007, 2008, 2009 and 2010.

4.2.3 The Cuban Experience

Since I published the amended 6th edition in 2007, I have experienced something that deserves its own sub-section in this book, and that is the work undertaken by the Cuban Government via the Finlay Institute in Havana, Cuba.

I first learnt of their wonderful work in December 2008 when I was invited to be a lead speaker at the NOSODES 2008 conference hosted by Finlay. They asked me to come and deliver my experiences to the very multinational audience who attended. In fact I quickly learned that they were the ones with the really interesting story to tell.

I kept in touch with Dr Gustavo Bracho, the Vice President of Finlay who planned and undertook the work under the leadership and inspiration of the Finlay President Dr Concepcion Campa.

I returned again for three weeks in April 2010 to renew acquaintances with Dr Campa and Dr Bracho, to further study their leptospirosis intervention in 2007 and 2008, to better understand their Swine Flu intervention in 2009/10, and to work with them on a possible trial of HP immunisation against Dengue Fever in an ASEAN country in 2010. I will now report on the three significant issues.

But firstly I wish to acknowledge the importance of having access to the Finlay data, without which much of this Section could not be written. This data was generated by the interventions managed by the Finlay Institute, and I wish to acknowledge and thank the President and Vice-President of Finlay for allowing me to use their data to prepare the graphs in this Section.

4.2.3.1 The 2007 and 2008 Leptospirosis Intervention

Leptospirosis is endemic in Cuba. It usually worsens during the high rainfall seasons from October to December each year, as the infection is usually spread via infected water, although rodent urine will also carry the disease.

The three eastern regions of Cuba, Las Tunas, Holguin and Granma (IR = Intervened Region), are usually the most affected by seasonal hurricanes and high rainfall, and thus have a much greater incidence of the disease per head of population than the rest of the country (RC).

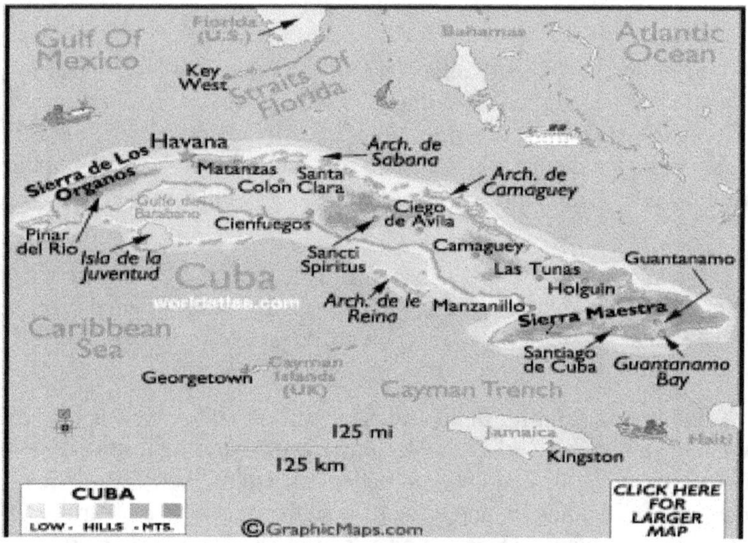
Gulf Of Mexico
Key West
Straits Of Florida
Atlantic Ocean
Havana
Sierra de Los Organos
Matanzas
Santa Clara
Colon
Arch. de Sabana
Arch. de Camaguey
Ciego de Avila
Cienfuegos
Pinar del Rio
Isla de la Juventud
Cuba
Sancti Spiritus
Camaguey
Las Tunas
Holguin
Guantanamo
Arch. de le Reina
Manzanillo
Sierra Maestra
Caribbean Sea
Santiago de Cuba
Guantanamo Bay
Georgetown
Cayman Trench
125 mi
125 km
Kingston
CUBA
LOW - HILLS - MTS.
©GraphicMaps.com
CLICK HERE FOR LARGER MAP

Ref: http://www.worldatlas.com/webimage/countrys/namerica/caribb/cu.htm

Figure 4-1 shows the average weekly incidence of leptospirosis for 2003-2006 in IR (2.4 million people) and RC (8.8 million people), weighted per head of population figure for both regions (Average x population in Cuba/population in region). It clearly shows that from Week 40 onwards (October to December) the IR suffers much more from the disease than RC per head of population.

In both 2007 and 2008 the RC was hit by severe hurricanes. In 2007 the Cuban Government, through the Finlay Institute which manufactures vaccines used in Cuba, decided to homeopathically immunise the bulk of the population in IR due to a severe spike in the incidence of the disease.

Figure 4-2 shows the Incidence of the disease in 2007, and the impact of the homoeoprophylaxis (HP) program which was conducted in Week 45. Once again a weighted per head of population figure is shown, which illustrates the impact of the intervention even more clearly. 2007 was already a worse-than-average year for residents of IR, and became dramatically so following the hurricanes. However the outbreak "broke" in IR in Week 47, 2 weeks following the HP intervention, although it continued in RC where there was no intervention.

Figure 4-1 Leptospirosis, IR and RC, 2003-2006 weekly average weighted per head of population

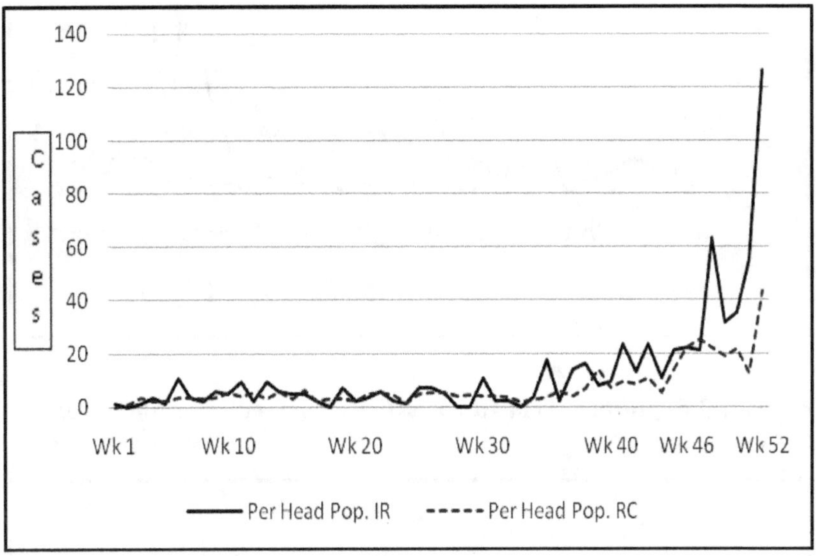
Cases
140
120
100
80
60
40
20
0
Wk 1
Wk 10
Wk 20
Wk 30
Wk 40
Wk 46
Wk 52
Per Head Pop. IR
Per Head Pop. RC

A second round of HP was administered in 2008 to the residents of IR, this time using a higher potency of the remedy (200C in 2007, 10,000C in 2008 – 2 doses a week apart). Figure 4-3 shows that the disease remained contained in IR (once again, the most at risk region), but continued as expected in RC with a significant single incident in Week 42.

Figure 4-2 Leptospirosis in IR and RC, 2007, weekly, weighted per head of population

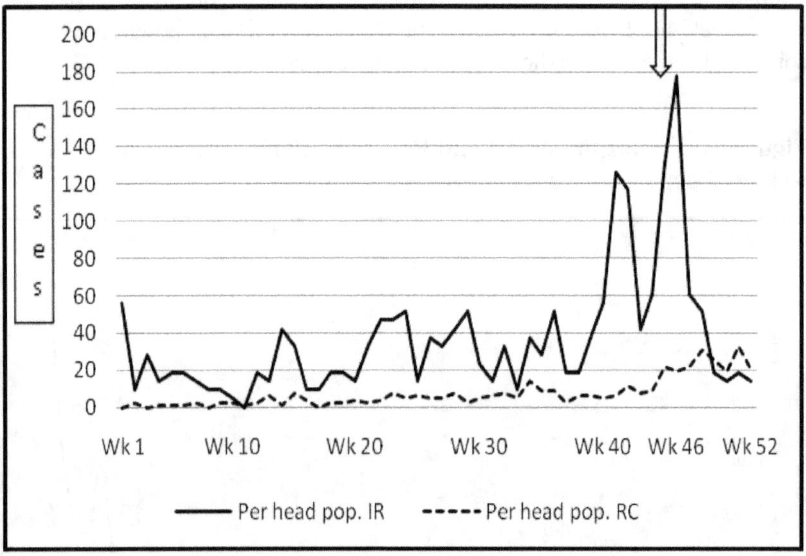

200
180
160
140
120
100
80
60
40
20
0
Cases
Wk 1
Wk 10
Wk 20
Wk 30
Wk 40
Wk 46
Wk 52
Per head pop. IR
Per head pop. RC

Figure 4-3 Leptospirosis in IR and RC, 2008, weekly, weighted per head of population

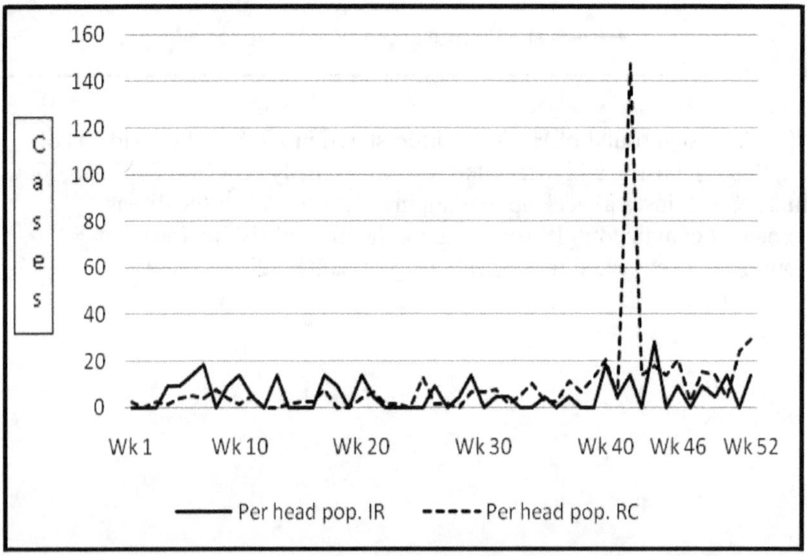

160
140
120
100
80
60
40
20
0
Cases
Wk 1
Wk 10
Wk 20
Wk 30
Wk 40
Wk 46
Wk 52
Per head pop. IR
Per head pop. RC

The impact of the HP intervention is clear from the above Figures, but was also demonstrated when comparing the progression of the disease in IR in 2007 to the expected number of cases derived using a predictive model based on rainfall experience over time, plus other factors. Figure 4-4 has been reproduced in other studies of the intervention (Campa C et. al., 2008; Bracho G et.al. 2010; Golden I, Bracho G, 2010).

Figure 4-4 Leptospirosis in 2007, actual and predicted incidence

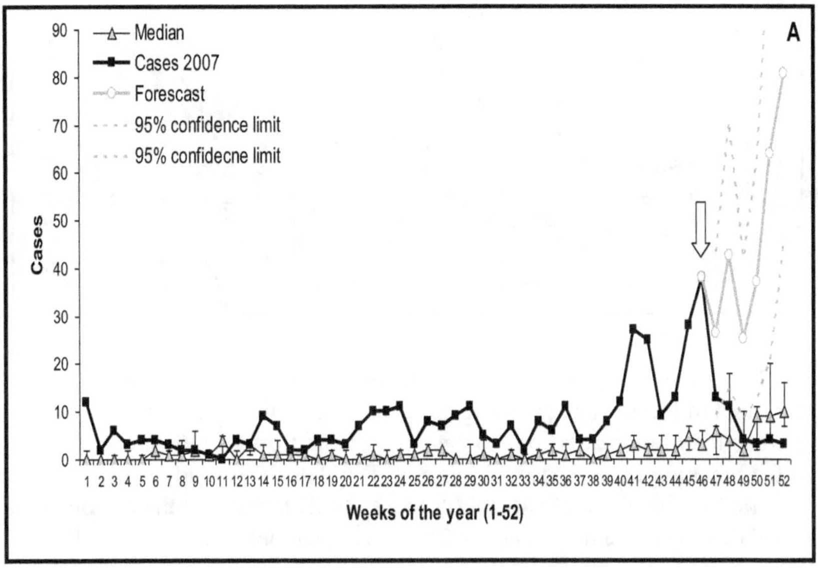
Median
Cases 2007
Forescast
95% confidence limit
95% confidecne limit
A
Cases
0
10
20
30
40
50
60
70
80
90
1 2 3 4 5 6 7 8 9 10 11 12 13 14 15 16 17 18 19 20 21 22 23 24 25 26 27 28 29 30 31 32 33 34 35 36 37 38 39 40 41 42 43 44 45 46 47 48 49 50 51 52
Weeks of the year (1-52)

One issue regarding this diagram was the reliability of the predictive model used. Further examination revealed that the model used was quite reliable in IR, but much less so in RC. Figure 4-5 shows actual rainfall figures from 2004 to 2008. These figures are only available monthly, so the data for leptospirosis was formed into monthly totals, and the predictive model for December was plotted onto the diagram.

This shows that the predictive model somewhat overestimated expected cases in IR, especially in December 2007 where the impact of the intervention was most clearly felt, but that the dramatic difference between predicted and actual figures shown in Figure 4-4 could be relied on. The predictive figures for 2008 factored in the effects of the intervention.

Figure 4-5 Leptospirosis cases (x10) and monthly rainfall in IR 2004-2008 with December predictive cases (x10)

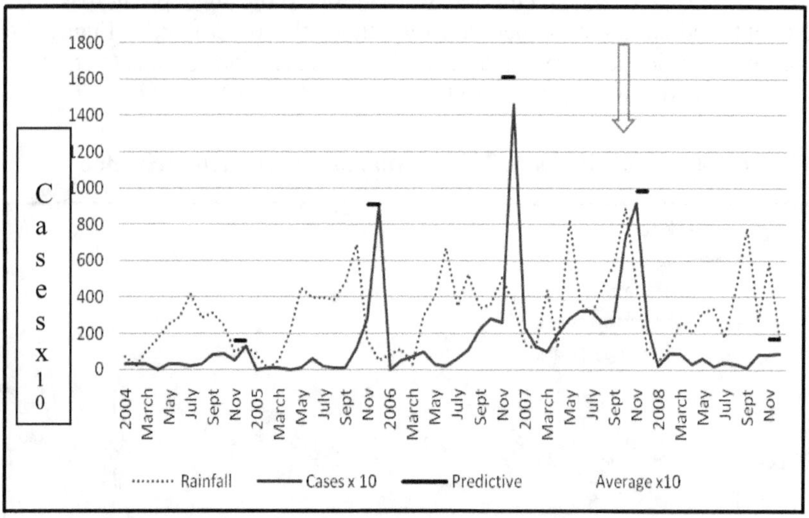
1800
1600
1400
1200
1000
800
600
400
200
0
C a s e s x 1 0
2004
March
May
July
Sept
Nov
2005
March
May
July
Sept
Nov
2006
March
May
July
Sept
Nov
2007
March
May
July
Sept
Nov
2008
March
May
July
Sept
Nov
Rainfall
Cases x 10
Predictive
Average x10

One final examination of the leptospirosis data from 2004 to 2008 is presented in Figure 4-6, showing the incidence of the disease for both regions. It shows clearly the seasonal peaks and troughs over the years, with a breaking of the seasonal trend in IR in late 2007, and the substantial reduction of the disease in IR in 2008 despite IR remaining the region most at risk due to severe hurricanes in 2008 as shown below in Table 4-10.

Table 4-10 Hurricanes in Cuba in 2008

Hurricane	Category	Week impact	Regions affected, **2008**
Fay	Tropical storm	Week 34	Central Region
Gustav	Hurricane, 5	36	Western Region but rains in Eastern Regions (including IR)
Ike	Hurricane, 4	38	Eastern (first impact on IR) and then western region but affecting almost all the country
Paloma	Hurricane, 4	46	Western region over IR

Figure 4-6 Leptospirosis cases in IR and RC from 2004 to 2008

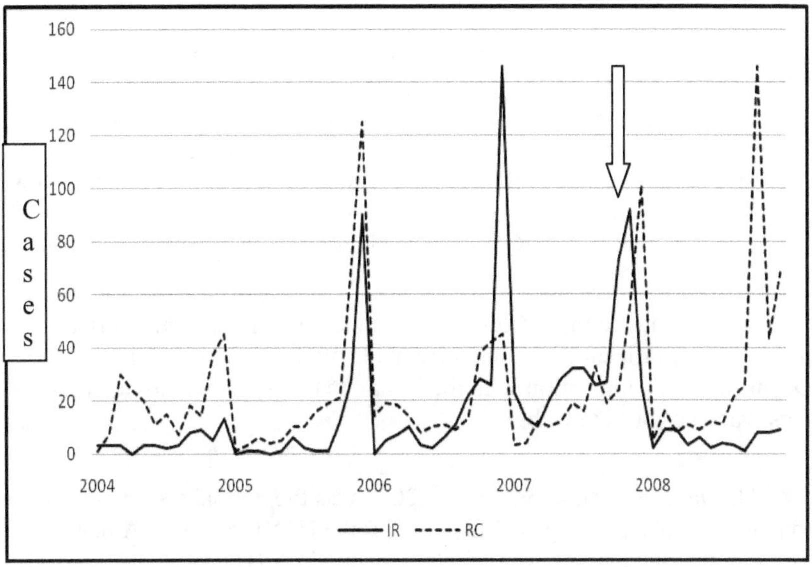
160
140
120
100
80
60
40
20
0
Cases
2004
2005
2006
2007
2008
IR
RC

Concluding Comments regarding the Lepto Intervention

The HP interventions against leptospirosis in IR in 2007 and 2008 have been an unqualified success. The details of the effective interventions was mentioned in the Cuban Assembly. Following on this experience, a decision was made to undertake a massive HP immunisation of the total population over 12 months of age against Swine Flu in 2009/10 involving over 9.8 million people. The results of this intervention will not be known until 2011 when data can be assembled and analysed.

The Cuban initiative proves that safe, effective, and low cost homoeopathic immunisation is possible. It will be followed with great interest by practitioners and public health scientists around the world. I revealed this initiative on Australian Television in late 2009. The station and reporters were attacked by members of the Australian Skeptics who clearly wanted to suppress an open discussion of factual scientific information which contested their narrow "pharmaceutical" view of the world which cannot understand energetic medicine. How scientific!!

4.2.3.2 The 2010 Swine Flu Intervention

An annual influenza vaccination program has been used in Cuba since 2002. The program typically targets high risk groups, and in the past has focused on elderly persons. The months typically showing the greatest incidence of influenza in Cuba are April and May (Spring), and in particular from October to December or January (Winter). The vaccination program usually takes place from September. The vaccines used are imported based on the WHO recommendations for the particular season.

In 2009, due to the world-wide outbreak of H1N1 (Swine Flu), a number of significant decisions were made by the Cuban Health Department in conjunction with the Finlay Institute (who manufacture most vaccines used in Cuba).

The vaccine used in September 2009 was the normal seasonal vaccine (due to the Cubans being unable to access the H1N1 vaccine). A new program was undertaken in April 2010 using the AH1N1vaccine from Novartis. The vaccination target group was expanded in April 2010 to include pregnant women and infants as well as the elderly. Acceptance of the vaccine was voluntary.

A decision was made to homeopathically immunize the majority of the Cuban population against influenza and other related respiratory diseases, and the program began from late November 2009 to early February 2010 (80% coverage), with some immunisation continuing into April 2010 (87.8% coverage).

The purpose of this brief outline is to describe the program undertaken by the Finlay Institute, and identify the methods of analysis that will be used once sufficient data has been collected. The following aspects of the intervention will be described:

The homoeoprophylaxis (HP) remedy used.

The HP program used.

The numbers of people immunised according to Province.

The proposed methods and timing of data collection.

The analytical techniques proposed.

The homoeoprophylaxis (HP) remedy used

The Cubans have extended the use of homoeopathic complexes (which contain more than a single potentised remedy) for immunisation. Whilst others have done this in a limited way for many years, the Cubans have found that when targeting a specific disease, the use of both the *Nosode* as well as *Genus Epidemicus* remedies and some treatments remedies produces a highly effective result. The remedies used are not random, but are selected carefully.

The Cubans have also perfected "antigen stripping" from orthodox vaccines – in effect a sophisticated filtration system where the large molecules of adjuvants, preservatives etc are filtered out leaving the pure antigenic material.

The Finlay Institute decided to prepare an HP complex containing:

Occilococinum 200CK

Influenzinum 200CK (From purified components* of AH3N2, AH1N1 and B influenza viruses – using antigen stripping)

Pneumococinum 200CK (From 5 inactivated strains of *Streptococcus pneumoniae*)

Aconitum napellus 30CH

Crotalus horridus 30CH

Eupatorium perfoliatum 12CH (in 30% hydro-alcoholic solution)

The Cubans, working with members of *Homeopaths Without Borders*, have also exhibited their preference for using complexes in their interventions. This may be disturbing for "classical" homeopaths (such as myself), but what they do works, and is still based firmly on the *Law of Similars* given that this is the basis for choosing the components of their intervention remedies.

The HP program used

The HP program was intended to be applied to the full population of the country over 1 year of age. The treatment schedule comprised 4 oral doses: starting with 3 doses in a period of 3 days (1 daily dose) followed by the last dose 7 days after. The massive application was achieved by doctor and nurses involved in the primary health care system. The Cuban health care system has a comprehensive health delivery system throughout the entire country, and was perfectly positioned to carry out this massive intervention. The resulting coverage is shown in Table 4-11.

The proposed methods and timing of data collection

The data will be collected from the National Program for Surveillance of respiratory diseases from the Minister of Public Health of Cuba. This program is based on the diagnosis and follow-up of patients attending primary care services, and by actively searching for cases within the community. The weekly data of the incidence of influenza, pneumonia and other respiratory diseases will be collected during 2010 to complete a year period at the beginning of 2011.

The analytical techniques proposed

The analytical techniques should be mainly focused on the comparison of incidence before and after the intervention by using historic data and trends of influenza throughout the country. Further comparison could be performed with other countries of the region. The results from this analysis are expected in 2011.

One of the consequences of using multiple nosodes in the HP complex is that the remedy should have a capacity to influence not just Swine Flu outbreaks but a whole range of respiratory symptoms.

As at September 2010, the administration of the HP immunisation has been completed with a nearly 90% coverage of the target population as shown in Table 4-11. It now comes down to a long period of observing, data collection, and finally data processing. The effectiveness of the intervention will not become clear until the end of 2010 and the beginning of 2011, but potentially will have profound international consequences within both the homeopathic and allopathic communities.

Table 4-11 The numbers of people immunised according to Province (to 9/4/2010)

Province	People	% of pop.
Pinar del Río	705,849	96.5
La Habana	515,420	69.7
Matanzas	667,019	97.5
Villa Clara	694,273	86.0
Cienfuegos	384,121	95.5
Sancti Spiritus	448,763	96.8
Ciego de Ávila	311,252	74.1
Camaguey	662,598	84.7
Las Tunas	461,314	86.4
Holguin	1,121,058	98.3
Granma	817,650	97.9
Santiago de Cuba	868,674	82.9
Guantanamo	498,642	97.2
Isla de la Juventud	69,414	80.1
Ciudad Habana	1,632,745	76.0
TOTAL	**9,858,792**	**87.79**

4.2.3.3 The Dengue Fever Trial 2010: Cooperation in Dengue Research

The Start

Links established between individuals, and then institutions, form the basis of cooperation in research. Figure 4-7 shows the initial relationships which were existing when the opportunity first arose. Figure 4-8 shows how it is hoped that the relationships will expand as described below.

In March 2010, senior officials of an ASEAN Government visited Cuba, and met with the President and colleagues from the Finlay Institute, saw Finlay's work on Dengue Fever, and offered Finlay seed funding to undertake a clinical trial of homoeoprophylaxis against Dengue Fever in the ASEAN country.

In April 2010 the CEO (Mr John Feenie) and Academic Business Manager from ECNH (myself) visited the Finlay Institute, and signed an MOU. The Dengue opportunity was discussed. ECNH advised Finlay of its existing MOU's with a University in the ASEAN country, and with the Mathematics School of Ballarat University in Australia (who have a capacity to process research data).

Figure 4-7 The First Relationships

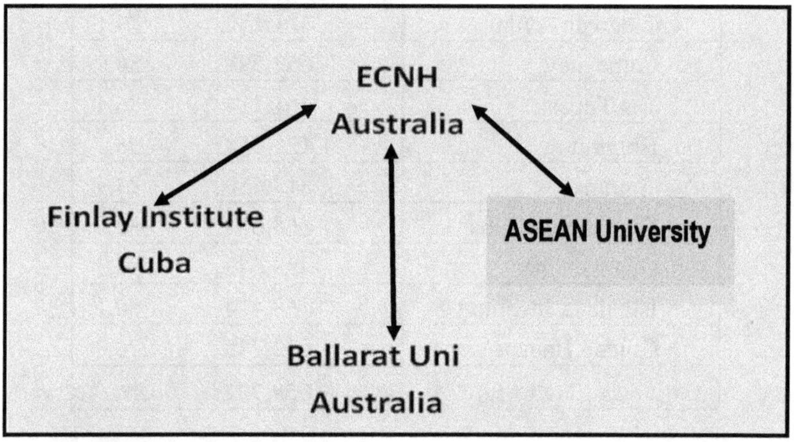
ECNH
Australia
Finlay Institute
Cuba
ASEAN University
Ballarat Uni
Australia

The Proposed Intervention

The relationships were proposed to be extended as shown in Figure 4-8. The proposed participants were:

EC = Endeavour College of Natural Health
FI = Finlay Institute
AU = ASEAN University
BU = Ballarat University

An initial plan was prepared, and a draft budget compiled.

Figure 4-8 Full Cooperation

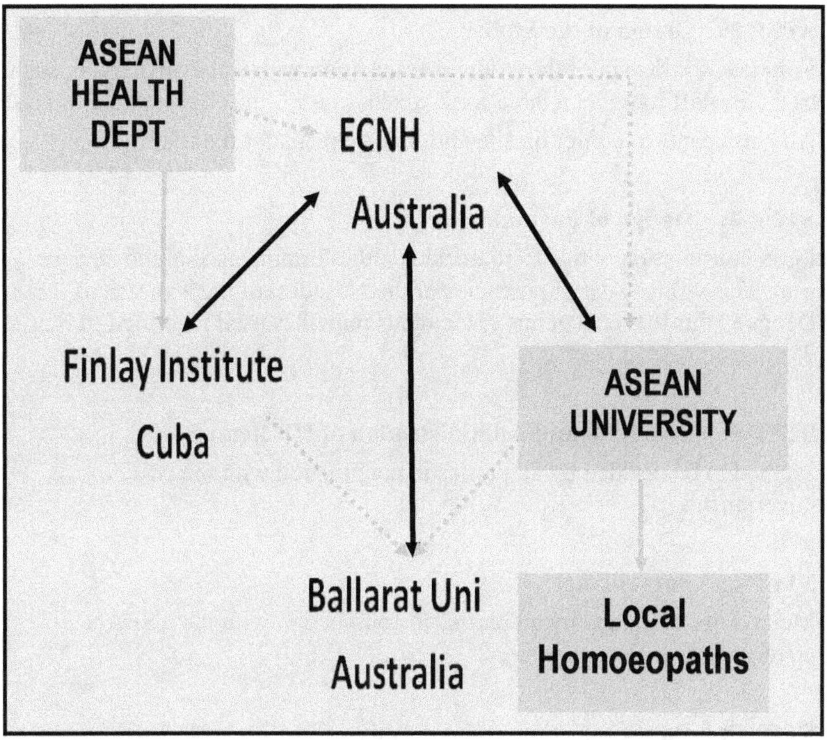
ASEAN
HEALTH
DEPT
ECNH
Australia
Finlay Institute
Cuba
ASEAN
UNIVERSITY
Ballarat Uni
Australia
Local
Homoeopaths

The Dengue Project

The project proposal was broken up into eight steps:

STEP 1: Selection of Region

AU personnel to consult with the ASEAN Health Department, and develop a profile of the Dengue outbreaks in the ASEAN country and suggest a particular region where the project might be best undertaken. Confer with FI and EC. Select the region to be studied.

STEP 2: Repertorisation of Regional Symptoms

EC staff visit the area, and consultat with AU staff, local homeopaths and medical practitioners develop an anamnesis of the Dengue outbreaks in the region. EC to undertake a repertorial analysis and confer with FI. Identify the genus epidemicus remedies associated with the disease in the region.

STEP 3: Design of the Study

FI to lead the design of the study in association with Cuban experts in such trials. FI staff to travel to area for 2 weeks, and EC and BU staff for 3 days. All particpants to confer on site and finalise plans for the trial.

STEP 4: Design of Formula

FI, in consultation with EC, to decide on the formula used in the Dengue trial. This will consist of potencies of the Nosodes of the 4 strains of Dengue, plus the local genus epidemicus remedies used identified in Step 2.

STEP 5: Provision and Administration of HP Remedy

Method to be decided by all parties in conjunction with the ASEAN government.

STEP 6: Surveillance

Method to be decided by all parties in conjunction with the ASEAN government.

STEP 7: Data Collection and Analysis

Once the trial is complete, staff from BU travel to area to collect data from AU staff. Process and analyse data in Australia, and provide a report to all participants

STEP 8: Recommendation to the ASEAN Government

FI to prepare a recommendation to the ASEAN Government based on the results of the trial. This will inform the possibility of undertaking a mass immunisation campaign against Dengue Fever in the ASEAN country.

At the time of writing in September 2010 it is unknown if this intervention will take place. Of course many people hope that it will, because it could offer to the world a model of dealing with infectious diseases which orthodox medicine cannot currently cope with. The information presented here is intended to show readers how practical research proposals aRE designed, and the complexity of arrangements needed for such projects to proceed.

4.2.4 HP Effectiveness v's Randomised Clinical Trials and Meta Analyses

The evidence I have presented from my own research is only one small part of the total range of evidence available, including 200+ years of recorded clinical experience, clinical trials in epidemic situations such as the meningococcal intervention in Brazil, and the massive interventions in Cuba.

Despite this significant body of data, orthodox critics will say that it is of no merit unless it includes randomised clinical trials (RCTs) which are the so called "gold standard" of orthodox research along with meta analyses of relevant RCTs. However this standard is far less reliable than orthodox sources suggest.

For a start, meta analyses are only as reliable as the clinical trials which they examine. When we find that data is manipulated to produce results which favour the biases of the researchers, then they lose all credibility. Homoeopathy has been subjected to such a biased attack via the now tarnished pages of the *Lancet* whose editors announced the "death of homoeopathy" in 2005 on the basis of an analysis by Shang and others which the *Lancet* published, and where the results were subsequently shown to be contrived by selective manipulation of the data (Shang et.al, 2005; Ludtke R, Rutten AL, 2008; Rutten AL, Stolper CE, 2008).

In fact the credibility of medical research in general has been compromised by numerous examples of how the massive financial influence of the multinational pharmaceutical giants has either directly or indirectly paid for corrupted research using RCTs, producing unreliable findings.

McGauren and colleagues have prepared a contemporary scholarly expose of dishonest research, and the implications it has on the release of unsafe or ineffective pharmaceuticals (McGauran et.al. 2010)

4.2.5 The general safety of homœoprophylaxis

The issue of whether HP is potentially toxic is a simple one to resolve. It is the one area where orthodox opponents of HP, and of homoeopathy in general, will agree. They say homoeopathically potentised substances cannot work because "nothing is there" of the original substance. Since "nothing" cannot be toxic, then homoeopathic potencies are not toxic.

However the matter is not quite so simple, for three reasons.

Firstly, homoeopathic potencies are carried in either a solution of alcohol and water, or in tiny pilules, usually made from either milk sugar, or maize starch. The carriers are medically neutral for the overwhelming majority of recipients, but very, very occasionally a recipient may be sensitive (allergic) to either alcohol or the base used to make the pillules. In such cases homoeopaths have techniques available to avoid this problem.

Secondly, we know with homoeopathic treatment that at times a patient who is not sensitive to the medicine carrier (they don't react to unmedicated pilules or to unmedicated alcohol and water), "reacts" to the medicine in a dynamic way. Explanations of why are given in homoeopathic texts (for example, Vithoulkas G, 1980). Similar reactions can also occur when HP remedies are administered. However, these reactions do not mean that the medicine is toxic, but rather that it has stimulated the recipient's own self healing mechanism, the *vital force* as it is called in homoeopathy, to act to remove disturbances in the mental/emotional/physical bodies of the recipient (refer to the example of Diphtherinum quoted in 4.2.5.1).

Thirdly, a few homoeopaths question the long-term safety of HP. They usually believe either (a) that homoeopathic medicines should only be used to treat diseases when they occur, (b) that HP should only be used in epidemics when a number of people have already become unwell, (c) that long-term use of high potencies and repeated doses can cause damage to the recipient in some energetic way.

Points (a) and (b) are more philosophical than evidence based, and I have addressed them in *Homœoprophylaxis – A Practical and Philosophical Review*, 3rd edition (Golden I, 2001). The third point was studied in my doctoral research, and a summary has been published in the homoeopathic literature (Golden I, 2004c). It will also be discussed below.

I can offer four pieces of evidence concerning the safety of my long-term HP program:

1. Physical – the remedies are non toxic, as discussed above.
2. The level of short-term reactions is very low, and the reactions are typically very brief and mild.
3. The long-term use of my HP program is generally associated with positive general wellbeing.
4. The long-term use of my HP program is statistically associated with lower levels of chronic illness than other methods of immunisation.

We shall now consider points 2, 3 and 4 in turn.

4.2.5.1 Short-term reactions to my HP program

Table 4-12 reports reactions to the medicines in the HP Program. The actual responses by parents reporting the reactions are reproduced in *Homœoprophylaxis – A Fifteen Year Clinical Study* (Golden I, 2004) for readers who would like to have that detail.

The majority of reactions were to the medicine Pertussin (as expected due to the recorded history of reactions to the pertussis vaccine). However, the number of reactions to the medicine Diphtherinum was significant. They suggest that there were a number of children whose parents or grandparents had contracted whooping cough or diphtheria, and not completely eliminated the effect of the disease. The Nosodes would have a balancing (healing) effect in such cases, and possibly explain the reported reactions.

In the latest series, Series 11-15, there was a relatively high level of reactions to Lathyrus Sativus (this remedy is not a Nosode), the remedy used as the poliomyelitis preventative. The reactions may be due to the likelihood of a fairly high level of exposure to the virus through contacts with recently vaccinated infants (the oral vaccine was used when these responses were being collected).

Table 4-12 Reactions to Remedies in Golden's Long-Term HP Program

	Definite Reactions to HP – per person		Reactions to HP – per dose (estimated) *
	No.	%	%
Series 1-5	51/708	7.2	1.2
Series 6-10	81/817	9.9	1.7
Series 11-15	81/817	9.9	1.7
Series 1-15	213/2342	9.1	1.5

* Note: the per-dose reaction rate is calculated by assuming on average 6 doses of medicine are administered each year. This takes into account the fact that many parents miss doses from time to time, and that in the later years of the program, doses are given more than one month apart.

The classification of the intensity and duration of the Series 11-15 reactions of my HP program is summarised in Table 4-13 below. Not all responses by parents showed their child's intensity or duration of reactions, and so the Table shows the figures for all responses, as well as the figures that exclude responses where no details were given.

Further, figures are shown for (a) all reactions that are classified as either "possible" or "definite", as well as (b) just for reactions classified as "definite". The "definite" figures are shown in brackets.

Note that the count in Table 4-13 is by respondent. The reason for this is that not all parents who reported a reaction to more than one remedy made clear which reaction was associated with which remedy.

There were 81 definite reports of reactions to kit remedies. However, 17 parents reported definite reactions to two diseases. That means that there were 64 questionnaire responses (children in the survey year) covering the 81 definite remedy reactions.

Table 4-12 reported that definite reactions were experienced in less than 1.5% of doses. The analysis of reactions in Table 4-13 shows (after excluding responses with no details) that most were mild (55.4%), and very few were strong (1.5%). The figures showed that 43.1% were classified as moderate in intensity.

If nothing else, this certainly shows that homoeopathic remedies containing only the "energy" of substances can produce definite and observable changes in infants and young children where the likelihood of a placebo effect is small.

The clear majority of respondents (87.8%) who reported the reactions stated that they were brief, lasting between 1-5 days. In fact, only 2 respondents who reported a reaction classified as moderate or strong also reported that the reaction was more than brief. Another 11 did not indicate the duration of the reaction.

The general comments of these 13 respondents were checked to see if there was any evidence of long-term health problems. One respondent (#11138) reported that her child had contracted whooping cough and was still unwell 6 months later. Two others (#14221 and #15110) repeated comments on the reactions that they had already reported. The others either made no comments, or positive comments about the health of their children.

Thus, it seems reasonable to conclude that whilst reactions to the remedies in the HP program are possible, the overwhelming experience of most children using the program shows that short-term reactions are very unlikely and those that do occur are usually mild and brief.

We can, however, clearly see that the use of triple doses in higher potencies has significantly increased the level of both definite and possible reported reactions to medicines in the kit, from 7.9% to 14.3% per person. The rise in the rate of definite reactions was from 7.2% to 9.9% per person. This emphasises the importance of precise parental instructions to ensure that any reaction to a medicine in a lower potency is followed by a suitable delay before administering higher potencies.

It should be noted that the above figures translate to a HP remedy reaction rate of less than 2% per dose of medicine, given the assumption of six doses from the program annually. As expected, the rate of reactions to medicines in the HP program is significantly less than that experienced with vaccination. For example, the National Health and Medical Research Council has stated that "Most vaccines have minor side effects" which "commonly follow immunisation with some vaccines and should be anticipated" (NH&MRC, 2008).

The results clearly demonstrate that an appropriate long-term HP program is very safe, as would be expected given that there are no toxic materials in the medicines, unlike vaccines which do contain toxic chemicals as well as antigenic material. Further information will be presented in section 4.2.5.2 and 4.2.5.3 below supporting this conclusion.

The time profile of reactions by respondent is shown in Table 4-14 below.

These profiles show that most reactions occur within the first year of the program, i.e., with the first doses of a new remedy. This result is expected by homoeopaths and, as with homoeopathic treatment, if a patient is sensitive to a substance (remedy) this will usually manifest most obviously with the first one or two doses, and so previous doses of HP remedies prepare the way for future doses.

Since the level of reactions falls throughout the program, this also suggests that the program is not recommending excessive doses of each remedy. If the doses were excessive, then we would expect reaction rates to rise.

The higher percentage of reactions in the first two years for Series 6-10 and Series 11-15 suggests that the use of triple doses has brought forward the reaction rate to the medicines in the program. Once again, this is expected from a classical homoeopathic perspective, given that a triple dose is a stronger challenge to the recipient than a single dose, and so a potential sensitivity will be activated more by a triple dose than a single dose. This is also why in my 2004 program I changed the first triple dose to three doses of the lower potency, rather than an ascending potency. I expect to see a lower reaction rate as a result. Data will be collected over the next five years to test and validate this assumption.

Table 4-13 A Summary of the Intensity and Duration of Reactions to the Series 11-15 HP Program, by Respondent

		Intensity/Duration of Reactions				
		All Responses				
		Mild/ Brief	**Moderate**	**Strong/ Long**	**No Details Given**	**Total Respon-dents**
Intensity	#	65 (36)	33 (28)	1 (1)	3 (1)	102 (66)
	%	63.7 (54.6)	32.4 (42.4)	1.0 (1.5)	2.9 (1.5)	100.0
Duration	#	46 (36)	7 (4)	1 (1)	48 (25)	102 (66)
	%	45.1 (54.6)	6.9 (6.0)	1.0 (1.5)	47.1 (37.9)	100.0
		Excluding Responses With No Details				
		Mild/ Brief	**Moderate**	**Strong/ Long**	**Total Respondents**	
Intensity	#	65 (36)	33 (28)	1 (1)	99 (65)	
	%	63.7 (55.4)	32.4 (43.1)	1.0 (1.5)	100.0	
Duration	#	46 (36)	7 (4)	1 (1)	54 (41)	
	%	85.2 (87.8)	13.0 (9.8)	1.9 (2.4)	100.0	

(1) The figures in brackets are for reactions classified as "definite". Other figures are for all reactions, classified as either "possible" or "definite".

(2) Classification of Duration of Reaction:

1 - 5 days – "Brief"; 6-13 days - "Moderate"; 14 + days - "Long"

(3) These 102 classifications are made by respondent, not by individual reaction (117), due to the nature of parental responses which did not always allow a clear classification by reaction. Two people reported definite reactions over 2 years.

In summary then, there are few (< 2%/dose) sort-term reactions to my HP program, and these reactions are typically mild and brief. In over 12,000 HP doses (2,342 x 6), only 34 reactions were more than mild, and of these no more than 13 were also more than brief. It is reasonable to conclude that the short-term safety of an appropriate HP program is high.

Table 4-14 Time Profile of Definite Reactions to Program Medicines by Respondent

Reactions occurred in	Series 1-5	Series 6-10	Series 11-15
1st year	64.3% (27)	76.8% (53)	83.3% (55)
2nd year	16.7% (7)	15.9% (11)	10.6% (7)
3rd year	11.9% (5)	4.4% (3)	4.6% (3)
4th year	7.1% (3)	2.9% (2)	1.5% (1)
Totals	100% (42)	100% (69)	100% (66)

Note: some respondents answered in more than one year

4.2.5.2 General comments by users of my HP program

At the end of each HP questionnaire, parents were invited to make comments if they wished to. Tables 14, 15 and 16 in the Appendix of the *15 Year Study* reproduce those parental comments which relate to the general health of their children.

One purpose of this analysis is to gauge whether there appears to be any evidence of a systematic weakening of children's immunity through using my long-term HP program.

While there are understandable biases in the figures, such as parents who were unhappy with the HP program not bothering to respond (although some clearly did), the figures seem to suggest quite clearly that children using the program enjoyed better-than-average medium-term health than their peer group.

This supports the proposition made in previous publications that a properly constructed and administered long-term HP program in no way weakens the general health and vitality of those children using the program (Golden I, 2004, page 8).

A classification of general comments made by Series 11-15 respondents to my HP program was made to assess the long-term wellbeing of children using the program. A summary of responses is shown in Table 4-15 below which shows the breakdown of all comments into "positive" and "negative" for three categories of response – "health related comments", "administration of the program" and "other comments".

There were a very large percentage of comments in the "neutral" categories (58.3%) which have been removed in Table 4-15 and only positive and negative comments are recorded. They provide a more accurate indication of the relative strengths or weaknesses of the program.

Three conclusions may be drawn from the data in Table 4-15:

1. Parents of children using the program who commented on the health of their child reported significantly more positive health experiences (92.3%) than negative ones (7.7%). This long-term figure, combined with earlier findings of a less than 2% reaction rate per dose, suggests that the program is safe both in the short and long terms.

2. Parents of children using the program who commented on the administration of the program reported a significant level of problems (72.5%). These problems mainly related to difficulties in administering the pilules, especially the need to dose between meals. There is little that can be done to change the method of administration, since giving doses with meals would antidote most doses. Fortunately, these administration difficulties were reported in only 3.55 % of total responses (29/817). Most will cease to be an issue when the child is older and does not require regular feeding.

3. Parents of children using the program who made general comments on their experience with the program were generally very happy (89.7%), with only a minority (10.3%) voicing discontent.

The comments by Series 11-15 parents whose children used my long-term HP program strongly suggest that these children experience very few long-term problems with their health, and in fact many positive comments are made about how well the children are.

This data suggest that the long-term safety of the program is high. This data are also totally consistent with the conclusions made using data from the General Health Survey for children who used HP and/or other methods of disease prevention.

Table 4-15 General Comments by Users of the HP Program

	Health Related Comments		**Administration of the Program**		**Other Comments**	
	#	%	#	%	#	%
Positive	72	92.3%	11	27.5%	52	89.7%
Negative	6	7.7%	29	72.5%	6	10.3%
Total	78	100.0%	40	100.0%	58	100.0%

4.2.5.3 Overall long-term safety of my HP program

As part of my doctoral studies at Swinburne University between 2001 and 2004, I collected a two page questionnaire (the General Health Survey) from parents of 781 children aged between 4 and 12 years of age.

This retrospective study used measures of the child's health experience such as the incidence of asthma, eczema, ear and hearing problems, allergies and behavioural problems, as well as the parents' evaluation of their child's general health. Cases of whooping cough, measles and mumps were recorded, as was each child's hospitalisation experience.

With both health conditions and infectious diseases, respondents were asked whether a diagnosis by a medical practitioner was made.

These indices of health were compared to a number of early childhood factors, as well as the method of disease prevention.

Four different types of immunisation history were questioned. They were: (1) Homoeoprophylactically protected with disease-specific medicines.

(2) Vaccine protected

(3) "Constitutionally" protected, (i.e., any general health measures intended to improve overall health, and thus improve overall immunity against all infectious diseases)

(4) No specific or general protection against infectious diseases.

NOTE: some respondents used 2 or 3 of the immunisation methods. We therefore define:

"**HP-only**" = persons who used HP as their sole method of immunisation against targeted diseases. Similarly for categories 2 and 3.

The findings of the General Health Survey were statistically significant, (P>95%), in regards to the safety of HP-only (this is the measure that excludes respondents who used both HP and one or more other methods of immunisation). The analysis was divided into measures of absolute safety, and measures of relative safety.

The Absolute Safety of HP

The data from the General Health Survey linked five health conditions – asthma, eczema, ear/hearing problems, allergies, behavioural problems - with the above four different methods of immunisation, including HP.

Two statistical measures of the absolute safety of HP were used in the analysis.

1. **Proportion (SHP1)** = $\dfrac{\text{Persons with the Condition (using HP only)}}{\text{All Persons (using HP only)}}$

The lower the value of SHP1, the more safe the method (HP). This proportion was compared to the national average for each condition, where available.

The figure was also calculated for conditions where a diagnosis was made by a GP, and this was compared with the total figures for all conditions. Whilst a GP diagnosis may not always be correct, and other diagnoses may not always be incorrect, it does give another insight into the reliability of the total figure.

Note that in order to minimise the influence of confounding variables (i.e. factors that may cause a distortion of results), the analysis considered those children who used HP-only, and excluded other children who used a variety of preventative methods together with HP.

2. **Odds Ratio (SHP2)** = $\frac{A1}{A2}$ where

$$A1 = \frac{\{\text{Condition (using HP-only)}\}}{\{\text{No Condition (using HP-only)}\}} \qquad A2 = \frac{\{\text{Condition (not using HP)}\}}{\{\text{No Condition (not using HP)}\}}$$

If the Odds Ratio was greater than 1, the method would be classified as unsafe. For a method to be regarded as very safe we would expect the Odds Ratio to be significantly below 1.

I constructed the following classification of degrees of safety as shown in Table 4-16. This classification provides a subjective guide only to the safety of a method.

Table 4-16 Definition of Degrees of Safety

0.00 < Odds Ratio <=0.25	– very safe
0.25 < Odds Ratio <= 0.50	– safe
0.50 < Odds Ratio <= 0.75	– moderately safe
0.75 < Odds Ratio <= 1.00	– not safe
Odds Ratio > 1.00	– unsafe

In addition to the Odds Ratio, the Chi Squared probability of the association between "the use of HP only" and "the observed condition" being a coincidence was calculated.

A measure will not be accepted unless its confidence level is at least 95%. This requires a Chi Squared probability of 0.05 or less. The lower the Chi Squared figure, the greater the likelihood that the association between the health condition (e.g., asthma) and the method of immunisation used (e.g., HP only) as reflected in the Odds Ratio is NOT a coincidence. These ratios and probability estimates are listed in Table 4-17 below.

The figure for SHP1 shows that the incidence of asthma among children who use only HP as a method of disease prevention (3%) is well below the national average of 19%. It further shows that the incidence of behavioural problems is extremely low, with very modest levels for the remaining conditions.

However, the Odds Ratio is the more reliable of the two figures. **It is less than 1 for every condition studied, which shows that HP-only is not linked with an increase in the incidence of any of the conditions examined**.

Further, we can say with a high probability (P>98%) that HP-only is associated with a lower than average chance of acquiring asthma and eczema; with a moderate probability (P=93%) of developing fewer allergies; and with a low probability of having fewer behavioural problems (P=83%) than children not using only HP. The result linking HP-only with ear and hearing problems indicated that HP-only was not safe based on the

Table 4-17 Ratio Analysis of the Safety of the HP-Only Immunisation Option

Condition	**Proportion (SHP1)***			**Odds Ratio (SHP2) ***	**Chi Squared Probability**	**Results**	
	No GP diagnosis	With GP diagnosis	National Average		P	**Measure of Safety**	**Level of Confidence**
Asthma	0.03	0.03	0.16** - 0.19*	0.117	0.0004	Very safe	Very high
Eczema	0.10	0.04	N/A	0.382	0.015	Safe	High
Ear/hearing	0.17	0.11	N/A	0.917	0.79	Not safe	Nil
Allergies	0.15	0.04	0.09 – 0.16**	0.550	0.07	Moderately safe	Medium
Behaviour	0.04	0.01	N/A	0.446	0.17	Safe	Low

References:

* (Australian Bureau of Statistics, 1999. *Health – Mortality and Morbidity: Asthma.* Australian Social Trends, 1999).

** (Australian Bureau of Statistics, 2003. *Summary of Results, Australia.* National Health Survey, 2003).

*** SHP1 = Safety of HP, measure 1; SHP2 = Safety of HP, measure 2.

classification described in Table 4-17; however, the result was not statistically significant.

Thus, in absolute terms HP-only is shown to be a safe method of disease prevention.

The Relative Safety of HP

A more precise measure of relative safety can be found by examining the relationship between HP and other methods of immunization, and the five different chronic health conditions covered by the General Health Survey questionnaire. This relationship is examined in Tables 4-17 and 4-18 below. **The measures for each condition that are statistically significant are shown in bold print.**

The relationship between the five conditions and HP programs supplied by me is also shown in Table 4-17. The difference between HP programs supplied by me and other HP programs is discussed fully in section 4.3 below. A significant difference is found.

We may summarize the statistically significant findings ($P<0.05$) for each condition using the above data as follows:

Asthma - we can say with 99% confidence that HP-only is 15 times safer than vaccination and 6 times safer than no method of protection.

Eczema - we can say with 98% confidence that HP-only is 1.8 times safer than no method of protection.

Ears/Hearing Problems, Allergies, Behavioral Problems - we are not able to draw conclusions about the safety of HP-only with a greater than 95% confidence that the conclusion is correct.

Thus, for the two conditions where statistically significant results were found, HP-only was the safest option in both conditions when compared with vaccination and the do-nothing option. This result also applied to HP programs supplied by me.

Table 4-18 The Relative Safety of HP – All Conditions

					Method	
Condition	**Measurement**	**HP only**	**Vaccination only**	**General only**	**Nothing**	**HP from Golden**
Asthma	Odds Ratio	**0.117**	**1.75**	0.464	**0.74**	**0**
	Chi Test P	**0.0004**	**0.0025**	0.102	**7.9E-40**	**0.017**
Eczema	Odds Ratio	**0.382**	1.315	0.781	**0.674**	**0.153**
	Chi Test P	**0.0146**	0.121	0.513	**5.3E-40**	**0.035**
Ear/ Hearing	Odds Ratio	0.917	1.149	0.585	**0.533**	0.393
	Chi Test P	0.792	0.459	0.222	**2.3E-40**	0.193
Allergies	Odds Ratio	0.550	1.220	0.653	**0.520**	0.60
	Chi Test P	0.074	0.239	0.254	**1.2E-40**	0.351
Behaviour	Odds Ratio	0.446	0.869	2.103	**0.397**	0
	Chi Test P	0.170	0.593	0.063	**2.7E-40**	0.123

Note: (1) Statistically significant figures are shown in bold type.
(2) $7.9E\text{-}40 = 7.9/(10^{40})$

The overall reliability of these measures can be tested by re-examining the above results, but only including those conditions that have been diagnosed by a medical practitioner. Of course, not all such diagnoses may be correct. Further, diagnoses made by non-medical practitioners or by parents themselves may be quite valid. These new figures are shown in Table 4-18 below.

It seems reasonable to assume that if the overall rankings of safety in the Tables 4-17 and 4-18 are consistent, then the results are reliable. We find that many more measures in Table 4-18 have P<0.05 than in Table 4-17.

We may summarise the findings using the GP diagnosed data as follows for each condition, including only those results with a confidence level of 95%:

Asthma - we can say with 99% confidence that HP-only is 15 times safer than vaccination and 5.6 times safer than no method of protection.

Eczema - we can say with 99% confidence that HP-only is 7.4 times safer than vaccination, with 97% confidence that HP-only is 0.06 times less safe than general protection, and with 99% confidence that HP-only is 2.8 times safer than no method of protection.

Ear/Hearing Problems - we are not able to draw conclusions about the safety of HP-only with a greater than 95% confidence that the conclusion is correct. However, we can say with 95% confidence that vaccination is 3.9 less safe than doing nothing

Allergies - we can say with 94% confidence that HP-only is 5 times safer than vaccination, and with 99% confidence that HP is 2 times safer than no method of protection.

Behavioral Problems - we are not able to draw conclusions about the safety of HP-only with a greater than 95% confidence that the conclusion is correct. However, we can say with 95% confidence that doing nothing is twice as safe as general protection. We can say with 94.5% confidence that HP-only is the safest option.

Examining the statistically significant results from both tables, we find that only once was HP-only shown to be less safe than another method, and that was only 0.06 times less safe in that instance.

Thus we may conclude that, with the exceptions of ear and hearing problems, we can say with a high level of confidence (>95%) that HP-only is a very safe method of disease prevention compared to other alternatives, especially vaccination.

Table 4-19 The Relative Safety of HP - All Conditions - GP Diagnoses Only

		Method			
Condition	**Measurement**	**HP only**	**Vaccination only**	**General only**	**Nothing**
Asthma	Odds Ratio	**0.124**	**1.89**	0.49	**0.69**
	Chi Test P	**0.0006**	**0.0007**	0.13	**6.5E-40**
Eczema	Odds Ratio	**0.239**	**1.76**	**0.225**	**0.665**
	Chi Test P	**0.0097**	**0.006**	**0.025**	**6.5E-40**
Ear/ Hearing	Odds Ratio	0.703	**1.517**	0.599	**0.401**
	Chi Test P	0.364	**0.04**	0.282	**9.4E-41**
Allergies	Odds Ratio	**0.307**	1.518	0.446	**0.608**
	Chi Test P	**0.038**	0.061	0.171	**5.8E-40**
Behaviour	Odds Ratio	**0.541**	0.784	**1.675**	**0.784**
	Chi Test P	**0.055**	0.613	**0.049**	**1.2E-40**

Note: Statistically significant figures are shown in bold type.

4.2.5.4 A summary of findings regarding the safety of long-term HP

The above findings are summarised in Table 4-20 below. The evidence clearly shows that the use of an appropriate long-term HP program is associated with no reduction in the general health of recipients, and in fact some positive association is suggested.

Table 4-20 Summary of Evidence of the Safety of Long-Term HP

15 Year Study – # = 2,342	**General Health Survey - # = 781**
	SAFETY
1. Short term safety – reactions to 1.5% of doses (Table 4-11). Reactions typically brief and mild (Table 4-12). **2. Long term safety** – General Comments by parents re: general health of child – 92.3% positive; 7.7% negative (Table 4-43).	**Long term safety of HP only** – 1. Absolute safety of HP only – (Tables 4-16) Odds ratio < 1 for every condition studied: Asthma = 0.12 (GP = 0.12) Eczema = 0.38 (GP = 0.24) Ear/hearing = 0.92 (GP = 0.70) Allergies = 0.55 (GP = 0.31) Behaviour = 0.45 (GP = 0.54) 2. Relative safety of HP only - Asthma - safest; P = 0.0004 (GP = safest; P=.0006) Eczema - safest; P = 0.015 (GP = 2nd s/t; P=0.001) Ear/hearing - 3rd safest; P = 0.8 (GP = 3rd sfst; P = 0.364) Allergies - 2nd safest;P = 0.07 (GP = safest; P=0.038) Behaviour - 2nd safest; P = 0.17 (GP = safest; P=0.055) (P = Chi squared probability) 3. Accumulated parental rankings of general health of their child - HP only is associated with the highest level of health over all rankings. (Thesis, Figure 5.19)

This material represents the first statistical evidence showing that an appropriate long-term HP program may be associated with a long-term improvement in the general health of recipients, as measured by a relatively lower incidence of asthma, eczema, ear infections, allergies and behavioural problems compared to vaccinated, constitutionally protected and unprotected children. The reason for this will be debated, but from a homoeopathic perspective, it appears consistent with the improvement in general health in people who participate in correctly designed homoeopathic provings. The subtle challenge to the immune system appears to mature and strengthen the immune system - a variation of the hygiene hypothesis discussed in Section 1.2. But not all HP programs are the same, and this will now be discussed.

4.3 A comparison of different HP programs

Respondents to the General Health Survey in my doctoral research who reported using an HP program used a variety of programs. It was possible, through matching respondents' names and addresses, to identify which respondents to the General Health Survey obtained their program directly from me, and those who did not.

Fifty-nine people responding to the General Health Survey used HP programs directly obtained from me (25 of these used no other method of immunisation). One hundred people in the survey used HP not obtained directly from me (47 of these used no other method of immunisation).

It is possible that some of the 100 respondents who did not obtain an HP program from me still used a program obtained from another practitioner who copied my program. It was not possible to identify these respondents from the data collected, but they are unlikely to be in the majority.

A comparison between respondents using HP programs obtained from me, and respondents using other HP programs, revealed noticeable differences. This has been analysed in some detail in *Homœoprophylaxis – A Fifteen Year Clinical Study* (Golden I, 2004a).

The results of the comparison are summarised in Table 4-21. The figures show conditions and diseases for all HP users (whether or not other methods of immunisation were reported), and those who used HP-only. The figures are further subdivided into people who obtained their HP program directly from me, and those who did not.

All but one comparison (allergies – HP-only) showed a better result for the programs supplied by me. However, the size of data collected does not allow the statistical significance of these comparisons to be calculated.

The results also show that using HP alone gives a better result than using HP combined with other forms of disease prevention. This suggests that some users may have had a bad experience with other forms of prevention and then switched to HP (something I regularly see in practice), but this cannot be proved from the figures.

In addition, Chi Squared tests were performed to compare programs which I supplied, and programs which I did not supply. An odds ratio >1 would show an unfavourable result for programs supplied by me, and a result <1 would be favourable to programs I supplied. The results presented in Table 4-21 were statistically significant. They showed that Asthma and the three diseases studied are all less likely to occur if a program supplied by me is used, compared to one not supplied by me.

Table 4-21 Comparison of HP Programs

	All HP		HP Only	
	Golden	Not Golden	Golden	Not Golden
Number of Respondents	59	100	25	47
CONDITIONS				
Proportion with Asthma	5.1%	16.0%	0.0%	4.3%
Proportion with Eczema	17.0%	20.0%	4.0%	12.8%
Proportion with Ear/Hearing	15.3%	26.0%	8.0%	21.3%
Proportion with Allergies	23.7%	29.0%	16.0%	12.8%
Proportion with Behaviour Issues	8.5%	12.0%	0.0%	6.4%
DISEASES				
Proportion with Measles	6.8%	18.0%	0.0%	12.8%
Proportion with Whooping Cough	10.2%	17.0%	0.0%	17.0%
Proportion with Mumps	1.7%	1.0%	0.0%	0.0%

The Chi-squared comparisons are now shown in Table 4-22.

The results confirm that the type of HP program used does make a difference. They indicate, with some degree of significance, that children using HP programs supplied by me acquired fewer infectious diseases and reported fewer adverse long-term health conditions, than children using HP programs that I did not supply. I was not able to collect details of the other programs used, but experience tells me that they often included lower potencies given at very frequent intervals for extended periods of time. This is an issue that needs to be taken up by professional homoeopaths.

Table 4-22 Comparative results of HP Programs: Golden and Not-Golden

	Use of HP All HP or HP only	Odds Ratio	Chi Squared Probability
Asthma	All HP	0.28	96%
Measles	All HP	0.33	95%
	HP only	0.00	94%
Whooping Cough	HP only	0.00	97%
Mumps	HP only	0.00	100%

4.4 The use of HP by Australian homoeopaths

As part of my doctoral research, I sent questionnaires to all Australian specialist homoeopathic associations. Most associations responded. The specialist associations surveyed all require dedicated training in homoeopathy, typically leading to a Diploma or Advanced Diploma in Homoeopathy. The results were reported to the profession in 2002 (Golden I, 2002a). Note that in 2010 an Advanced Diploma is the minimum entry standard to practice, and in time it will become a degree.

It was decided not to survey naturopathic associations, who have relatively few members who specialise in homoeopathy, because results might have been significantly influenced by a great number of responses from non-specialist homoeopaths whose knowledge of HP would have been much less than those practitioners whose qualifications allowed them to join a specialist homoeopathic association.

Practitioners were surveyed via their associations, as mailing lists are confidential, and the associations usually have up-to-date addresses. In all, 532 questionnaires were sent out. Practitioners who belonged to more than one of the associations surveyed received multiple questionnaires. It was impossible to determine the exact number of multiple questionnaires sent to these practitioners, as Associations did not disclose membership lists. However, an allowance has been made for the 5 multiple responses found in the responses received. Further, associations tended to order questionnaires in rounded figures, and it is likely that some questionnaires would not have been used due to over-ordering.

210 responses were received, representing a response rate of 39.5% of questionnaires sent. The effective response rate would thus have been greater than 40% given multiple association membership and the over-ordering by associations.

Nationally, the response rates were varied. NSW, Victoria and Tasmania recorded responses over 50%, whilst responses from WA and Queensland were below 30% and the response from SA was 8%.

Responses from different associations were also very mixed. Response rates exceeding 40% were received from members of the Australian Medical Faculty of Homoeopathy and the Australian Homoeopathic Association. Less than 20% of members of the Australian Association of Professional Homoeopaths Inc responded. A third of all members contacted who belonged to the Homoeopathic Education and Research Association [HERA] responded. The latter association was the only one whose executive did not assist the research, and members of HERA were identified in Yellow Pages listings and contacted directly. This may have affected the response rate.

In order to analyse a "majority" view (i.e., States where more than 50% of eligible practitioners responded), the data were examined in three batches: (1) all 210 responses; (2) 156 responses from N.S.W., A.C.T., Victorian and Tasmania (States where the response rate was above 50%); and (3) 54 responses from Queensland, W.A. and S.A. (States where the response rate was below 50%).

In addition, two other profiles in the data were examined, (1) 100 responses from experienced homoeopaths who had been in practice for eight or more years; (2) 48 responses from practitioners who were not certain about their use of HP, or who said they would not use HP.

The following conclusions may be drawn from the survey:

1. **Knowledge of HP**. Whilst just 3% of respondents have never learned about HP, only one third **had** read Hahnemann's essay first describing his use of HP. Interestingly, of the 8 respondents who said they would never use HP, 6 had not read Hahnemann's essay. Further, of the 5 respondents who said it was not appropriate for a homoeopath to assist in the prevention of infectious disease if requested by a patient, none had read Hahnemann's essay.
2. **Use of HP**. Half of all respondents currently use HP; another quarter intend to use it in the future with 19% being unsure concerning future use.
3. **HP and the Law of Similars**. A majority of respondents believed that HP is based on the Law of Similars, 17% were unsure, and 24% believed it was not. Of the 51 respondents who believed HP was **not** based on the Law of Similars, 38 had not read Hahnemann's essay on HP.
4. **Type of Prevention.** Two thirds believed that HP should be used for both long-term and short-term prevention, 16% would use it only for short-term prevention, and 3% would never use it in any circumstance.
5. **Opposed to any use of HP.** 11 respondents (5.2% of the total respondents) answered "yes" to at least one of the following questions in the survey, thus indicating their opposition to the use of HP.
   - (i) Never use HP in any circumstances (Question 6)
   - (ii) It is not appropriate for a homoeopath to assist in the prevention of infectious disease if requested by a patient (Question 7)
   - (iii) A homoeopath should only treat infectious diseases once they have appeared, and should never assist in the prevention of infectious diseases (Question 8)

   Four of these eleven respondents answered "yes" in two of the three questions, and one in all three. Of these eleven, one said he/she currently used HP, five said they would prevent diseases if requested, and four of these said they would prevent and not just treat.

   Thus only four practitioners were unambiguously opposed to the use of HP under any circumstances.

Even though just under half of specialist homoeopaths responded, it is clear that HP enjoys considerable support among Australian homoeopaths, and is used by a majority of practitioners who completed the survey. To suggest that all of the non-responding practitioners were opposed to the use of HP is grossly unrealistic (such people usually take any opportunity to express their opposition). It certainly may be possible that many who did not respond were uncertain or did not understand the issue, but this is more a reflection on the quality of homoeopathic education in some Colleges than reflecting an opposition to the use of HP.

4.5 Suggested homoeopathic prophylactics for overseas travel

I am frequently asked to provide prophylactics for overseas travel. I can state with confidence that for almost every disease there is a homoeopathic remedy which has proven to be effective in providing protection from that disease.

At the turn of the century, homoeopathy was widely used because of its effectiveness in both treating and preventing the plagues of infectious diseases which swept Europe, India, and (to a lesser extent) America during the late 1800's. There is no reason why the remedies which proved effective then should be less effective today. It is to the discredit of medical science that historical facts such as these have not been acknowledged and utilised to the benefit of all people.

In deciding which homoeopathic remedies to take overseas, three excellent references are recommended:

- Dr P Sankaran, *Prophylactics in Homoeopathy*. The Homoeopathic Medical Publishers, Bombay, 1972. (This publication includes a very comprehensive bibliography of Homoeopathic sources from the earliest masters to contemporary authors.)
- K Thompson, E Miksevicius, *Vaccination - Research, Information and Guidelines for Homoeopathic Practitioners*. Australian Institute of Homoeopathy, 1988.
- Dr Colin B Lessell, *The World Traveller's Manual of Homoeopathy*. C W Daniel Co Ltd, 1993.

Travellers should also purchase the booklet, *International Travel and Health* (ISBN 924 158 017 8), available from any World Health Organisation Office. It contains excellent travel hints. In Australia, the web site www.smarttraveller.gov.au is a valuable resource, and leads to a WHO web site showing infectious diseases active in different countries around the world.

While not every country's health authorities will accept the use of the homoeopathic alternative, the following list of remedies can certainly be considered for use overseas. (Remember that people such as Christian Scientists, who refuse to be vaccinated for religious reasons, are still allowed into most countries). Yellow Fever appears to be the one disease where vaccination is needed to prevent possible quarantine restrictions upon return from certain African and South American countries. Other than that, vaccination is not compulsory for most overseas travel.

The list below in Table 4-23 covers infectious diseases for which vaccination is usually given. Recommended dosages are based on the assumption that exposure will be relatively brief; for example, during a holiday or working visit to a country of from one to three months. If longer periods of exposure are anticipated, it would be preferable to commence with the doses as listed, followed by less frequent doses (i.e. every four to six months) of much higher potencies [(M) and (10M) potencies]. Experience and research suggests that triple doses (i.e., three doses within 24 hours) are best in these cases.

Table 4-23 Homœoprophylaxis for Overseas Travel

Disease	Remedies and Doses
Cholera	Cuprum Metallicum (200) - one dose every two weeks while in Cholera-prone areas. Camphor (200) has been used specifically in treating the early stages of Cholera, and would therefore be an effective prophylactic; however, since this remedy is also an antidote to many other homoeopathic remedies, it would not be suitable if other diseases need to be covered.

Dysentery	Arsenicum Album (30) for amoebic dysentery; Merc. Cor (30) for bacillary dysentery - one dose weekly should be sufficient for short term protection. The nosode Giardia (M) is a useful prophylactic, used locally by the author in preventing a range of gastro-intestinal infections; it appears to have a very broad range of protective action.
Malaria	Nat. Mur. (200) or Cinchona Officinals (200) - one dose every two weeks, beginning at least two weeks before travelling in Malarial areas; two further doses on returning home are also recommended. The Malaria nosode can also be useful, but may be too specific to cover some strains of Malaria, while the two remedies listed [particularly Nat. Mur. (200)] cover all strains.
Smallpox	Malandrinum (M) - a triple dose (three doses in 24 hours) every month for three months. Variolinum is also commonly recommended, and all classical Homoeopaths would consider Thuja as well. Note: Smallpox vaccination is not usually required these days.
Tuberculo sis	Tub. Bov. (M) - one dose monthly while visiting suspect areas.
Typhoid/ Typhus	Baptisia (200) - one dose every two weeks during exposure.
Yellow Fever	Arsenicum Album (30), Crotalus Hor. (30), or Phosphorous (30) - one dose weekly during exposure (these remedies have been recommended by Dr Grimmer).
Hepatitis A, B, C	The Hepatitis Nosode for each type in an M potency is recommended, one dose every 2-4 weeks during exposure.
Meningitis	Meningococcinum M every 1-4 weeks depending upon the intensity of exposure.
Jap. B Encephalitis	The Nosode M should be used. If not available, Belladonna 200 weekly should be used.

4.6 A response to the homoeopathic sceptics

The use of potentised substances for protection against infectious diseases (homœoprophylaxis) is still a matter of debate among some homoeopaths, especially in countries where HP is not discussed fully in teaching Colleges. This debate has at times created confusion and concern, especially for parents faced with the decision on whether or not to vaccinate their children.

In responding to those homoeopathic practitioners who are sceptical about the use of homoeopathic prophylactics, my intention is also to reassure readers that the information contained in this book attempts to present parents with a full range of opinions, and not just ones that suit my personal viewpoint.

4.6.1 Criticisms by medical homoeopaths

A letter from a New Zealand mother to the author enclosed a quotation from a senior homoeopath at the Royal London Homoeopathic Hospital, Dr D Spence, President of the Medical Faculty, who stated that: "We do not have the research data showing the persistence of satisfactory antibody levels after using homoeopathic preparations for immunisation, and this is why the advice is to use the 'conventional' vaccines if at all possible". This quotation was also used by an allopathic doctor to advise his colleagues that: "It seems that our homoeopathic colleagues support and encourage the use of [conventional] immunisation" (Hindle RC, 1991).

The homoeopath quoted above would appear to show an apparent ignorance concerning the use of potentised medicines. However, the context in which this statement was written is detailed in Section 8.6.4. It is clear when one reads the full text of Dr Spence's letter that the Medical Faculty gave its members the option to use homœoprophylaxis if they believed that vaccines were contraindicated. The letter also mentioned the efficacy of homœoprophylaxis. The letter was written following threats by the UK health authorities to withdraw Nosodes from use unless the medical homoeopaths issued a statement supporting vaccination.

In Australia, the Medical Faculty also issued a statement supporting vaccination, and this statement was subsequently used by some orthodox authorities to attack homœoprophylaxis.

The Australian statement followed reports of threats against homoeopathic doctors. For example, under the large headline, **"Doctors warned on child vaccines"**, the Melbourne *Herald Sun* of 18 April 1994 reported that "Medical practitioners who give children homoeopathic preparations instead of proven standard vaccines could be sued". It further reported, "The Australian Medical Association's president, Dr Brendan Nelson, said some doctors gave homoeopathic vaccines and if they came to his attention he would refer them to medical boards". In 1995 Nelson threatened "We are gunning for people who behave in this way" (Herald Sun, 9/3/95).

It must be stressed that if any homoeopath gave unqualified support to vaccination and unqualified opposition to homœoprophylaxis on the basis of the absence of antibody production, it would show clear ignorance of homoeopathic method for the following reasons:

- Firstly, it has never been claimed that the potencies confer immunity by stimulating antibody production. How, for example, could a potency of the herb Belladonna (Hahnemann's first prophylactic application) be expected to stimulate antibodies to scarlet fever?
- Secondly, such practitioners must be unaware of the reported efficacy of HP that we do have, or for some reason choose to ignore this evidence.
- Thirdly, before recommending the injection of toxic material into infants, could such practitioners attest to the existence of any double blind, placebo controlled trials of conventional vaccines (the scientific community's own standard of proof) that would unambiguously support vaccination as being either completely safe or completely effective? Long term trials showing vaccine safety to the whole person simply do not exist.
- Finally, no experienced homoeopath could reasonably ignore the miasmic problems caused by conventional vaccination.

But not all concerns with homœoprophylaxis come from medical homoeopaths. A number of prominent homoeopathic colleagues in the UK and the USA are vigorously opposed to the use of potentised medicines for prophylactic purposes, although not all of these recommend conventional vaccination. One example is a leaflet sponsored by the Society of Homoeopaths in England, entitled *Vaccination - A Difficult Decision*, which states: " . . . the patterns of illness in a child may change for the worse after vaccination". However, in discussing alternatives to vaccination, this leaflet only mentions the use of homoeopathic remedies for treating an illness, not for preventing it (Society of Homoeopaths, 1990).

In recent years, I have had a number of disagreements with prominent homoeopaths both in Australia and internationally. In particular, the disagreements with American homoeopath and oriental medicine practitioner Dr Randall Neustaedter, and well known online homeopathic teacher David Little are worth further consideration.

4.6.2 The Neustaedter claims

Our disagreements began in the literature (Neustaedter R, 1990a, 1995; Golden I and Neustaedter R, 1996), and have continued in the 2nd edition of Neustaedter's book *The Vaccine Guide*.

Let me first say that I believe that Neustaedter's book is generally well written and researched, and a valuable resource for parents. However, when it comes to his Chapter titled *Alternative Vaccine Methods* where he discusses homœoprophylaxis, Neustaedter exhibits a lack of balance, and clear double standards. For example:

- He expects HP to pass standards of proof that homoeopathic treatment has not yet passed. There certainly have been some randomised clinical trials of homoeopathic treatment, but the results are very mixed. But more to the point, our greatest homoeopaths over 200 years chose to practice NOT because there were clinical trials available, but because the method was clearly effective, and satisfied fundamental Laws of Nature. This is precisely why practitioners like me choose to use HP – because it is clearly effective, and satisfies fundamental Laws of Nature. So Neustaedter's criticism of HP as being scientifically unproven, but apparent suggestion that homoeopathic treatment is scientifically proven, is inconsistent and undermines both homoeopathic treatment and homoeopathic prevention.

- Neustaedter appears to accept the use of HP in short-term epidemic situations, but not for long-term prevention. But according to his own book, there are no randomised clinical trials for short-term protection either (although a few substantial trials do exist, as referred to in Section 4.1.2), so why accept one but not the other on the basis of evidence?
- Neustaedter concludes his Chapter by saying, "Homoeopaths would do well to present the facts to parents, and assume that parents have the intelligence and good judgement to come to their own educated opinions. Consumers deserve to have access to all the information available, so that their choice about vaccines, conventional or homoeopathic, can be an informed one" (p. 107). I totally agree!! I only wish that Neustaedter had lived up to his own rhetoric. (i) His book was published in 2002, five years **after** the publication of my *Ten Year Clinical Study* describing 1,305 questionnaire responses from parents of children using my HP program. Yet he only refers to 879 questionnaires; (ii) he states that "Golden does not specify which diseases the exposure entailed" (p. 104). In fact, all these details were given in the Tables in my 1997 study; (iii) if Neustaedter had contacted me in 2001, prior to preparing the 2nd edition, he would have been advised that the count was nearing 2,000, that my doctoral research had started at Swinburne University, and that far from being "an informal study of customers" (p. 103), a number of rigorous statistical analyses of the data were being carried out; (iv) his claims that there is no evidence of the long-term safety of long-term HP, and that there is no evidence of dynamic damage, are now clearly outdated.

In early 2005, I sent Neustaedter a (complimentary) copy of my *Fifteen Year Clinical Study*, which examined 2,342 responses in an effort to promote discussion between us on this issue. Unfortunately, some months later I have not received a response from Neustaedter commenting on the data. His recurring claim that "there is no evidence" for the efficacy of long-term HP is simply untrue. He may not accept the evidence presented here, but he cannot say it doesn't exist. My personal preference is to have a reasoned and collegial debate with Neustaedter about this material. I know he is not an unreasonable person. I hope that distance will not prevent our discussion continuing.

I also hope that if he prepares a 3rd edition of his book, Neustaedter will "present the facts to parents" so that they will "have access to all the information available, so that their choice about vaccines, conventional or homoeopathic, can be an informed one". Hopefully, he will also refrain from talking about "homoeopathic vaccines" – we do not vaccinate!

4.6.3 David Little's criticisms

David Little has published a most impressive web site that shows a massive scholarly devotion to Hahnemannian principles (web site: www.simillimum.com). He has also contributed, and may still do so, to homoeopathic chat rooms where a lot of interchange takes place. Personally I find that I just don't have the time to actively participate in chat rooms – however well constructed and hosted. There are some people who must devote hours every day to making lengthy contributions. I just don't have the time.

Unfortunately my contact with Little has been unsuccessful. He said in a chat room post some years ago that he had emailed me and that I had not replied, yet I have never received any personal emails from him. Also some years ago, I sent Little copies of my three books on the topic. They were never returned, but I received no acknowledgement from him of their receipt. Finally, there was some discussion between us on a chat room via postings by a friend of mine, as I was not a member of the chat room. This made effective discussion very difficult, and unfortunately I only have a printout my friend sent me without any reference site or date. But the following points appear to be relevant:

1. Little and I agree that HP is part of the history of classical homoeopathy.
2. He seems to think that I encourage parents to protect against every infectious disease. This is simply not true as can be seen from my comments in Section 4.
3. He disagrees with me that parents have the right to choose to prevent diseases that he and I may see as being mild, and easily treated. He states that "he believes the 'fear' of the parent is

enough reason to give remedies to the child". However, I personally never recommend prevention of, for example, rubella in a healthy child. But if the parent was sincerely concerned about their child acquiring the disease then I would help them, knowing that appropriate HP is safe. Little and I must agree to disagree regarding parental rights.

4. He once stated that I would let the parents choose the remedies to use. This was an obvious misunderstanding as I have never stated this.
5. He stated that "The long term effects of such massive doses of so many remedies is unknown", when discussing my HP program. Firstly, I do not give massive doses of each individual remedy – a single dose, then if no reaction a month later a triple dose, then repeated doses spaced a year or more apart. Secondly, the long term effects now are known as a result of my doctoral studies as reported earlier in Sections 1 and 4.
6. Related to point 5, he states "We humbly request that the principle of minimal dose and minimal intervention be reintegrated into Isaac's system". My reply above stands.
7. He stated that using my HP program would delay constitutional treatment for 5 years. As I have previously stated, I always give constitutional treatment priority over HP remedies, except where immanent exposure to a serious disease is likely. I agree with Little that constitutional treatment offers great advantages to all people, whatever age. However, the fact is that most of the people who use my program have never previously heard of homoeopathy. Many live in remote areas where attendance at a clinic of an experienced homoeopath is impossible (Australia is a BIG country), and therefore even if they have any interest in constitutional treatment, it is not feasible. The use of an appropriate HP program, however, is.
8. He criticises my program for offering protection against unnecessary diseases. This is somewhat different to points 2 and 3 above. This problem relates to the question of when do we decide whether a disease is sufficiently active in a community to warrant preventative measures to be taken. One of the reasons I modified my main program in late 2004 was to adjust for severity and relevance. However, many parents don't want to wait until many children are falling ill before they commence protection – some diseases are continually present in our community.

I may have inadvertently missed some other of Little's points. However I hope I have represented the main ones fairly, and answered them. I greatly respect David Little's contribution, and his contribution deserves to be answered. Some of the above points would have been easily resolved if communications had been better. I would like to finish this part with an interesting quote he made on his web site on 20/4/2000.

"I think this editor's point about prophylaxis being similar to provings is well taken as they are both performed on the healthy human organism. If the posology of the proving is administered in a careful manner the effects of the proving only strengthen the general constitution to diseases. Hahnemann attributed some of his long life and health to the proving of his remedies over a 50 year period. In homœoprophylaxis the same principles come into play. The problem is that those who need protective remedies the most are those who are most susceptible to proving the symptoms. If a remedy is used in too large a dose, too high a potency, and repeated when not needed, there is a chance that too many signs and symptoms will be produced. If such over medication is continued there is a chance of producing a remedy miasms in that individual. Some mishandled provings did produce pathology and remedial diseases. Best to be conservative in such matters."

I completely agree.

What most of my homoeopathic critics have not done is carefully look at what I do before criticising. They do not consider the instructions that come with the program that tell parents that if a child reacts to a remedy, then stop the remedy until I can be contacted and direct them as to the appropriate action to take. I agree that there are less-than-appropriate HP programs, which use too many doses of the same remedy. The evidence for this is in Section 4.3 above. I believe that my program uses the minimum doses needed of each individual remedy to achieve effective protection against the targeted disease. The evidence concerning the safety of my program is presented in Section 4.2.3 above.

4.6.4 Types of homoeopaths

In an attempt to assist parents to understand the range of homoeopathic opinions that are possible, I will identify three types of homoeopaths in relation to their attitude towards homœoprophylaxis:

- *Type A - the 'purists':* They don't prevent any disease other than by increasing general vitality, but treat the disease if acquired. This position must be respected, provided that parents know their position and are supported if they disagree.
- *Type B - the 'pragmatists':* In practice, they believe it is better to prevent some diseases, and the homoeopathic alternative is clearly preferable to vaccines. Three classes of 'pragmatists' may be defined:

  Class 1 Believe HP is comparatively effective to vaccines and totally safe dynamically. They use HP without hesitation.

  Class 2 Believe HP is comparatively effective to vaccines and acceptably safe dynamically. They use HP.

  Class 3 Believe HP is not as effective as vaccines, but they are sufficiently effective (and safe dynamically) to be of value. They generally use HP.
- *Type C - the 'sceptics':* They believe that specific protection is necessary, but have no confidence in the homoeopathic alternative. They believe that vaccines are safer than the diseases they are used to prevent, and therefore recommend vaccination.

When you speak with a homoeopath about HP, try to determine which of the above type they are to better understand the advice they might give you.

4.6.5 Conclusions

The above analysis suggests that as homoeopaths, we can confidently stand as 'purists' or 'pragmatists' and still claim to follow the Organon in the tradition of our greatest prescribers.

Whether the 'sceptics' can make such a claim is questionable. Their position is identical to the allopaths (orthodox practitioners), and as such, they deny the wisdom of the masters of their own field. Their claim that we do not have scientific proof of the efficacy of HP (as measured in the laboratory) is meaningless: if we relied on laboratory results, none of us would practice homoeopathy.

To ignore both the physiological *and* dynamic dangers of vaccines shows that the 'sceptics' are, yet again, ignoring the wisdom of our master prescribers. Hahnemann and Kent had words to describe such people, and rather than repeat them, suffice it to say that those words still apply today. As a fellow homoeopath, all the author asks is that the 'sceptics' do not presume to speak for our profession.

As far as the 'purists' are concerned, their position must be accepted and respected. As long as parents are happy to accept their view, it is appropriate to rely on treatment after the disease has occurred. Nevertheless, they have not made a case against the 'pragmatists' in whose illustrious company (Hahnemann, Boenninghausen, etc), the author is happy to stand. The 'purists' have not proven that HP causes dynamic damage. To ignore the value of HP, however, places those patients who would otherwise vaccinate at a disadvantage. And to be openly antagonistic towards colleagues who are doing no more than following in the footsteps of the master prescribers is as foolish as it is divisive.

In terms of prevention and treatment of disease, homoeopaths have a great deal to offer this planet. Agreeing to some differences will still enable us to offer parents the best options available in what must, ultimately, be the parents' choice for the prophylactic treatment of their children.

Note: Those practitioners or parents who wish to read more about the objections to HP, and the relevant responses, will find the 3rd edition of the author's publication, *Homœoprophylaxis - A Practical & Philosophical Review*, of great value. The cost is $15.00 (including postage and packaging), and orders enclosing payment should be sent to PO Box 695, Gisborne Victoria, 3437.

4.7 Conclusions regarding the homoeopathic option

Many in orthodox medicine are immediately dismissive when homoeopathy is mentioned, and become agitated when homoeopathic immunisation as an option to vaccination is suggested. Reactions like this are a product of ignorance and arrogance (two qualities that often co-exist). The responses from "pseudo-scientists", self titled intellectuals who belong to organisations like the Skeptics Society, are even less rational.

Unfortunately it can work both ways, as I know a few homoeopathic colleagues who have no time at all for anything pharmaceutical.

What we need is information, and a preparedness to examine it objectively. **Only a hopelessly biased person can suggest that a method that has been used for 200 years in every continent on our planet, mainly by people with orthodox medical qualifications, can be a total sham.** I have done my very best to provide factual information. My data is not perfect (no data ever is), but it comprehensively supports the experience of homoeopaths over two centuries.

It also strongly suggests that if a significant number of people used homœoprophylaxis rather than vaccines, that the incidence of chronic conditions such as asthma could fall, and benefit the entire community.

It is up to you, the reader, to decide if my data is sufficient to give you confidence in homœoprophylaxis.

I have absolutely no doubt that homoeopathy can offer a safe and reasonably effective means of immunising against targeted infectious diseases. It gives parents choice, and that is all it should do. I have patients who choose to vaccinate, and they have my full support. The decision is theirs, not mine, not their doctor's.

Homœoprophylaxis has stood the test of time. It has a great deal to offer every national public health system. It has a great deal to offer every individual on the planet both as a method of treatment as well as a means of infectious disease prevention.

PART 3: CONCLUSIONS

5 QUESTION 5: What are the comparative risks and benefits of the disease prevention options?

5.1 The comparative effectiveness of vaccination and homœoprophylaxis

Because the vaccination debate has at times been both emotive and irrational, with fear employed as often as facts, many people are left with the impression that there are no areas of agreement between practitioners who use homœoprophylaxis and the orthodox medical community. This, however, is not the case.

Approaching the issue logically, there are four important points to consider, and there is substantial agreement on the first three.

1 **Some infectious diseases should be prevented:** It is generally agreed that it is preferable to prevent certain severe diseases rather than have to treat a very distressed patient. There is, however, some disagreement about the need to prevent milder diseases, and some natural therapists (including some homoeopaths) believe that it does no harm to allow healthy people to acquire at least some infectious diseases and then be treated for the disease.

2 **Disease-specific prevention is the most effective method:** There is substantial agreement on this point, although some natural therapists believe that the most effective form of disease prevention is to strengthen the general constitutional health of patients. While optimum health does have a significant bearing on disease prevention, there are numerous examples of healthy, stress-free people acquiring infectious diseases (e.g. south-sea islanders exposed to Europeans for the first time in the 1800's). Furthermore, statistics show that disease-specific protection is more effective than general protection.

3 **Vaccines are more toxic than homoeopathic medicines:** This point is generally accepted; in fact, many doctors criticise homoeopathic substances because they do not contain any molecules of the original substance used. They say that "nothing" is there, and "nothing"

cannot be toxic. Vaccines, however, contain a number of toxic substances. For example, the triple antigen vaccine contains molecules of diseased material modified with formaldehyde, together with an adjuvant (usually aluminium phosphate) and a preservative (previously thimerosal, a mercury-based chemical, and now another chemical).

4 **Vaccine efficacy is comparable with that offered by the homoeopathic option:** While there is considerable disagreement on this point, if debate could focus on this critical issue, parents would be better able to make informed decisions. We shall now examine this point in more detail.

An analysis of the material drawn from the medical journals clearly demonstrates that the medical community itself acknowledges that vaccination is not completely effective. The best measures of vaccine efficacy range from about 75-98%, depending on which vaccine is being examined (the whooping cough vaccine is generally regarded as the least effective common vaccine, the measles vaccine as one of the most effective).

Some of these measures of efficacy have been obtained through controlled clinical trials (which are the scientific community's own standard); some, through field trials. We saw in the material presented in Section 3 that the difference between the efficacy of vaccines in clinical trials and the efficacy experienced in the field can vary considerably

Other measures of efficacy have been obtained through *large epidemiological studies* which analyse communities of vaccine recipients. When conducted without bias, epidemiological trials provide information about the short-term toxicity of vaccines because they show how many children were vaccinated and how many of these had short-term reactions. They are, however, not reliable measures of effectiveness because although we know how many children were vaccinated, we do *not* know how many children were *exposed* to the disease being examined.

For example, if 100,000 children were vaccinated and 5,000 of these children acquired the disease, it would appear that the effectiveness of the vaccine is 95%. However, if only 50,000 of the 100,000 vaccinated children were exposed to the disease, the effectiveness is actually 90%; if

25,000 of the 100,000 vaccinated children were exposed, the effectiveness is 80%; if 10,000 of the 100,000 children vaccinated were exposed, effectiveness is only 50%. Since the epidemiological studies do not (and in fact cannot) include data for how many children were exposed to the disease in question, these studies are poor measures of effectiveness.

In the statistical studies of the homoeopathic method reported in Section 4, the key measure of effectiveness is arrived at only *after* attempting to eliminate children whose parents believed the children were *not* exposed to the target diseases, leaving only children who appeared to have been definitely exposed to a disease covered by the homoeopathic program in the analysis. While the analysis has weaknesses, it does attempt to eliminate the major bias affecting all 'after-the-event' analyses, such as epidemiological studies and questionnaires.

So the vaccine efficacy of 75-98% benchmark against which to compare the homoeopathic alternative is almost certainly an overstatement of the actually efficacy in the community.

The single measure of effectiveness of the homoeopathic method derived from my 2004 analysis was 90.4%. This figure not only gives a general indication of efficacy, but, more importantly, supports the historical experience with the homoeopathic method over the last 200 years. Nearly all other research attempting to quantify the efficacy of HP has produced a figure of around 90%. When we add to this the latest experience from Cuba involving millions of people and conducted by orthodox scientists employed by the Government's vaccine manufacturing facility, we see that the effectiveness of HP is now established beyond reasonable doubt.

Clearly, both history and current research support the conclusion that, **while no method of disease prevention is completely effective, vaccination and homoeopathy offer similar levels of protection against infectious disease.**

5.2 The comparative safety of vaccination and homœoprophylaxis

Vaccines contain a variety of toxins, and therefore are clearly potentially toxic. Homœoprophylaxis remedies do not contain toxic materials and are not toxic.

The analysis of my doctoral research presented in Section 4 has provided material on which to make a more direct comparison between the safety of vaccines and homœoprophylaxis. The relevant data presented in Tables 4-17 and 4-18 is summarised in Table 5-1.

Table 5-0-1 Comparative Safety of Vaccination and Homœoprophylaxis

		All Diagnoses		GP Diagnoses	
Condition	**Measurement**	**HP only**	**Vaccination only**	**HP only**	**Vaccination Only**
Asthma	Odds Ratio	**0.117**	**1.75**	**0.124**	**1.89**
	Chi Test P	**0.0004**	**0.0025**	**0.0006**	**0.0007**
Eczema	Odds Ratio	**0.382**	1.315	**0.239**	**1.76**
	Chi Test P	**0.0146**	0.121	**0.0097**	**0.006**
Ear/Hearing	Odds Ratio	0.917	1.149	0.703	**1.517**
	Chi Test P	0.792	0.459	0.364	**0.04**
Allergies	Odds Ratio	0.550	1.220	**0.307**	1.518
	Chi Test P	0.074	0.239	**0.038**	0.061
Behaviour	Odds Ratio	0.446	0.869	**0.541**	0.784
	Chi Test P	0.170	0.593	**0.055**	0.613

In every case, Odds Ratio measures show that there is less chance of a child who uses homœoprophylaxis acquiring the chronic conditions listed than a child who is vaccinated. Many of the figures are statistically significant (shown in bold type). In some cases the ratio difference is significant (for example, the 15 times greater chance of acquiring asthma if vaccinated rather than using HP).

5.3 A general summary of comparative risks and benefits

Homœoprophylaxis and vaccination are comparably effective, but homœoprophylaxis is by every measure much safer both in the short and long term.

5.4 The economics of immunisation options

Not only is HP a comparably effective and non-toxic option to vaccination, but it is a very inexpensive one.

We now have data from Cuba on which to base some useful analysis. In 2007 the Cubans immunised 2.4 million people with 2 doses of medicine each for around $400,000US. On these figures, the Australian Government could immunise the entire country at a base cost of $4,500,000A – let's double it and say $10m. In 2009 the Government paid $200m for sufficient Swine Flu vaccine to vaccinate the country (they have still a lot of unused stock on hand).

America could have been homoeopathically immunised against Swine Flu for under $100m instead of paying $3billion dollars in R&D and production costs. The pharmaceutical industry and offshoots benefited by $2,900,000,000 which the country could have saved by using a comparably effective and safer option. And these figures do not include delivery costs, which would further widen the gap, and they do not include the costs of repairing vaccine damage.

The Australian government has identified the potential blowout in future Federal budgets from the aging population – a problem common to most western developed countries. It can be seen that hundreds of millions of dollars can be saved simply through using a different immunisation option. Even more could be saved through an appropriate integration of complementary and conventional medicine in treatment and preventative health care.

The economics are simple to see, as are the reasons why they have been resisted. One day politicians will break free from their pharmaceutical/medical minders and see what savings are possible. That will be a great day for us all for many reasons, only one of which is economic. In September 2010 Australia's leading economic analysts, Access Economics, released a report showing that the Government could save hundreds of millions of dollars annually by using natural medicine in treating just 5 different conditions. If we looked at all health conditions, plus vaccination, the potential savings to Government would reach billions in just one small country (Access Economics, 2010).

As discussed in Section 4.2.3 above, in 2009/10 the Cubans homeopathically immunised over 9,800,000 people against Swine Flu. This and other massive interventions will allow us to even more closely map cost of vaccines compared to HP.

6 QUESTION 6: Which option is best for my child?

We now have arrived at the point where it is necessary to try and bring all the above information together, and answer this most difficult, yet most important of all the questions asked so far – *which is the best option for my child?*

Some of the possible options are:

1. Vaccinate as suggested by orthodox health authorities.
2. Vaccinate only against diseases which you feel are potentially very dangerous. For some parents this would mean omitting the MMR vaccine, and Hep B (unless in a high risk category).
3. Vaccinate against some diseases, and use HP against the rest.
4. Use HP only against diseases which you feel are potentially very dangerous.
5. Use HP against all the diseases suggested by orthodox authorities.
6. Only use general methods to constitutionally strengthen your child in order to provide disease specific immunity.

Note: (a) Options 1-5 may all be used with constitutional treatment as well.

(b) Options 1-3 may be used together either with treatment in advance to attempt to lessen vaccine damage, or treatment afterwards to address any identified vaccine damage.

(c) A 7th option of doing nothing at all exists, but if you have taken the trouble to read this book it is unlikely that you will fall into this category.

It is your right to choose the option that you think is best. I am often asked what I do for my own children and my grandchildren. I prefer option 4 together with constitutional treatment. But this is only my personal preference, my own opinion. At this point, my opinion doesn't matter; neither does that of your GP. The decision must be yours. I hope that Table

6-1 below may assist you in considering further relevant points in the debate.

I have tried to keep my own biases out of the Table, but no doubt some intrude. For example, I don't regard saying that "HP is effective" as a bias, I regard it as a statement of fact. But you may disagree with my view. Therefore I suggest that you start with a blank sheet of paper, and fill in the Table as you believe is appropriate. If you like, this is the one bit of "homework" I recommend that you complete before you finish your research. Once you do this, then hopefully you can answer the question - *which is the best option for my child?*

Take all factors into account. The effects of criticisms by others that I have put into Table 6-1 are very very real for some parents. If the approach you choose leads to bitter family disputes, and considerable stress, then that factor alone is capable of lowering your level of immunity and that of your children. I know some parents who have felt unable to deal with such a stress, and have chosen to vaccinate as a result. I don't believe that such a decision should be criticised as a "cop-out" – we all live with different pressures, and to ignore them is foolish.

In an ideal world there would be no such pressures because both viewpoints would be understood and respected, and a decision to use HP would be just as supported by orthodox authorities as a decision to vaccinate. This is the health system that I am calling for, and I hope you will too, whatever your personal preferences. But now it is time to put your ideas down on paper and prepare your own comparison of the 6 options listed above , and make a decision!

Table 6-1 A Comparison of the Options

Option	Point For	Points Against
1	Your child will be substantially protected against all of the diseases in the vaccine program. You will have the support of the orthodox health system. You will not be criticised by uninformed people.	Your child will be at risk of both short-term and long-term damage vaccine damage.

2	Your child will be substantially protected against the diseases you believe are potentially the most dangerous. You have the support of many in the orthodox health system.	Your child will be at risk of both short-term and long-term damage vaccine damage, but the risk will be reduced because you have avoided some vaccines. You will be criticised by some in the orthodox health system, and by some uninformed people.
3	Your child will be substantially protected against the diseases you choose to cover. You have the support of a few in the orthodox health system.	Your child will be at risk of both short-term and long-term damage vaccine damage, but the risk will be reduced because you have avoided some vaccines. You will be criticised by many in the orthodox health system, and by many uninformed people.
4	Your child will be substantially protected against the diseases you choose to cover. The effect on your child's general health will be positive.	You will be criticised by most in the orthodox health system, and by most uninformed people.
5	Your child will be substantially protected against all of the diseases in the vaccine program. The effect on your child's general health will be positive.	You will be criticised by many in the orthodox health system, and by many uninformed people.
6	Your child will be partially protected against all of the diseases in the vaccine program. Your child will be given an excellent opportunity to enjoy a high level of general health, given their unique individual constitutional characteristics.	You will be criticised by most in the orthodox health system, and by most uninformed people.

7 CONCLUDING COMMENTS

Official statistics showed in 1994 that over 2,216,000 Americans were seriously damaged by toxic reactions to correctly prescribed pharmaceutical medications and as a result 106,000 died in hospital in that year (JAMA, 15/4/1998, and JAMA 26/7/2000). Over 200,000 people a year die from "adverse reactions" from drugs, and another 80,000 die from medical malpractice, according to the pharmacy industry magazine *Drug Topics* (October 23, 1995, pp. 14-16). In 2010 it was estimated that 48,000 patients die in US hospitals each year from health care associated sepsis and pneumonia alone (Eber MR et.al. 2010).

In the UK, an estimated rate of adverse events of 5-10% of admissions in UK hospitals has been made (BMJ Editorial, 2001b). Further, 2-4% of all hospital admissions are medication related, and most are preventable (Runciman WB et al, 2003). Despite these deaths and injuries, the pharmaceutical dominance of politicians and therefore governments continues.

In Australia the figures are just as bad – over 60,000 serious adverse events, and over 15,000 deaths annually from prescription drugs.

The people advising public health authorities in developed countries are almost entirely advocates of pharmaceutical medicine (doctors and medical scientists). Thus our politicians only ever get to hear one side of most medical debates. The number of drug company lobbyists continues to increase, along with the amount spent on lobbying activities. In the US alone in 2002, the drug industry spent $30 billion in advertising, including close to $13.2 billion lobbying doctors and hospitals, and $15.7 billion on drug promotions (Deya RA, Patrick DL, 2005, pages 71, 78).

All this expenditure comes despite the fact that in 2003, Dr Allen Roses, worldwide Vice President of Genetics at GlaxoSmithKline and a pre-eminent figure in the field, stated that **more than 90 percent of drugs only work in 30-50 percent of people** (http://icfda.drugawareness.org/Archives/4thQtr_2003/record0012.html).

His comments were supported by estimates the *British Medical Journal* Clinical Evidence centre which showed the following outcomes of all medical interventions, only a third of which provide definite benefits (http://clinicalevidence.bmj.com/ceweb/about/knowledge.jsp)

7-1 BMJ Effectiveness of Clinical Interventions

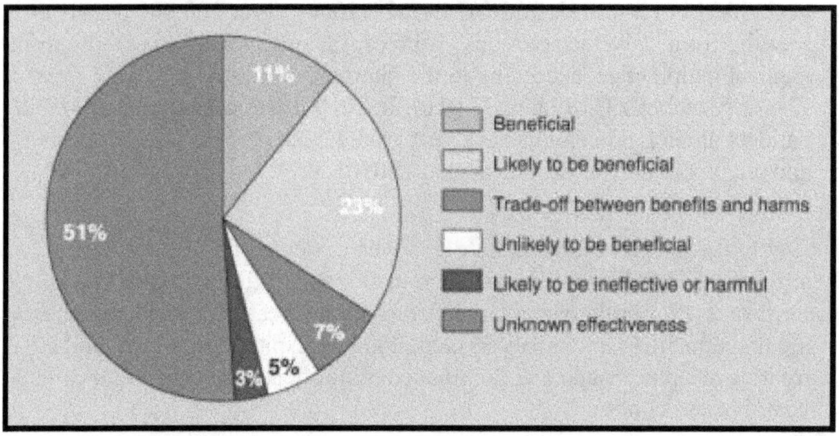
11%
23%
7%
5%
3%
51%
Beneficial
Likely to be beneficial
Trade-off between benefits and harms
Unlikely to be beneficial
Likely to be ineffective or harmful
Unknown effectiveness

Only individuals with a capacity and a willingness to think independently are prepared to look beyond the officially supported reaches of the pharmaceutical media machine. Orthodox researchers have found repeatedly that the main users of natural medicine are generally better educated and from higher socio-economic groups than those who rely totally on drugs (Eisenberg DM et al, 2001). This doesn't mean that those with higher education or a higher income are the only people who can think for themselves, but that they often have more access to information, and more economic opportunity to act on their choices. I know from 25 years experience that the parents who use my homœoprophylaxis program come from a broad range of socio-economic groups, but the factor they all have in common is that they have searched out information on which to make their decisions. They have chosen to take responsibility for their own health, and the health of their children.

Pharmaceutical medicine does have a place. At times it offers the best treatment (especially emergency medicine and surgery in some conditions). However, it is often generally ineffective in curing long-term health conditions as it relies on the chemical suppression of symptoms which may move the results of the illness to a deeper and more serious level.

The ideal health system is surely one where people are free (both by preference and economically) to use the best of both pharmaceutical and natural medicine. We have a LOT to learn from the Cuban medical system which has developed free from multinational pharmaceutical influence due to the USA embargo against that country.

When we come to immunisation, most people want to prevent certain infectious diseases. Nothing can guarantee prevention, but vaccines have been shown to provide a significant level of protection. However, there are risks of possible short-term and long-term damage with vaccines. Mild short-term reactions are common; severe short-term adverse events don't happen all that often, and we don't really know the true incidence of long-term damage from vaccines because it has not been sufficiently studied.

However we are assured by most doctors that the potential risks of the diseases we want to prevent definitely outweigh the potential dangers of the vaccines. Such a statement is unscientific simply because all the facts including long-term health impacts have not yet been assembled which permit such a claim to be made.

A growing number of people are not satisfied with their doctor's reassurance, and are not convinced that the risks of vaccination really are as infrequent as the doctors suggest, so they choose to investigate for themselves.

They find that there is an option to vaccination. It certainly appears to be safe. It has been used successfully for over 200 years. Recent research supports the historical evidence that it provides a significant level of protection against the diseases they are worried about.

So they decide: if there is such a viable alternative, then why take the risk of vaccine damage, let's use the safer alternative.

If you are, or intend to be one of those who thinks and acts independently, you will probably then find that many people begin criticising you – your doctor, the infant welfare nurse, some members of your family, some parents at play group, etc. They say that what you are doing is not proven, and doesn't make sense. None of them have actually examined the evidence which exists about the alternative you have chosen, but the doctor was told by his professor, and the nurse was told by the doctor, and the family and friends and acquaintances were told by the doctor, the nurse and the government department (who were told by the professor and the pharmaceutical companies).

All this conflict may put you under great stress – what should you do?

My suggestion – look at the evidence for yourself, make up your own mind about what is best for your child, taking everything into account (including stress and pressure from others), **make a decision, act on it, and know that you are doing the very best you can for your child**.

Whether you vaccinate, use homœoprophylaxis, use constitutional treatment, or do nothing specific, if you have made such an effort to become informed, then no one can do better than that.

Know that you have done more, out of care and concern and love for your child, than any of your critics have done. Be proud that you have done your best, whatever may happen.

We don't live in a perfect, risk free world. Uncertainty is part of life. At least you have not avoided your responsibilities as so many do. You deserve support, and you deserve congratulations!

A FINAL NOTE FOR POLITICIANS

My doctoral research, supervised as it was by a Professor of Medicine and a medical epidemiologist, and examined by Doctors of Medicine who also had PhD's, as well as training in homoeopathic medicine, has shown the following:

(1) Use of appropriate homœoprophylaxis programs has the potential to improve the national coverage against potentially serious infectious diseases due to increased coverage for children who will not otherwise be vaccinated.

(2) At the same time, use of appropriate homœoprophylaxis programs has the potential to reduce the incidence of chronic debilitating illnesses in our community.

This is a win-win situation for both individuals and the community. It also provides these benefits at significantly less cost than vaccination.

We need politicians who are not bound by advice from people who are locked into pharmaceutical medicine, who will investigate and think for themselves, and act for the good of our entire community.

Economically, practically and morally, a dual system of immunisation where parents are supported to choose between vaccination and homœoprophylaxis makes complete sense.

Its time has come. Let's make it happen.

8 GENERAL APPENDICES

The following topics are covered in the General Appendix:

8.1 Vaccination, school entry and conscientious objections

8.2 Vaccine damage register

8.3 Examples of changes in vaccine law

8.4 The treatment of vaccine damaged children

8.5 Reported criticisms of the homoeopathic method
- NH&MRC criticism
- Choice magazine
- The British medical faculty quote
- The Roden paper
- Whooping cough in the north coast of NSW
- A Current Affair
- MJA review of the homoeopathic alternative
- The Australian Skeptics

8.6 Special topics
- Economics of health care
- Vaccination in third world countries
- My experience with the health establishment

8.7 The earlier homœoprophylaxis programs: 1986, 1991, 1993

8.8 Parents' support groups

8.9 Summary of available reference material

8.1 Vaccination, school entry, and conscientious objections

Many Australian parents have been led to believe that their children must be vaccinated before entry into primary school will be allowed. In fact, they have been misled.

While State laws in Australia regarding vaccination vary, the most any State requires is that your child has a Vaccination *Certificate* prior to school entry. This certificate indicates whether or not your child has received routine vaccination.

If a child has not been vaccinated, he or she may be required to stay away from school in the event of an outbreak of one of the infectious diseases covered by the conventional program. The irony in this is that unvaccinated children may be required to stay at home when an outbreak occurs among vaccinated children.

A copy of the Vaccination Certificate I obtained prior to enrolling one of my own sons into primary school in 1991 is shown in Figure 8-1. The Health Officer involved simply ticked the box indicating 'Immunisation Not Complete'.

Unfortunately, some public health officials have taken it upon themselves to pressure parents (particularly mothers) when obtaining their certificate. Since parents have the right to choose whether or not to have their children vaccinated, they are legally entitled to lodge a formal complaint against anyone acting in a deliberately uncooperative or aggressive manner. Fortunately, not all health officials adopt such a negative position; in my own case, the person involved was both courteous and helpful.

Interestingly, *the Vaccination Certificate did not specify Whooping Cough* among the diseases listed for "complete" or "incomplete" immunisation. The following official response was given to a concerned parent who wrote to Dr G J Rouch, Chief Health Officer of Victoria in 1992:

"Whooping cough is still an important and dangerous disease for our young children. The vaccine available is very safe and is known to be about 80% effective in protecting against the disease. Those children who do contract the disease after being vaccinated are less severely affected. The vaccine does, however produce some short-term side effects in many children, such as swelling and redness at the injection site, and fever. It is thought that these side effects become more pronounced the older the child is at vaccination. In fact, the National Health and Medical Research Council does not recommend giving the vaccine to any child over the age of 4. This disease is most dangerous in very young babies.

For these reasons, whooping cough vaccines is not a requirement on the immunisation certificate. If parents had delayed immunisation of their children until the age of five, just before school entry, then whooping cough vaccine would not be able to be given . . . ".

Letter from Dr G J Rouch, dated 25.2.1992.

From this letter, it appeared that our Governments back then believed that the Pertussis vaccine was dangerous in a 5 year old child, but not in a 2 month old child! This represents a remarkable admission concerning the danger of the vaccine, as well as a disturbing conclusion that a 2 month old infant can safely take a vaccine which becomes toxic in an older child whose immune system is more mature.

Interestingly, DTPa is now recommended at 4 years of age. It would be suggested that the current use of an acellular vaccine rather than a whole cell vaccine is what makes the difference in recommendations. It must be asked whether, in another decade, it will be said that the current acellular vaccines are not so safe, and how something safer has become available. There is no certainty with this issue.

The obvious solution to the problem of a potentially dangerous vaccine and a dangerous disease in infants is to give infants safe yet comparably effective protection using the homoeopathic alternative described in Section 4 above.

The Victorian Government states that school entry immunisation status certificates can be obtained from:

• the Australian Childhood Immunisation Register (ACIR). Telephone 1800 653 809. Email acir@medicareaustralia.gov.au

http://www.medicareaustralia.gov.au/public/services/acir/index.jsp

• Medicare Australia Office. Online at www.medicareaustralia.gov.au

• your GP

• your local council immunisation service.

Figure 8-1 A School-Entry Vaccination Certificate

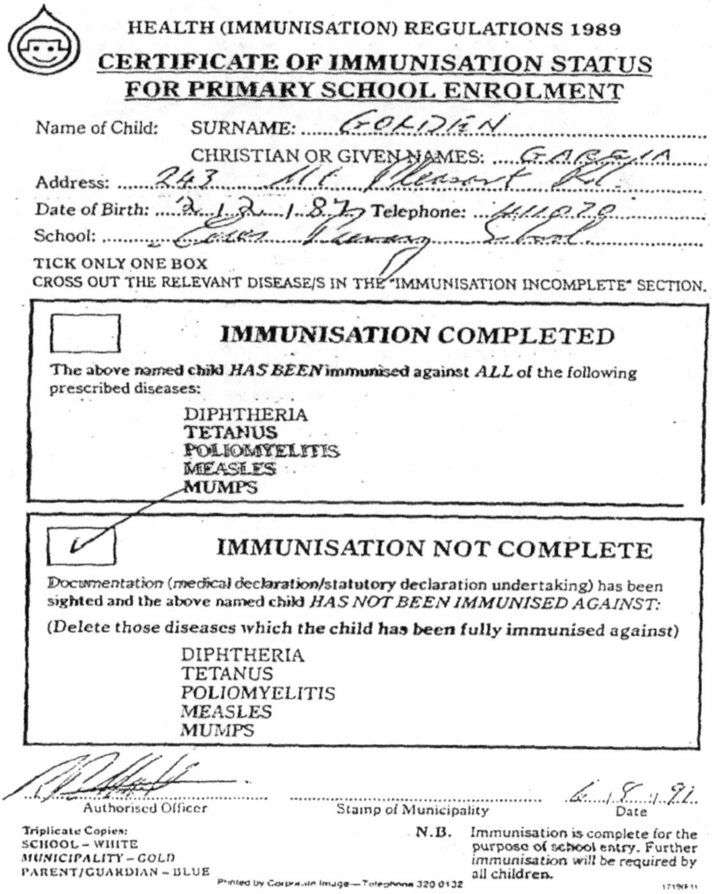

HEALTH (IMMUNISATION) REGULATIONS 1989

CERTIFICATE OF IMMUNISATION STATUS FOR PRIMARY SCHOOL ENROLMENT

Name of Child: SURNAME: ....

CHRISTIAN OR GIVEN NAMES: ....

Address: ....

Date of Birth: 2.2.87 Telephone: ....

School: ....

TICK ONLY ONE BOX

CROSS OUT THE RELEVANT DISEASE/S IN THE "IMMUNISATION INCOMPLETE" SECTION.

☐ **IMMUNISATION COMPLETED**

The above named child *HAS BEEN* immunised against *ALL* of the following prescribed diseases:

DIPHTHERIA
TETANUS
POLIOMYELITIS
MEASLES
MUMPS

☑ **IMMUNISATION NOT COMPLETE**

Documentation (medical declaration/statutory declaration undertaking) has been sighted and the above named child *HAS NOT BEEN IMMUNISED AGAINST:*

(Delete those diseases which the child has been fully immunised against)

DIPHTHERIA
TETANUS
POLIOMYELITIS
MEASLES
MUMPS

Authorised Officer | Stamp of Municipality | Date 6.8.91

Triplicate Copies:
SCHOOL – WHITE
MUNICIPALITY – GOLD
PARENT/GUARDIAN – BLUE

N.B. Immunisation is complete for the purpose of school entry. Further immunisation will be required by all children.

Printed by Corporation Image—Telephone 320 0132

Figure 8-2 Conscientious Objection Form

Australian Government
Medicare Australia

Australian childhood **immunisation** register

Immunisation exemption
Conscientious objection form

Important information

This form must be completed by a recognised immunisation provider and the parent/guardian of the child.

Assistance

For additional information or enquiries about the Australian Childhood Immunisation Register (ACIR) call **1800 653 809****

Lodgement

Send completed and signed form to:

Medicare Australia
GPO Box 295
Hobart TAS 7001

or fax to: **03 6281 0555**

Tick where applicable ☑

** **Call charges apply from mobile and pay phones only**

Child's details

1 Medicare number | Reference number

2 Surname

First given name | Initial

3 Postal address

Postcode

4 Date of birth
/ /

5 Sex

☐ Male

☐ Female

Provider declaration

6 **I declare that:** I have explained the benefits and risks associated with immunisation to the parent or guardian of the child named, and have informed him/her of the potential dangers if a child is not immunised.

7 Medicare provider/ACIR registration number

Signature

Date
/ /

Parent/guardian declaration

8 **I declare that:** I have discussed the benefits and risks of immunisation with the provider named above and have considered the information given. I have also been given the opportunity to discuss any concerns about immunisation with the provider.

I have a personal, philosophical, religious or medical belief involving a conviction that vaccination under the National Immunisation Program should not take place. On this basis, I choose not to have my child immunised.

Parent/guardian name (please print)

Signature

Date
/ /

Privacy note

The information provided on this form will be used by the Australian Childhood Immunisation Register to record a conscientious objection to vaccination by a parent or guardian. Its collection is authorised by the *Health Insurance Act 1973*. This information may be disclosed to the Family Assistance Office, a parent or guardian of the stated child and to authorised immunisation providers and bodies as authorised or required by law.

Page 1 of 1 IMMU-12.14.10.08

Figure 8-2 shows the conscientious objection form that is used for parents who do not wish to vaccinate their children, but remain eligible for the child support payments. It has to be signed by a licensed vaccine provider (usually a GP). **It is important that parents realise that they will not be financially penalised if they don't vaccinate PROVIDED they fill in this paperwork**. The form is available online at http://www.medicareaustralia.gov.au/public/files/ma_conscientious_objection_form.pdf.

8.2 Vaccine damage register

The work of establishing a register of vaccine damage is essential for many reasons, not the least of which is to provide factual information concerning vaccination.

In the UK there has been a program of compensation payments for vaccine damage since 1965. A similar program was introduced in the United States in 1986, partly as a consequence of the documentation of vaccine damage presented in the book, *D.P.T. - A Shot in the Dark* (Coulter HL & Fisher BL, 1985). The Japanese Government provides compensation for severe vaccine damage, as do some other governments.

The Australian government has established a mechanism in 1970 to report adverse events when taking drugs and vaccines – the Adverse Drug Reactions Advisory Committee (ADRAC). In 2010, ADRAC was replaced by the Advisory Committee on the Safety of Medicines (ACSOM) (http://www.tga.gov.au/committee/acsom.htm). Adverse reactions can be reported by phoning the Adverse Medicine Events Line: Ph 1300 134 237, or by following advice at http://www.tga.gov.au/adr/bluecard.htm.

However, there have been serious questions concerning the reliability of the register given the perceived reluctance of many GP's to acknowledge vaccinations as the cause of adverse events.

The Australia Vaccination Network has established its own vaccine damage register, which may be accessed by ticking the "report a reaction" option on their website - http://www.avn.org.au/.

The need for a properly maintained register is shown in the following material:

The NVIC/DPT investigation was featured on the March 2 NBC News' "Now with Tom Brokaw and Katie Couric" show. At the end of February, NVIC/DPT also conducted a survey of 159 doctors' offices in seven states, including Arkansas, California, Georgia, Illinois, Maryland, New York, and Texas. When asked the question "In case of an adverse event after vaccination, does the doctor report it and, if yes, to whom?" only 28 out of 159 or 18 percent said they make a report to the FDA, CDC or state health department. In New York, only one out of 40 doctor's offices confirmed that they report a death or injury following vaccination.

(Blatant Propaganda PO Box 1327 Woden 2606 Australia)

In the United States of America

A total of 54,072 reports of adverse events following vaccination were listed in a 39-month period from July 1990 to November 1993 with 12,504 reports being associated with DPT vaccine, including 471 deaths.

From 1988 to 2002, almost 1,800 families have received more than $1.3 billion in compensation from the program. Since 1988, almost 7,000 petitions for claims have been filed. Almost 3,800 were dismissed, and more than 1,300 cases still are in the pipeline, according to the program's Aug. 9 report.

The following figures to 2008 are shown in my *Vaccine Damaged Children* book, including Table 8-1 showing that the compensation paid for vaccine damage now exceeds $2billion – averaging over $40,000,000 per year since 1988:

USA Government official statistics, March 2008

http://www.hrsa.gov/vaccinecompensation/statistics_report.htm

Table 8-1: NVICS Compensation Payments 1988 to March 2008

	Post 1988 Claims		**Pre 1988 Claims**	
Petitions Filed	8,167		4,264	
	Compensatable	**Dismissed**	**Compensatable**	**Dismissed**
Adjudications	948	1,519	1,189	3,070
Awards Paid	944	758*	2,542**	
	$840.92m	$16.18m	$902.52m	
Total Paid to March 2008 = $1,759.62m USD				

* - compensation not awarded, but legal fees paid

** - includes compensation, plus legal fees only

The average time for a successful case to progress from filing a claim to the award of compensation is seven years. A child injured by a vaccine must file a claim within three years after the first symptoms appear. The family of a child who dies must file within two years of the death. No lawsuits concerning vaccine injuries can be filed in a civil court, the law says, until after a claim has been filed with the vaccine compensation program and the litigant has decided to reject its award. As a result, the number of lawsuits filed against vaccine manufacturers has plunged since the fund's inception: four suits against DTP makers in 1997, compared with 255 in 1985.

In the United Kingdom

“The government has paid out £3.5m to patients left disabled by vaccinations since 1997, it has been revealed.

Since then, any claimant who is successful in their claim has received a tax-free lump sum of £100,000.

Thirty-five such payments have been made, the Department of Work and Pensions said, but could not reveal which jabs were involved in the claims. It was also revealed that a total of 917 payments have been made since the Vaccine Damage Payment Scheme was introduced in 1979”. (BBC News 16/3/05).

Material released through UK Hansard by Anne McGuire covering the period 2000/01 to 2006/07 showed that the Scheme had received 1,164 claims, but had approved only 21, a significant difference to the USA scheme where roughly 1 in 4 claims are approved (TheyWorkForYou.com, 16/6/2006).

8.3 Examples of change in vaccine law

8.3.1 The Japanese Experience

One of the most revealing episodes in the history of vaccination occurred in Japan. In 1975, following 37 infant deaths linked to vaccination, the Japanese Government decided to raise the minimum age for vaccination from 3 months to 24 months, in an attempt to minimise the immediate and severe risks associated with giving the DPT vaccine to tiny infants whose immune systems had not yet matured.

The official Japanese figures, shown in Table 8-2, have confirmed that vaccine damage is significantly reduced by delaying the onset of vaccination (Cherry et al, 1988). The figures account for episodes for which compensation was paid by the Japanese Government, and are not the total figures for damage. In fact, we can assume that they represent only the exposed edge of a large group of damaged children.

Most importantly the figures show that by delaying the onset of vaccination, the category of Sudden Infant Deaths disappears from the compensation statistics. We expect this result, as SIDS generally only occurs in infants. However, this is clear evidence that vaccination is one cause of SIDS, without being in any way the only cause. Other deaths and complications fell dramatically after the minimum age was increased.

Table 8-2 Comparison of Deaths and Notifications

Year: Period:	1970-1974 61 months	1975-1981 79 months	1981-1984 40 months
Type of vaccine	Whole cell	Whole cell	Acellular
First given	3-5 months	24 months	24 months
Doses (Million)	25.1	19.8	20.4
S.I.D.	11	0	0
Other deaths	26	3	2
Other reactions	102	39	17

Some commentators have stated that it was inevitable that the vaccine-related SIDs deaths would fall when the minimum vaccination age rose to 24 months, as SIDs is no longer a problem at that age. But that is the point! If infants are not vaccinated, they will avoid the risk of any vaccine-related death.

Figure 8-3 below charts the official Japanese Government figures for notifications and deaths from Whooping Cough from 1965-1991. The figures were kindly supplied by the Director, Statistical Standards Department, Statistics Bureau, Management and Coordination Agency, Tokyo, Japan, 15 April 1993.

Unfortunately, the Japanese figures begin with the commencement of vaccine use in 1951, and thus cannot tell us whether the introduction of vaccination changed the incidence of Pertussis or, as in other countries, made little difference to an already declining trend.

Figure 8-3 does suggest that when the minimum vaccination age was increased to 24 months in 1975 that the incidence of the disease rose markedly. However, it should be noted that the figures later returned to pre-1975 levels without a subsequent reduction in the minimum vaccination age. This would suggest that Japanese doctors were sensitised to pertussis rates and, while some increase in the disease did occur, there probably was over-reporting of the disease - as occurred in the UK in the 1970 "epidemics" (see Section 3.6.13).

This conclusion is supported in part by Figure 8-3 which shows, as with the UK experience, that the ratio of notifications to deaths increased during the period of the Japanese "epidemic" (1975-1984), indicating excessive notifications of the disease (since the severity of the disease as measured by relative mortality would not suddenly fall and then suddenly increase again without reason).

The Japanese experience shows clearly that vaccinating tiny infants is a potentially dangerous, high-risk, low-benefit policy, and that the medium term incidence of the disease is largely unaffected when the minimum age for vaccination is increased from 3 months to 24 months. All governments would do well to note the evidence that delaying the onset of vaccination significantly reduces its toxic consequences.

Figure 8-3 Whooping Cough in Japan 1965-1991: Notifications and Deaths and Ratio of Notifications to Deaths

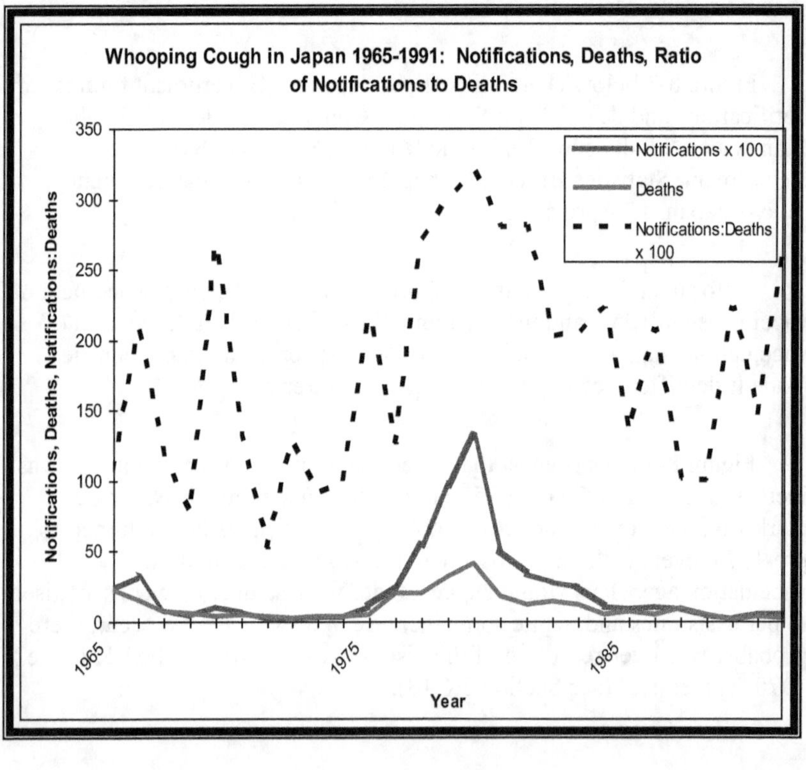
Whooping Cough in Japan 1965-1991: Notifications, Deaths, Ratio of Notifications to Deaths
Notifications, Deaths, Notifications:Deaths
350
300
250
200
150
100
50
0
1965
1975
1985
Year
Notifications x 100
Deaths
Notifications:Deaths x 100

It should be noted that current Japanese law now recommends immunisation of infants for polio, diphtheria, tetanus and BCG, and older children for measles, rubella and Japanese encephalitis. Whilst other vaccines are optional, this is a significantly smaller list than most developed countries. The Japanese government must be commended for the responsibility with which they approach vaccination (Nakatani H et.al. 2002).

8.4 Reported criticisms of the homoeopathic method

8.4.1 Introduction

A number of criticisms concerning homoeopathic disease prevention are regularly aired in the media, by health authorities, and through infant welfare centres. This section examines a number of the more persistent criticisms in detail to assess both their accuracy and usefulness as evidence against the homoeopathic option.

8.4.2 NH&MRC criticism

The National Health and Medical Research Council (NH&MRC) reported in 1993 that one of their members had proven the ineffectiveness of the homoeopathic method. This report was based on a doctor's examination of blood samples of 20 children who had used homoeopathics, which revealed no antibodies for the disease covered. No specific details of the study were given.

According to the orthodox medical model, absence of antibodies means lack of immunity, although this does not explain why some people in so called "virgin" populations (i.e. where a disease has never appeared before) do not acquire a disease despite the fact they have no antibodies to that particular disease.

Nevertheless, the NH&MRC finding is meaningless in terms of providing evidence against the homoeopathic option, since the homoeopathic method of disease prevention does not rely on antibody stimulation (refer Section 4).

8.4.3 Choice Magazine

The April 1990 issue of *Choice* contained a 'Special Report' on Immunisation.

The *Choice* report contained almost every commonly cited justification for vaccination. For example, in quoting figures for deaths from whooping cough, diphtheria and tetanus for the years 1925-35 and 1975-85, the report implied that the reduction in deaths was due to vaccination. They did not report the actual decline in deaths before and after mass vaccination programs (as shown in Section 3.4.1 of this book), which clearly show that vaccination had little impact on an already improving situation.

The report also referred to the "passing of Smallpox from our world" (p. 8), and attributed this to vaccination; section 3.6.21 of this book shows this assumption to be incorrect. Also repeated were the fear-inspiring messages that are typically used by all health departments, such as "no adult who has seen first-hand the ravages of polio or measles would ever consciously refuse to immunise their child" (p. 10), completely ignoring the fact that homœoprophylaxis is a form of immunisation.

Choice, however, failed to present examples of medical opinion and research denouncing specific aspects of routine vaccination, as provided in this book. The absence of counter arguments demonstrates a lack of any objective research into the subject.

8.4.4 The medical faculties of homoeopathy quotes

A statement frequently quoted by opponents of the homoeopathic option was made by Dr D S Spence, then President of the Faculty of Homoeopathy, who stated that:

> "we do not have the research data showing the persistence of satisfactory antibody levels after using homoeopathic preparations from immunisation, and this is why the advice is to use 'conventional' vaccines if at all possible" (Hindle RC, 1991, p. 171).

On the basis of this quote, it appears that Dr Spence shares the NH&MRC's limited understanding of the homoeopathic option, since the homoeopathic method does not rely on antibody stimulation.

However, when one reads the full text of Dr Spence's letter, it becomes apparent that his support is not unqualified. Dr Spence also said:

"Where there is no medical contraindication, immunisation should be carried out in the normal way using conventional tested and approved vaccines. Where there is a medical contraindication and/or a patient would otherwise remain unprotected against a specific infectious disease, it may be appropriate to consider the use of the relevant homoeopathic preparation applicable to the disease.

"There has been a small epidemiological study done using the Pertussin medicine, which seemed to show a degree of protection to be imparted and was thus deemed to be 'better than nothing' for patients that would otherwise be totally unprotected".

Letter from Dr D S Spence (President of the Faculty of Homoeopathy) to Dr R C Hindle (Community Paediatrician, New Zealand), 22 February 1989. [Reproduced in full in the *IAS Newsletter*, Vol.7, No. 2, Nov 94 - Jan95.

At the time, the British Medical Faculty was responding to the considerable pressure from the Health Department to support vaccination, while offering its members the option to use homœoprophylaxis if they felt that vaccination was medically contraindicated - which for classical homoeopaths is all the time.

Evidence of this pressure was shown in a letter by Dr Peter Fisher, Director of Research at the Royal London Homoeopathic Hospital, to my solicitor (collected during my defamation action against *A Current Affair*). He said that "the British Department of Health responded by restricting the product license of pertussin, and other "nosodes" so that they could not be prescribed for prophylaxis, although they continue to be available for other applications"

The fact that the Faculty also acknowledged the value of homœoprophylaxis whilst being under such pressure shows their (quiet) support for the method. We know that many doctors who worked at the

Royal London Homoeopathic Hospital and who were members of the medical Faculty (e.g., Dr Shepherd, Dr Clarke, etc.) used homoeopathic preventatives.

The quote from Dr Spence has been widely misused. For example, Bedford and Elliman stated that "Some parents believe that there are ways of protecting a child against infection that work equally as well as vaccines, one of the commonest being homoeopathy. There is no evidence that homoeopathy can prevent a child from becoming infected with a disease that is preventable by vaccination or that it can reduce the severity of a disease. The Faculty of Homoeopathy acknowledges this *(ref 1)* and recommends the use of conventional vaccines. *(ref 2)* Hahnemann, the founder of homoeopathy, was a supporter of smallpox vaccination". *(ref 3)* Note: the three references used by Bedford and Elliman are discussed below.

Homoeopathic historian Peter Morrell replied that "Bedford and Elliman discuss some of the concerns about immunisation. The Faculty of Homoeopathy speaks for a medically qualified minority. The more numerous medically unqualified homoeopaths belong to the Society of Homoeopaths, the Institute of Complementary Medicine, or the Homoeopathic Medical Association, totalling some 2000 practitioners. None of these bodies supports vaccination. The Society of Homoeopaths, in a leaflet, encouraged parents to seek advice about it. Currently the Homoeopathic Medical Association has no policy on vaccination. The Institute of Complementary Medicine, which has a register of "classical homoeopaths," opposes vaccination" (Morrell P, 2000, p. 108).

Further examination of the three references given by Bedford and Elliman shows that they apparently didn't expect many homoeopaths to read their article.

Ref 1: "The Faculty of Homoeopathy acknowledges this" – they reference an article by Dr JM English. (English J M, 1987). English actually showed that HP remedy Pertussin had an efficacy ranging between 87.0 and 91.5%.

Ref 2: "and recommends the use of conventional vaccines" – they reference a letter by Dr P Fisher who is a member of the Faculty of Homoeopathy, but wrote as an individual, not the Faculty itself (Fisher P, 1990).

Ref 3: "Hahnemann, the founder of homoeopathy, was a supporter of smallpox vaccination" – smallpox vaccination had just been introduced, and to Hahnemann it initially appeared to be helpful. It also appeared to be consistent with the idea of giving minute doses of potentially causative agents to produce either cure or prevention. But the point is; if Bedford and Elliman are seriously suggesting that we should use what Hahnemann recommends, then we would be using homœoprophylaxis today instead of vaccines (Hahnemann S, 1982).

It should also be noted that the Commonwealth Department of Human Services and Health issued a press release on 19.10.94 where it "welcomed an announcement by the Australian Medical Faculty of Homoeopathy that it does not support homoeopathic immunisation over conventional immunisation". Once again, this statement must be considered in the light of calls to de-register medical practitioners who use homœoprophylaxis reported in Section 4.6.1 above.

It also is interesting that the then president of the Medical Faculty who made the statement had earlier said that "It is foolish and unscientific to ban something which may actually work, simply because we don't understand why" – "On that basis much of modern medicine would remain unused" (Australian Doctor, 6.8.93).

It is not unreasonable to ask the question: **if the various health departments and medical bodies have nothing to fear from the truth, why do they need to threaten medically trained homoeopaths to "maintain the orthodox line" on vaccination?**

8.4.5 The Roden paper

At the third National Immunisation Conference in Melbourne (1993), Ms Janet Roden presented a paper, *Immunisation: A Natural Part of Health?*, which has since received wide circulation through its appearance in a number of journals (primarily nursing journals) and through photocopying and distribution to parents by infant welfare staff (Roden J, 1993).

Ms Roden claimed to have examined the case for "homoeopathic immunisation" and had done some appropriate reading on the subject.

However, the numbers of errors contained in her explanations of homoeopathy suggest that she has not clearly understood her subject.

In attempting to attack the claim (as made in earlier editions of this book) that government statistics prove that the introduction of mass vaccination did *not*, in most cases, significantly influence already declining trends in deaths and notifications of most infectious diseases, Ms Roden claims that "Golden's graphs, however, are difficult to interpret as they are incompletely labelled".

The graphs in the 5th Edition showed actual trends in deaths and notifications over time, with arrows indicating the introduction of mass vaccination programs; this information was supplied by the health authorities concerned.

Although accepting her criticism in part regarding unclear labelling (it is difficult to determine exact dates and figures from the graphs alone, since time periods are generally given in ten year increments and deaths/notifications given in increments of hundreds and/or thousands), the graphs do clearly show that most of the diseases concerned were already declining or virtually eliminated prior to the introduction of vaccines.

Ms Roden also noted that "Golden (undated) states that measles should not be regarded as a serious disease". This is a misleading quotation, since section 3.6.10 of the 5th Edition actually stated that "it is often fatal and otherwise serious" in malnourished children, as well as acknowledging that, in our community, "significant complications, including SSPE and sometimes deaths do occur".

Ms Roden further wrote that "the anti-immunisation lobbyists such as Golden are convinced that a healthy lifestyle and a balanced diet are an adequate defence against serious childhood diseases". While Section 2 of the 5th Edition strongly supported adherence to a healthy diet and lifestyle, it also stated that "even the healthiest of people may succumb to specific infectious diseases, which is why other homoeopaths (the writer included) believe that specific protection for the more serious infectious diseases is desirable".

In attacking homoeopathy as being unscientific and unproven, Ms Roden refrains from making any objective evaluation of the evidence to the contrary, the painstaking clinical records maintained throughout the two centuries of homoeopathic use.

The paper concludes with references to the statements made by the NH&MRC, *Choice* magazine, and Dr Spence of the Medical Faculty quote, which have already been examined and found wanting.

In summary, her review was incomplete and biased, and her conclusions unsustained. It was a poor piece of research.

8.4.6 Whooping cough in the North Coast of NSW

A report on an outbreak of whooping cough in the North Coast of NSW has also received wide circulation since 1993. The report claimed to examine the efficacy of the triple antigen vaccine and homoeopathic immunisation (Furber S, 1993). The report was based on questionnaire responses from 79 people with the following immunisation status:

Triple Antigen (TA)	46	58%
Homoeopathic	8	10%
None	9	11%
Unknown	16	20%
Total	**79**	**100%**

Thirty-five survey respondents reported an illness consistent with whooping cough (although clinical confirmation was not obtained in the majority of these cases). Of these, the following immunisation status was reported:

Four doses of TA	2	6%
Less than 4 doses of TA	16	46%
Homoeopathic	5	14%
None	4	11%
Unknown	8	23%
Total	**35**	**100%**

The study concluded that: "People fully immunised were five times less likely to contract whooping cough compared with people with other immunisation status", and that "homoeopathic immunisation was not effective in preventing whooping cough". Dr John Beard (one of the report's authors) has since suggested that the homoeopathic method may have increased the risk of acquiring the disease (refer 8.6.7. below).

Although these conclusions have been both embraced and widely quoted, a further conclusion of the study remains unacknowledged, that "The sample size was too small to demonstrate possibly significant results". So, while authors of the report themselves acknowledge that the scope of the study was insufficient to support the foregoing conclusions (including possible evidence against the homoeopathic option), the report is being used both to promote the cause of routine vaccination and to denounce the homoeopathic option.

Another aspect of the study reveals the hypocrisy of reporters who attack homoeopathy and other forms of traditional medicine in the name of science: The authors made a point of accepting only children vaccinated four or more times as being "fully immunised". This suggests that younger children, who receive the routine course of vaccination and are (according to age) fully vaccinated at the time of exposure, are inadequately protected; for example, a child of seven months who has been vaccinated three times for whooping cough, but will not receive the fourth course for many months.

While the study provided a filter for 'partially vaccinated' children, no filters were established to allow for incomplete homoeopathic cover in the non-vaccinated children. Effective filtering of the children who had received the homoeopathic option would have involved an assessment of the remedy, potency, and timing of doses received: the authors did not make such an assessment and were probably unaware of the need to do so.

Ironically this study, based on 79 questionnaires completed by parents assessing their children's exposure and reaction to the disease, has been approved and used as evidence by the medical/scientific community, yet the same people refuse to give any credence to the study reported in this book, which also involves parental assessment of exposure and reaction to disease, but has been ongoing since 1986 and involves 2,342 survey responses to date.

8.4.7 A Current Affair

On 25 May 1994, *A Current Affair*, hosted by Ray Martin ran a segment attacking the homoeopathic option and myself in particular; the reporter was Chris Smith.

Again, the usual quotes were produced - the Medical Faculty quote and the ANTA quote from *Choice* - with a number of amendments: In quoting Dr Spence, the reporter added my name to the original statement; it appeared that Dr Spence was attacking me personally. The *Choice* statement was presented as the current position of ANTA, rather than (as it was) an alleged personal statement by an ex-president.

The facts were further distorted in discussing the NSW North Coast experience (refer section 8.4.6 above), which clearly stated that 58% of respondents had been vaccinated. Mr Smith stated that "a health department survey showed that just six percent (6%) of people here had been fully immunised using conventional vaccination. Fourteen percent (14%) used homoeopathic vaccination, and the rest, well most of them had never been immunised at all".

This deliberate alteration of facts by the media, which is by no means an isolated example, illustrates the need for discernment, especially where commercial interests may be involved. It is a tragedy that in most developed countries the mainstream commercial media are so beholden to big-money interests (advertisers). It stifles free thinking and independent journalism.

8.4.8 MJA review of the homoeopathic alternative

An article, *Homoeopathic vaccination - what does it mean?*, was published in the Medical Journal of Australia, 5 September 1994. The article reported on a survey of sixteen homoeopathic practitioners in Sydney (Sulfaro F et al, 1994).

Unfortunately, the research did not extend to practitioners who were specialists in the use of homoeopathy for the prevention of specific diseases. Had they done so, the survey would have revealed that there is no such thing as 'homoeopathic vaccination' - we do not *vaccinate* children with homoeopathic medicines. While this may seem insignificant, it illustrates that 'scientific' review of the homoeopathic method comes from a position of ignorance, which is further exacerbated by inadequate research.

While using the above mentioned popular quotes (from the Royal London Homoeopathic Hospital, NH&MRC, and *Choice*), the authors did not include an adequate review of the historical evidence for the efficacy of the homoeopathic method.

8.4.9 The Australian Skeptics

I have been somewhat undecided whether to make a comment about attacks on homœoprophylaxis by the Australian Skeptics. In many ways their views are of little consequence to independently thinking people. Further, I have no doubt that many of their members are sincere and well meaning people, unlike some in their organisation. But they do make the headlines from time to time, send off numerous complaints to official bodies, they stalk online chat rooms, and their members write emotive and misleading letters to editors, etc. Their aim is often to stifle free speech unless the speaker agrees with them. So some comment should be made.

They state; "The Australian Skeptics Inc. is a group that investigates the paranormal and pseudo-science from a responsible scientific viewpoint". In fact, they frequently release totally inaccurate allegations and misinformation in the name of science, as the following few extracts from a speech given by their leader, Peter Bowditch, show. He stated:

- There are some principles of alternative medicine that you might like to keep in mind throughout this talk and the demonstrations of devices and potions. One is that the body is incapable of regulating itself and consequently becomes polluted with many toxins.
- In alternative medicine there is no such thing as mental illness or somatization or anxiety disorders.

- Another principle is that clinical trials of alternative treatments are not necessary, because all you have to know is that things work.
- The one overarching principle of alternative medicine, however, is that science is unnecessary, closed of mind, knows nothing and wants to know nothing.

From a speech given by Peter Bowditch to a dinner meeting of the Australian Skeptics on Saturday, 22 February, 2003. http://www.skeptics.com.au/ F:\Aust Skeptics\Quackery.htm

I have been a natural therapist for over 25 years, and not one of these statements is true. Yet Bowditch claims to be both responsible and scientific.

After reading the material on their website, I decided that it would be pointless responding to it in detail. I doubt if any intelligent person could read the material without realising that a great deal of it is totally unbalanced. There are some good references to orthodox medical material, but the rest is written without any scientific objectivity, and often with venom that approaches hatred. And as is so common with obsessions, there is just so much of it!!

So I have decided to leave it alone – if any readers want to check it out, the web site is referenced above. You can make up your own mind about it. All I can say is that if I was a serious scientist, I would be embarrassed by having this irrational organisation on my side. I have received a few letters from distinguished orthodox medical professors over the years concerning my work. They are characterised by their dignity and balance, even while agreeing to disagree. These latter two characteristics are badly needed in the Skeptics material.

It is also worth remembering that homoeopathy is practised around the world. In Europe, most homoeopaths are also medical practitioners. In the UK, there are five homoeopathic hospitals under the National Health system. The list goes on and on, yet the Skeptics believe in their blind ignorance that these tens of thousands of medically trained people have been somehow hoodwinked. **The Skeptics do prove one thing - that truth can never enter a closed mind!**

8.4.10 The Adelaide Advertiser, 2010

The misinformation and shoddy journalism that is unfortunately typical of much of the mainstream health media in this country surfaced again on 18/9/2010 when the *Adelaide Advertiser* ran an article titled "**Herbs no cure for fatal cough**", discussing homoeopathic treatment and prevention of whooping cough during a current outbreak in the region. The following are some of the errors that were made:

(a) The article began "Homeopaths are recommending "unproven herbal remedies including belladonna and phosphorous..." The remedies recommended by homeopaths are neither herbal (this is why they are not called "herbalists"), nor unproven, being used and studied for over 150 years. Phosphorous is a mineral.

(b) "Drosera and pertussinum are other herbal remedies…". The basis of the latter is not herbal, and the former is a herb before it is potentised into homeopathic form, but is not administered in herbal form by homeopaths.

(c) They quoted an AMA spoksman saying "anyone recommending homeopathic "vaccinations" or treatments was not legitimate". In fact there is no such thing as a homeopathic vaccine, and homeopathic treatments are legitimate, and the remedies approved by the government's TGA.

(d) The AMA spokesperson continued that the evidence supporting the homeopathic option "is complete rubbish". I wonder if he has read the evidence, especially the evidence from Cuba? I am sure he has not. Therefore his unresearched opinion is unscientific. Why would a genuine journalist allow such unscientific statements go unchallenged – unless of course the article writer had done no research himself.

(e) A genuine journalist would also have asked – was the child who tragically died from whooping cough vaccinated? The article writer did not mention that point.

It is greatly disappointing that the quality of debate in this and many other countries is so poor. I understand that the mainstream media receives hundreds of millions annually in advertising revenue from Big Pharma, and this would also explain why, on numerous occasions over the past 10 years, I have received a call from an eager young journalist asking to do a story on the homoeopathic option, only to either never hear from them again, or be told that their Editor has told them not to do the story.

Once again, this is why parents have chosen to take matters into their own hands and seek their own information. They can't trust Health Department spin, they can't trust the media, they can't trust AMA officials, they certainly can't trust advertising by Big Pharma whose toxic influence pervades the other bodies.

If there are fearless and committed journalist out there, then please make it one of your aims to correct the misinformation which continues to circulate about the homoeopathic option. Parents deserve truthful resporting and they generally don't have it yet.

Finally, the article quoted the mother of a child who tragically died from whooping cough giving support to the parents involved in the reported incident. This mother has become a well meaning but ill informed crusader for vaccines, often repeating the health department line that unvaccinated children create a pool of infection which impacts on the rest of the community. In fact, this pool of infection can also be created by vaccinated children, as the following research shows.

"The effects of whole-cell pertussis vaccine wane after 5 to 10 years, and infection in a vaccinated person causes nonspecific symptoms. Vaccinated adolescents and adults may serve as reservoirs for silent infection and become potential transmitters to unprotected infants. The whole-cell vaccine for pertussis is protective only against clinical disease, not against infection. Therefore, even young, recently vaccinated children may serve as reservoirs and potential transmitters of infection" (Srugo I et.al, .2000).

Blaming parents who choose not to vaccinate for community-wide problems is as thoughtless as it is inappropriate.

8.4.11 Conclusions

Examination of the above, frequently-reported criticisms of the homoeopathic option clearly indicates that statements about homœoprophylaxis are often misquoted, misleading, irrelevant, or even completely untrue.

While examples used to denounce the homoeopathic option are clearly refutable, and sometimes knowingly false, positive evidence is generally ignored and little genuine effort is made to thoroughly research the topic. To date, no convincing evidence has been presented to refute the effectiveness of the homoeopathic option.

For those readers who feel that my own bias in favour of homoeopathy has distorted my analysis, just remember that whatever arguments we may use for and against homoeopathy, there is one bottom line here – it works!

8.5 Special Topics

In addition to comments on health care economics, this section includes information on the problems associated with vaccination in Third World countries.

8.5.1 Economics of health care

In Australia, we are fortunate that both Federal and State Governments have substantially resisted the economic and political pressure from pharmaceutical companies in their efforts to have legislation introduced to prevent the widespread distribution of natural medicines. So far, their efforts have been unsuccessful, principally due to the massive popular support for natural medicine. As voters, we need to continue to lobby our politicians to ensure that our freedom of choice in this vital area is maintained.

In time, the Ministers responsible for finance and health care will realise that they can save millions of dollars each year by simply accepting properly trained and accredited natural therapists into the health care system. Continued failure to do this will only perpetrate the steady increase in chronic disease in this country, as discussed in Section 3.5 above. This is starting to happen through government initiatives to support allied health practitioners.

Research into the potential monetary savings from an increased availability of appropriate natural therapies is starting to happen, such as the 2010 Access Economics study mentioned earlier. Further studies should quantify the reduction in the costs of medications and professional visits as well as a general improvement in health producing considerable savings in the medium term. It should certainly take into account the implications of the possible links between vaccination and other pharmaceutical drugs, and chronic illness.

8.5.2 Vaccination in third world countries

Children in so-called Third World countries urgently need adequate and balanced nutrition, improved hygiene and sanitation, and comprehensive nursing care. They need this much more than they need vaccines.

It is a well established fact that malnourished children are most at risk when exposed to an acute challenge to their immune systems. Such a challenge can occur through exposure to infectious disease *or* vaccination, both of which stress the child's already depleted immune system.

The obvious solution is to redirect the millions spent on vaccination in these countries to the improvement of health care, nutrition, and sanitation facilities, as well as to education in better hygiene. In order to provide protection against infectious diseases, homoeopathic prophylactics could be distributed. Unlike conventional vaccines, these are inexpensive, safe and simple to administer, and free from harmful side effects. The only disadvantage involved is that it would not yield the enormous profits for the pharmaceutical companies that the current vaccination programs do.

The following facts will dispel any doubts concerning the fact that vaccines can kill malnourished children.

- Dr Archie Kalokerinos' publication, *Every Second Child* (1974), details his work with Aboriginal children in the Australian outback. Although ridiculed at the time by most medical 'experts', his work saved tens of thousands of children's lives.

  Dr Kalokerinos discovered that Aboriginal children were being killed by Government-issued vaccination programs - in some areas, up to 50% of the children vaccinated - and he saved their lives by administering massive doses of Vitamin C. In his own words:

"A health team would sweep into an area, line up all the Aboriginal babies and infants and immunise them. There would be no examination, no taking of case histories, no checking on dietary deficiencies. Most infants would have colds. No wonder they died. Some would die within hours from acute vitamin C deficiency precipitated by the immunisation. Other would suffer immunological insults and die later from 'pneumonia', 'gastro-enteritis' or 'malnutrition'. If some babies and infants survived, they would be lined up again within a month for another immunisation. If some managed to survive even this, they would be lined up again. Then there would be booster shots, shots for measles, polio and even T.B. Little wonder they died. The wonder is that any survived." (Kalokerinos A, 1974).

- In the 1980's, this story was repeated in Africa. Word of this came back with engineers from New Zealand, who were working in Africa. They told of vaccination teams moving through villages, and some few days after the teams left, of many children dying. The deaths are recorded as being from malnutrition, because the children had no actual 'disease'. The cause of death should have been shown as: Immune system collapse - precipitated by vaccination.
- The World Health Organisation (WHO) conducts massive vaccination programs in Africa. While we assume that the purpose of these programs is to save lives, others suggest that economic and political pressures are the silent partners.

No matter what the *real* truth is, the fact remains that these vaccination programs have done enormous harm to African children (some evidence to support this statement was provided in Section 3).

In September 1987, Dr William C Douglass published an article entitled, *WHO Murdered Africa*, in which he claims that WHO vaccination programs: "murdered Africa with the AIDS virus". (Douglass W C, 1987).

- In this disturbing, but obviously carefully researched article, he claims that the AIDS virus could not have developed accidentally in African Green Monkeys, but was deliberately manufactured by WHO scientists, who combined a number of animal retroviruses and grew them in human tissue.

- Dr Douglass demonstrated statistically that, rather than AIDS starting with occasional bites from Green Monkeys, "a large number of people had to be infected at the same time".

  He further claims that, in Africa, this occurred as a result of deliberate contamination of the Smallpox vaccines. This claim is independently supported by 'leaked' WHO figures which show that, in both Africa and South America, the progress of the AIDS virus closely correlates to the WHO vaccination programs (refer Section 2.3).

- Dr Douglass also states that US Hepatitis B studies, in which only males between 20 and 40 years who were not monogamous participated, caused a sudden spread of the AIDS virus, particularly among homosexual groups. (*Note:* In Africa, AIDS is a heterosexual disease - the Smallpox vaccine is given to both males and females.)

  He states: "The Centres for Disease Control reported in 1981 that 4% of those receiving hepatitis vaccines were AIDS infected. In 1984 they admitted to 67%. Now they refuse to give out figures because they don't want to admit that 100% of hepatitis vaccine receivers are infected with AIDS"

While Dr Douglass' claims may not be totally correct, the evidence he presents, combined with other available material, show that there is a substantive basis to his allegations.

A similar piece of investigative journalism was published in 1992 titled, *Was this science's biggest blunder*? It began "In Africa in 1957-58 thousands of children were given polio vaccine grown in a culture made from the kidneys of African monkeys. A controversial new theory now claims this program was the origin of the AIDS epidemic" (Cribb J, 1992).

The idea was also discussed in medical journals (Kyle WS, 1992).

Whatever the final truth about AIDS, it is certain that we cannot trust international organisations such as WHO, pharmaceutical companies, or 'official' scientific research to provide us with completely factual information concerning vaccination programs.

Instead, we must determine this truth for ourselves and reject unnecessary and invasive procedures (such as vaccines) to protect our own health and that of our children.

Well meaning people (like Rotarians) who are working hard to raise money for vaccination programs in other countries, need to re-evaluate their position so that their gifts and personal efforts are directed to saving lives, and are not (unknowingly) contributing to further death and suffering. They now have a clear option presented by the Cubans to offer effective prevention without the risk of toxic damage to people in economically disadvantaged countries.

We have the means to achieve world peace, world health, and the elimination of poverty and suffering. However, before these goals can ever be realised, we need to recognise the forces working against them.

8.5.3 My experience with the health establishment

Since I began in the mid 1980's, five major official investigations have been undertaken against me. My understanding is that they were all instigated by individuals who opposed my work. Since the 5th edition of the book, I have been warned against revealing all the details that I have about these investigations.

The following is a summary of all major events to date:

1 *29.6.89* - I was investigated by an officer from the Victorian Health Department because an anonymous doctor had filed a complaint against me for my work in the immunisation field.

   The officer also informed me that I might have committed a criminal offence. An Act of Parliament was shown to me and I was advised that I might not be allowed to continue to dispense medicines.

   Result: No follow-up from the Health Department.

2 *4.7.90* - In response to a complaint from another anonymous doctor, I was again investigated by the same Health Department Officer. On this occasion, the Act of Parliament was read to me in great detail with the clear suggestion that I was practising

illegally with illegal substances.

Result: No follow-up from the Health Department.

3 *24.12.92* - I received a letter from the Pharmaceutical Adviser to the New South Wales Health Department (refer item [a] following), claiming that I had breached Schedule 4 of the Poisons Act 1966 and certain labelling requirements of this Act as well as the Therapeutic Goods and Cosmetic Regulations (Regulation 23). I was told either to refute these claims, correct breaches, or cease supplying Kits to NSW patients unless they had a doctor's prescription.

Results: In replying (refer item [b] following), I pointed out that, since the remedies did not contain any toxic material, they could not be regarded as poisons; no reply from the NSW Health Department to date.

4 *12.1.93* - An article by Professor John Dwyer appeared in a suburban newspaper chain, attacking me in rather emotive terms. Professor Dwyer used information supplied by a "Cheryl" whom he described as "my detective". Cheryl apparently makes a habit of trying to debunk anyone not using pharmaceutical drugs. She had purchased a book and a Kit from me (pretending to be someone she was not), presumably with the intention of 'exposing' these new homoeopathic developments (unfortunately, she is 200 years late).

Result: Although I wrote a reply to the newspaper, I believe it was not published.

5 *13.1.93* - A letter received from the Therapeutic Goods Administration (refer item [c] following) advised that I would be fined $24,000 for any Kit mailed interstate. Apparently, when the attempt to suppress my work mentioned in point 3 (above) failed, it was passed onto the TGA. Upon phoning the TGA in Canberra, I was advised that they were preventing the sale of the Kits, *not* because they were unsafe, but because the 'intention' was to prevent infectious diseases.

Result: Since contesting their decision or complying with the TGA's request would impose enormous costs, I was forced to reply that I would cease supplying Kits interstate by mail.

6 *22.1.93* - A further attack by Professor Dwyer appeared in The Australian Doctor journal.

Result: In March 1993, my reply was published (refer item [d] following).

7 *1.2.93* - I received a letter from the Complaints Unit of the NSW Health Department, notifying me that I was under investigation following a complaint. Official confidentiality requirements mean that details of this investigation cannot be provided to readers.

Result: Although not officially covered by their jurisdiction, I replied in detail. There was no case to answer.

8 A series of public attacks against me in the Newcastle Herald were started by a person who signed the letters as "Miss Cheryl Freeman, Gardner St., Dudley". These attacks lasted for two years from 1993 to 1995. Sounds very much like the person referred to by Professor Dwyer as his "detective" in point 4 above. This Miss Freeman also wrote letters against me to natural health journals such as Grass Roots, and to homoeopathic pharmacies such as Martin & Pleasance. Interestingly, she was awarded the 1999 Australian Skeptic of the year award.

8 6.8.93 – It was reported in the *Australian Doctor* that the NSW Health Department was analysing a Kit with a view to banning "homoeopathic vaccination kits".

9 24.8.93 - This proved incorrect when the pharmaceutical adviser from the Victorian Department of Health and Community Services asked to purchase a Kit to send to NSW. I was, of course, happy to donate a Kit in the interests of research; no follow-up to date.

10 25.5.94 - The Current Affair program featuring Professor Dwyer was aired.

11 24.10.94 - The last official investigation, to date of publication, commenced when I received a letter from the Health care Complaints Commission of NSW. Official confidentiality requirements mean that details of this investigation cannot be provided to readers.

Result: A number of letters were exchanged, and the investigation closed on 20.7.95 – no case to answer.

In the attacks between 1993 and 1995, and others, I have been accused of being "irresponsible", "mischievous", "dangerous", "a quack", etc; *yet no evidence has ever been given that the Homoeopathic option is either unsafe or ineffective.*

The items referred to above [a-d] are reproduced below:

Figure 8-4 Item [a] - Letter from the Pharmaceutical Adviser to the New South Wales Health Department.

NSW HEALTH
DEPARTMENT

PUBLIC HEALTH SERVICES BRANCH

Dr Isaac Golden
Aurum Healing Centre
PO Box 1198
GEELONG VIC 3220

Ph.S.S./DB:sdbt

(02) 887-5678

10.DEC.1992

Dear Dr Golden,

It has been reported to the Department that your organisation is supplying by mail order into NSW, therapeutic goods - namely "Homoeopathic Immunization Pills" which would be classified in the Poisons List as vaccines and therefore would fall within Schedule 4 of the List. Therapeutic goods included in Schedule 4 must only be supplied on a medical Doctor's prescription, supply otherwise is a breach of the Poisons Act 1966.

In addition it appears that the items supplied are not labelled in accordance with the requirements for Schedule 4 substances or in accordance with the requirements of the Therapeutic Goods and Cosmetic Regulations (Regulation 23).

In view of the above you are requested to provide, within one month of the date of this letter, information which will refute the foregoing or, if it is an accurate reflection of your activities in NSW a written undertaking to correct any breaches of NSW Regulations or to cease supplying the products in NSW.

Yours faithfully

D Buckley
Pharmaceutical Adviser
Pharmaceutical Services Section

Macquarie Hospital
Wicks Road North Ryde NSW 2113
PO Box 380 North Ryde NSW 2113
Telephone (02) 887 5608 Facsimile (02) 888 7210

Figure 8-5 Reply to the Pharmaceutical Adviser to the New South Wales Health Department

Aurum Healing Centre,
P.O. Box 1198.
GEELONG. 3220.
25.12.92.

Dr David Buckley,
Pharmaceutical Adviser,
Pharmaceutical Services Section.
Public Health Services Branch.
N.S.W. Health Department.
P.O. Box 380.
NORTH RYDE. 2113.

Dear Dr Buckley,

Thank you for your letter Ph.S.S./DB:sdbt dated 18.12.92 concerning the Homoeopathic prophylactic kit I provide to patients in your State.

I do not prepare any of the Homoeopathic preparations used in my kit, but purchase them from a licensed Homoeopathic pharmacy. I then prepare the kit as requested by patients.

I have been advised that since the Homoeopathic preparations used in the kit have been potentised well past the point where any molecules of any toxic material remain, that they cannot be Poisons, and certainly cannot be considered vaccines. The dilutions range from 10^{-400} to 10^{-20000}. I believe that Avogadro's number is close to 10^{-24} so there is just no possibility that any material substance remains in the Homoeopathic preparations I use.

I had assumed that this advice was correct since every Homoeopathic and most Naturopathic practitioners in your State are using these potentised substances every day in their practices, without action against them by the NSW Health Department.

I had assumed that I was not contravening any labelling requirements under the poisons schedule, since I am not supplying poisons. If I am contravening any other labelling requirements then I would of course be pleased to amend the instructions and labelling I use with my Kit in accordance with your advice.

I perhaps should also advise you that I do not place advertisements for the kit. It has been mentioned in articles I have written for some professional journals, but I am paid for these articles, they certainly are not advertising. Mostly I am contacted through personal recommendation.

I trust that this information is what you require. I look forward to your reply to clarify the above points. I of course remain willing to co-operate fully with the Health Department and any appropriate legal requirements which apply to my profession.

Yours sincerely,

Isaac Golden.

Figure 8-6 Letter from the Therapeutic Goods Administration

TGA Therapeutic Goods Administration

PO Box 100, Woden, ACT 2606, Australia
☐ Woden Telephone: (06) 289 1555. Fax: (06) 289 8709
☐ Mawson Telephone: (06) 286 0222. Fax: (06) 286 1386

COMMONWEALTH DEPARTMENT OF HEALTH, HOUSING AND COMMUNITY SERVICES

Dr Isaac Golden
Principal
Aurum Healing Centre
P.O.Box 1198
GEELONG VIC 3220

Dear Dr Golden

HOMOEOPATHIC VACCINATION PRODUCTS

It has been brought to the attention of the TGA that you are supplying interstate, homoeopathic vaccination products as part of a Homoeopathic Prophylactic Kit and publicising this kit via your publication, 'Vaccination? A Review of Risks and Alternatives.'

You should be aware that in Australia these products appear to be Therapeutic Goods requiring entry on the Australian Register of Therapeutic Goods (ARTG). Under Section 20(1) of the Therapeutic Goods Act 1989, it is an offence for a person who is the sponsor of therapeutic goods to knowingly or recklessly import, export, manufacture or supply the goods in Australia for use in humans, unless those goods are listed or registered on the Australian Register of Therapeutic Goods or are exempt goods or are subject of an approval under Section (19) of the Act.

"Sponsors" include persons who import or arrange for the importation of the goods, or who manufacture or arrange for another person to manufacture the goods for supply. Sponsors are subject to the requirements of the Act if they are trading corporations or, in the case of individuals and corporations generally, trade the goods between Australia and another country or among the States within Australia. The maximum penalty is $24,000 for an individual in respect of each offence.

Our records indicate that these products are not entered on the Register. You are requested therefore to cease promotion and supply interstate immediately of these and any other unregistered or unlisted therapeutic good which is not exempt from this requirement.

In addition, under Section 35(1) of the Therapeutic Goods Act 1989 "a person must not, at premises in Australia, knowingly or recklessly carry out a step in the manufacture of therapeutic goods for supply for use in humans unless:

(a) the goods are exempt goods or the person is an exempt person in relation to the manufacture of the goods; or

(b) the person is a holder of a licence that is in force that authorises the carrying out of that step in relation to the goods at those premises."

Manufacturing includes "engaging in the processing, assembling, packaging, labelling, storage, sterilising, testing or releasing for sale of the goods".

It would appear therefore, that you are required to hold a licence to manufacture those products which are being supplied interstate. The maximum penalty in this case is also $24,000 for an individual in respect of each offence.

You are requested also to provide written confirmation within 5 days of receipt of this letter that interstate supply will cease until such time as the product has been included in the Register.

Application forms for Listing (Registration) of Drugs are available from the TGA Information Officer at the above address or by phoning 062398634. Copies of the Licence Application Form may be obtained from Ms S. McGregor of the GMP Section of the TGA by phoning (06)2398628.

Failure to comply may result in enforcement action without further notice.

Yours sincerely

Val Johanson

Val Johanson
Head of Surveillance
13th January 1993

cc Mr Keith Moyle
Victorian Health Department

Figure 8-7 Response to Professor Dwyer article in the *Australian Doctor.*

Dr Isaac Golden, Ph.D.(M.A.).
P.O. Box 1198.
GEELONG. 3220.
(052) 411 070.
4.2.1993.

The Editor.
The Australian Doctor.
P.O. Box 5487.
CHATSWOOD WEST. 2057.

Dear Madam,

HOMOEOPATHIC PREVENTION OF INFECTIOUS DISEASE

In a recent article to your Journal, Professor John Dwyer has attacked my use of Homoeopathic prophylaxis as being "extremely irresponsible", and has referred to "nonsense preparations" which are "clinically unproven alternative methods".

Most readers of your Journal would have had little opportunity to access facts concerning the Homoeopathic option. The following is the rationale behind it's use:

1. Conventional vaccines are neither completely safe, or completely effective (ref. various medical Journals and clinical experience).
2. The decline in deaths from most infectious diseases were mostly unaffected by the introduction of mass vaccination programs. Notification rates were influenced with some diseases and not with others (ref. statistics for deaths and notifications from health departments in U.S.A., U.K., and Australia).
3. It follows that vaccination is not a perfect solution. Thus it is reasonable to examine other tested options to see if they have merit.
4. Homoeopathy was founded 200 years ago by a German physician Dr Samuel Hahnemann. It rapidly became popular throughout Europe for one principal reason - it was effective in both treating and preventing the many infectious diseases which swept Europe at that time. It is surprising that Prof. Dwyer failed to find the many references to this fact when he was researching Homoeopathy prior to criticising it so vehemently!
   Dr Hahnemann first used a potency of Belladonna to prevent Scarlet Fever. He and other doctors used other remedies to prevent Cholera, Typhoid etc. They have been used frequently and successfully since then. This is a matter of historical fact.
5. Homoeopathic medicines do not guarantee 100% protection. However they are non toxic, and in particular no adjuvants such as Aluminium compounds are necessary.
6. Clinical evidence over 200 years suggests that the efficacy of Homoeopathic prophylaxis is comparable to that of vaccination. Once again I am suprised that Prof. Dwyer did not find this in his research of the subject. It is also supported by the statistical evidence which I collect annually from parents who use the program which I have published.
7. Thus it is reasonable and logical to consider the Homoeopathic method as an alternative to vaccination.

Most Homoeopaths would welcome further objective evaluation by independent review committees, but to suggest that our method is "clinically unproven" is based purely on ignorance of our method.

Prof Dwyer implies that vaccines have been subjected to the "rigorous method of approval" used to "get a new drug onto the market". He is of course referring to double blind, placebo controlled trials. I invite Prof. Dwyer to advise readers where such trials of the commonly used vaccines are reported in the medical literature. The few placebo controlled trials of vaccines which I have seen have been rather unsuccessful (e.g. Lancet, 30.4.88).

My involvement with this issue over the last seven years has been to offer parents facts, and an alternative if they so wish. I have never demanded that vaccines be banned. I have never written outside traditional medicine circles. I have never paid to advertise my Kit. The recent public attention to this issue has been generated by Prof. Dwyer.

The Homoeopathic option to vaccines has stood the test of time in the clinic. It has proved to be safe, and relatively effective. I believe it should be freely available those those relatively few parents who see it as a preferred option. The final aim should be, after all, the the protection of our children.

Yours sincerely,

Isaac Golden.

8.6 Parents' support groups

A number of support groups exist in most countries, whereby experiences and concerns relating to vaccination may be shared. Some national groups do exist, and some are listed below. For anyone wanting an excellent summary of available links, I recommend the following Australian Vaccination Network (AVN) site - http://www.avn.org.au/links.htm#1

Australia

Australian Vaccination Network (AVN) - www.avn.org.au

Australia's longest standing parent support group. Has been attacked in media and by orthodox authotrities in 2010, but still maintains a valuable web site and provides information for parents on which to make informed choices.

PO Box 177 Bangalow NSW 2479. Ph. (02) 66871699

Vaccine Information South Australia (VISA) - www.visainfo.org.au

Vaccination Information South Australia formed on the 11th of February 1997, out of a need to respond to the government push to raise immunisation levels, and a need to provide alternative factual information about vaccination, including the dangers. We are a voluntary, non-profit, membership funded organisation.

PO Box 643 Magill SA 5072. Ph. (08) 8336 5236.

Email: visa@adelaide.on.net

Vaccination Awareness and Information Service (VAIS)
http://www.vaccinationawareness.com.au/Default.html

V.A.I.S. is a non-profit, volunteer organization dedicated to supplying factual information on vaccinations so parents can make an informed choice on this issue. We have a comprehensive health library and support groups in many areas so like-minded, health conscious parents can get together and support each other. Call Stephanie on 07 3821-5454 or 0412671922 for information or a support group near you. Email: growingawareness@hotmail.com

Vaccination Information Service - www.vaccination.inoz.com

For comprehensive information sourced from extensive literature including over 100000 pages of medical research articles on vaccination collected by internationally recognised expert Dr Viera Scheibner, who has published a number of scientific papers in reputable scientific and medical journals. Also supportive information on legal rights and how to build strong immunity. Books, videos, DVD, colour information brochures and packs available.

PO Box 4 Turramurra NSW 2074. Ph. (02) 9144 6625.

Email: vaccinfo@bigpond.com

Healthy Families of Illawarra.

http://sites.google.com/site/healthyfamiliesofillawarra/

A site to provide information about vaccines

Wollongong, Ph. (02)4284-6143. Kiama (02) 4232 1761

Association for Prevention of Cot Death, 26 Ada Street, Blackheath NSW 2785

Humane Research Australia,

Suite 205, 19 Milton Parade, Malvern, Vic. 3144. Ph: 03 8823 5705.

http://www.aahr.org.au/index.html

Campaign Against Fraudulent Medical Research, PO Box 128, Cabramatta NSW 2166.
http://www.pnc.com.au/~cafmr/online/research/index.html

New Zealand

Immunization Awareness Society (IAS) - http://www.ias.org.nz/

United States

National Vaccination Information Centre (NVIC) -
http://www.909shot.com/

512 W. Maple Ave, Suite 206, Vienna, Virginia 22180, United States.
Phone (703) 938-0342

A brilliant resource by Barbara Lou Fisher, a world leading authority on the topic, who was partly responsible for the introduction of a vaccine damage compensation scheme in the USA.

Thinktwice Global Vaccine Institute
PO Box 9638
Santa Fe, NM 87504.
505-983-1856 (Telephone & Fax)

http://www.thinktwice.com/support.htm

This website will provide links to all the other vaccine support groups in the USA.

United Kingdom

VaccineVictim Support Group
27 Malcolm Grove, Rednal, Birmingham . B45 9BS. Tel: 0121 243 7759

http://www.webhealth.co.uk/support_groups/Vaccine_victim_support_group.asp

Cry Shame
www.cryshame.com

Justice Awareness and Basic Support
http://www.jabs.org.uk/pages/single.asp

Vaccine Information Service (VIS) - http://www.vaccine-info.com/

8.7 Selected list of available reference material

The following selected list of reference material relating to vaccination includes publications specifically recommended for parents, as indicated by the notation (REC).

8.7.1 Books

Australian Vaccination Network. *Vaccination Roulette: Experiences, risks and alternatives*. 1998.

Barham-Floreani J. *Well Adjusted Babies*. Vitality Productions Pty Ltd, Mt.Macedon, Victoria. Australia. 2nd Edition. (REC)

Chaitow L, *Vaccination and Immunisation: Dangers, Delusions and Alternatives*.

Coulter H L, *Vaccination, Social Violence and Criminality. The Medical Assault on the American Brain.*

Coulter H L & Harris B, *D.P.T. - A Shot in the Dark.* (REC)

Kalokerinos A, *Every Second Child.* (REC)

Kirby D, *Evidence of Harm: Mercury in Vaccines and the Autism Epidemic: A Medical Controversy*. St Martin's Griffin, New York. 2005.

Mendelsohn R S, *Confessions of a Medical Heretic.* (REC)

Mendelsohn R S, *How to Raise a Healthy Child ... In Spite of Your Doctor*. Contemporary Books, Chicago, 1990. (REC)

Mothering Magazine. *Vaccinations. The Rest of the Story*. PO Box 1690, Sante Fe, NM 87504, USA. (REC)

Neustaedter R, The Vaccine *Guide: Risks and Benefits for Children and Adults.* 2002.

Nossal G J V, *Antibodies and Immunity.* Nelson, 1968.

Olmstead D, Blaxill M. *The Age of Autism – Mercury, Medicine, and a Man-Made Epidemic.* Thomas Dunne Books. New York. 2010.

Scheibner, V, *Vaccination: The Medical Assault on the Immune System.* 1993.

Wakefield AJ *Callous Disregard: Autism and Vaccines – The Truth Behind a Tragedy*. 2010.

NOTE: Many of these books are available from the AVN bookshop

8.7.2 Journals

Australian Wellbeing, PO Box 249, Mosman Junction NSW 2088.

Nature & Health, PO Box 170, Willoughby NSW 2068.

The International Vaccination Newsletter, Krekenstraat 4, B-3600 Genk, Belgium; Fax: 32 89 304 982.

Informed Choice (Official Journal of the Australian Vaccination Network).

8.7.3 Other resources by Dr Isaac Golden

Isaac Golden
PUBLICATIONS

Other books written and published by Dr Isaac Golden PhD, as at 1.11.2010
(prices inc p&p to Victoria, Australia)

(Quantity discounts are available on request)

BOOKS ON HOMŒOPROPHYLAXIS

Vaccine Damaged Children: Treatment, Prevention, Reasons. 2010.

This book examines what is possibly the most unrecognised public health problem in our community; the long-term impact of vaccination on the general health of children and adults. The book provides data which shows that vaccines cause damage, and details the findings of Isaac's new "reverse" research quantifying the symptoms caused by vaccines. Homoeopathic treatment of vaccine damage is described, including cases of both long and short term treatment are shown. This is a book for practitioners of all modalities, but especially homoeopaths. It is also a book for parents, and an Appendix introducing homoeopathic method is provided. $35.00 inc. p&p (interstate $3.00, overseas $12.00)

Homœoprophylaxis - A Fifteen Year Clinical Study: A Statistical Review of the Efficacy and Safety of Long-Term Homœoprophylaxis. 2004.

An in-depth statistical analysis of 2,342 responses from parents whose children used my homœoprophylaxis program from 1986-2003. Includes written responses from parents describing reactions and diseases. Also data from 4-year General Health Study on long-term health, comparing effects of different methods of immunisation. A4 size, 150 pages. $34.00 inc. p&p (interstate $3.00, overseas $16.00).

Homœoprophylaxis-A Practical and Philosophical Review. 4th edition.2007. Examines the philosophical and practical arguments for and against homœoprophylaxis. A book for practitioners who are evaluating their options, and the points for and against using homoeopathic option. A5 size. $18.00 inc. p&p (interstate $3. 00, overseas $12. 00).

SIMPLE HOMOEOPATHIC PRESCRIBING

Australian Homoeopathic Home Prescriber - Part 1 - Treatment of Simple Everyday Conditions. 3rd edition. 2007. A very simple, uncomplicated prescriber for parents. Quick and easy to use. Used by Martin & Pleasance in their First Aid kits. A5 size. $14.00 inc. p&p (interstate $3.00, overseas $12.00).

Australian Homoeopathic Home Prescriber - Part 2 - A Simple Materia Medica of Common Remedies With Repertory. 2001. An easy to read Materia Medica of common first-aid remedies, with a very simple, uncomplicated Repertory for parents- Quick and easy to use. A5 size $16.00 inc. p&p (interstate $3.00, overseas $12.00).

Australian Homoeopathic Home Prescriber - Part 3 – Basic Homoeopathy. 2006. A very simple, uncomplicated explanation of homoeopathic prescribing. Quick and easy to use. A5 size.

$13.00 inc. p&p (interstate $3.00, overseas $12.00).

DETAILED HOMOEOPATHIC BODY-SYSTEM PRESCRIBING

Homoeopathic Body-System Prescribing - A Practical Workbook of Sector Remedies. 2nd Ed. 2002. Homoeopathic analysis of major diseases from every body system. A major rewrite of this manual has just been completed. The 2nd Edition of the Workbook 10 new diseases, and substantially reworks 29 diseases that were in the 1ST edition A4 size. 420 pages. $66.00 inc. p&p (interstate $5.00, overseas $16.00- $30.00).

NEW DEVELOPMENTS IN HOMOEOPATHY

Homoeopathic Treatment of The Energy Bodies - Traditional Strategies And New Developments. 2002.

Homoeopathic medicines are energetic substances that interact with the energy bodies of the patient. An explanation of the bodies is given. The healing models of homoeopathy and theosophy are compared, and integrated. A new approach to remove negative material in the energy bodies of patients is introduced, using new equipment called the *Auric Replicator*- The use of potentised medicines in both chronic and acute cases is discussed B5 size, 99 pages. **OUT OF PRINT IN 2010**

Visit our web page at www.homstudy.net

THE AURIC REPLICATOR

A world first - designed to make potencies of the negative (lower sub-plane) material in the energy bodies of patients. Shown to be effective in both short and long term cases. Useable by practitioners, or at home by those wanting to help themselves, family and friends. $350.00 plus p&p.

EDUCATION IN HOMOEOPATHY AND NATURAL MEDICINE

(1) Correspondence Courses written and supervised by Dr Isaac Golden, and taught through the *Australasian College of Hahnemannian Homoeopathy*

An Intermediate Course in Homoeopathic Medicine

This course is designed for those who wish to learn how to prescribe accurately for the basic health problems of their family or friends. It gives credits for the Professional course if students continue with their studies. The 6 Tutorials are understandable and practical. The cost of $340.00 (inc. books) is spread over the length of the course. Suitable for parents, students, or therapists who want a basic knowledge of practical homoeopathy.

An Introductory Course in Natural Medicine

This three Tutorial course costing $155.00 introduces students to the use of herbal medicine, homoeopathy, flower essences, tissue salts, diet, and colour healing. A simple, "how to do it" course.

Certificate in Homoeopathic Case Taking

Practitioner Certificate in Homoeopathy

For people wishing to expand their basic homoeopathic prescribing skills. These are not accredited courses, but are practical and relevant.

(2) On-Line Courses in Homoeopathy and Natural Medicine, written and supervised by Dr Isaac Golden, and taught through the *Homeopathic International Online College*

Visit our web page at www.homstudy.net

HOMOEOPATHIC SOFTWARE

ISIS Vision Homoeopathic Software - the best value-for-money available. Easy to use, reasonably priced, with a full back-up. Cara was the first on the market, and has shown a commitment to innovation and thoroughness, now demonstrated in the latest ISIS software. Contact Isaac for current prices. Substantial student discounts are available.

CONTACT: P.O. Box 695. Gisborne. Victoria. 3437. Australia.
Ph. (03) 5427 0880. Email: admin@homstudy.net

9 APPENDICES TO QUESTIONS 1, 3 AND 4

9.1 Appendix to Question 1: The Characteristics of Each Infectious Disease

9.1.1 Chicken Pox (Varicella-Zoster)

1. The Organism

The disease is caused by the varicella-zoster virus (VZV). It is also known as human herpes virus 3 (HHV-3), or herpes zoster (possibly causing shingles at a later date). Transmission is through direct contact of droplets, or a recently used handkerchief. The disease is highly contagious, with an attack rate of up to 90% (Davies et.al. 2001; page 240). The incubation period is from 11-20 days. A person is infectious for 1-2 days prior to the rash until 5 days after onset, or while new lesions appear. A person generally becomes immune for life following infection.

Chicken pox is typically a mild disease in healthy children, but can be serious and occasionally fatal in people of any age with a weakened immune system. It is generally more distressing in adults than in children. The disease is potentially very serious during pregnancy for both the mother and the foetus.

2. Clinical Symptoms

Chicken pox usually begins with a runny nose that is followed by a fever and the appearance of a vesicular rash (an eruption filled with clear fluid), which is very itchy. Groups of vesicles appear more frequently on the chest and back than the arms and legs. After some days the vesicles often break open and form crusts. The active lesions may continue for a week in children, or at times for months in adults. The infection can become very distressing if mucus membranes (e.g., eyes) are infected. A common complication is a staphylococcal infection of the skin.

Following infection the virus persists, as do other herpes viruses, as a latent infection that remains in the nerve ganglia. In some individuals it later reappears as shingles (herpes zoster). Herpes zoster may also occur in children who have not had chicken pox, but whose mothers had the disease during pregnancy.

Very occasionally other severe complications occur, such as Reye's syndrome (a serious form of encephalitis causing convulsions and coma). The risk of death from chicken pox in healthy children has been estimated at 14 in 100,000 (Preblud, 1986).

3. Orthodox and Homoeopathic Treatment

Generally, creams are used externally to help reduce itching. Varicella-zoster immunoglobulin may be given to high risk individuals, and acyclovir (an anti-viral drug) may be used if infection has already occurred.

Homoeopathic treatment for both chicken pox and shingles is very effective if well chosen. The remedy Rhus Tox is commonly indicated, but as with all homoeopathic treatment, an appropriate remedy needs to be chosen based on the individual presenting symptoms for each patient.

4. Summary

Chicken Pox is an unpleasant but relatively benign disease in a healthy child. It is potentially more serious in adults, especially pregnant women, or in children or adults with weakened immune systems. Vaccination may only delay the onset of the disease to a later and potentially more serious time in life, which would seem to be rather counter-productive.

It would appear to make sense to allow healthy children to acquire the disease, as this will give the most certain likelihood of immunity for life. Appropriate homoeopathic treatment will lessen both the duration and severity of the disease.

If it is decided that prevention is required, the homoeopathic option is available as an option to vaccination.

* * * * * * *

9.1.2 Cholera

1. The Organism

Cholera is a widespread epidemic disease, caused by *Vibrio cholerae*, a bacterium. There are a number of serogroups (different types of the organism). *V. cholerae* can exist in water, depending on the temperature, pH, salinity and availability of nutrients. It is a tenacious organism that can survive under unfavourable conditions.

The very few annual cases of cholera in Australia almost always occur in individuals who have been infected in endemic areas overseas. However rare cases of cholera may follow contact with river water in northern Australia. The disease is usually transmitted via food and water contaminated with human excreta. The use of waste water to irrigate vegetables can be a cause. Shellfish obtained from contaminated waters have also been responsible for outbreaks. Good sanitation and personal hygiene greatly reduce the likelihood of endemic cholera.

The incubation period of the disease may last for 5 days. Stool cultures can be used to confirm infection if required. Food handlers should not be allowed to return to work until 2 consecutive stool samples, taken at least 24 hours apart, are negative. Contacts should also be advised to maintain high standards of personal hygiene to avoid becoming infected.

2. Clinical Symptoms

Asymptomatic and mild infections are very common, but unlike many diarrhoeal diseases, cholera can develop quickly and has a high fatality rate if not treated appropriately. It is characterised by sudden onset of painless, effortless, profuse, watery "rice water" diarrhoea, followed by vomiting.

Dehydration (loss of water from body tissue due to the profuse diarrhoea), metabolic acidosis (accumulation in the blood of keto acids causing deep, regular, but difficult breathing, and a fruity smelling breath) and hypotension (low blood pressure) may soon follow. Hypoglycaemia (low blood sugar causing confusion and eventually coma) and convulsions are common in children. Severe muscle cramps rising from the legs are common. If untreated, more than half the severe cases will die.

3. Orthodox and Homoeopathic Treatment

Orthodox treatment is usually highly effective. It includes oral rehydration therapy (ORT), or intravenous rehydration, which can be used if dehydration is severe. Antibiotics are also used to remove *V.cholera* from the gastro intestinal tract.

Homoeopathic treatment has been used for 200 years. Remedies such as Camphor (in homoeopathic potencies), Veratrum Album, Cuprum Metallicum and Carbo Veg are indicated in the progressive stages of the disease. Professional advice is essential.

4. Summary

Cholera is a potentially serious disease that is unlikely to occur in regions where there is good sanitation and hygiene, etc. It is easily treated if orthodox medical facilities are available. Proven homoeopathic treatment is also available.

Prevention is mainly needed if travelling in areas where cholera is active. If exposure is likely, then prevention makes sense. One must decide whether to rely on hygiene alone, or to also use vaccination or homoeopathic prevention.

* * * * * * *

9.1.3 Diphtheria

1. The Organism

Diphtheria is an acute bacterial illness caused by toxigenic strains of *Corynebacterium diphtheriae*. The exotoxin produced by *C. diphtheriae* acts locally on the mucous membranes of the respiratory tract to produce an adhesive membrane which makes breathing very difficult. The exotoxin may affect the heart, the nervous system, causing paralysis, and the adrenals. The incubation period is 2 to 5 days. The disease can be passed on for up to 4 weeks or longer. It is spread by droplets or by direct contact with sores or with articles contaminated by infected persons.

Diphtheria has been almost eradicated from Australia, but sporadic cases continue to occur, principally through contacts with overseas travellers.

2. Clinical Symptoms

Diphtheria primarily affects the upper respiratory tract, but the skin can be involved. Symptoms often begin with a low-grade fever for a few days with a sore throat. The infection then causes an inflammatory discharge which forms a thick, adhesive, grey/white or green membrane in the upper respiratory tract. This can cause an acute severe obstruction of the respiratory tract making breathing very difficult. The membrane may also appear in the nose.

Diphtheria toxin can cause neuropathy (any disease of the nervous system) and cardiomyopathy (a sub-acute or chronic disorder of the heart muscle), which may be fatal.

3. Orthodox and Homoeopathic Treatment

Orthodox treatment with diphtheria antitoxin reduced the death rate to about 10%, which has remained stable even after the introduction of antibiotics and other modern treatments, but treatment does render the patient non-infectious after 24 hours. It is not considered useful to treat diphtheria of the skin with the antitoxin, and wound cleansing and antibiotics are recommended. Benzylpenicillin is often used as the preferred antibiotic.

Homoeopathic treatment is also available; the remedy selection depends on the individual presenting symptoms of the patient.

4. Summary

A potentially serious disease that is unlikely to occur in regions where there are no current outbreaks. It is reasonably well treated if orthodox medical facilities are available. Proven homoeopathic treatment is also available. Prevention is mainly needed if travelling in suspect areas. If prevention is required, vaccination or the homoeopathic option may be considered.

* * * * * * *

9.1.4 Haemophilis influenzae type b (Hib)

1. The Organism

Haemophilis influenzae is a bacterium that is a normal part of upper respiratory tract flora (bacteria). There are 6 capsular types, although type b is the most common, and potentially the most troublesome. It was first isolated in 1892. Hib resides in the throats of around 30% of healthy individuals, and is associated with many common infections. Hib is the major cause of meningitis (inflammation of the membrane covering the brain and spinal cord) and epiglottitis (infection in the throat) in children aged less than 5 years, but also affects the elderly. The meningitis peak is between 6 and 15 months of age, and the epiglottitis at 2.5 years of age. Despite originally being named due to being found in people with the flu, Hib is not related to influenza.

Before Hib vaccination, invasive disease (bacterial invasion of the blood and nervous systems) caused by Hib rarely occurred after the age of 5 years. This was because of the existence of antibodies to Hib, which progressively increased from the age of 2 years, thought to be related to exposure to Hib (or cross-reacting organisms) which survive in the nasopharynx (the space behind the nose and mouth) or other sites. Children less than 2 years of age are usually unable to mount an antibody response to the type b organism, even after an invasive disease, and they used to be the group most at risk before vaccination.

Hib can cause very serious health problems, including death. It has been estimated in the U.S. that 60 out of every 100,000 children will get Hib-caused meningitis, of which 3-6.5% will die, and 14% will have continuing problems (WDDTY, 1991, p.18). Breastfeeding can provide some protection (Cochi et al, 1986; Silfverdal S A et al, 1997 and 1999).

2. Clinical Symptoms

Clinical categories of invasive disease caused by Hib include meningitis, epiglottitis and a range of other infections such as septic arthritis, cellulitis (a painful infected swelling within solid tissues, usually in the loose tissue beneath the skin), pericarditis (inflammation of the membrane surrounding the heart), pneumonia (acute inflammation/infection of the lungs) and permanent hearing loss.

The classical clinical signs of meningitis – neck stiffness, seizures and photophobia (sensitivity to light) – are often not detected in infants, who initially present with drowsiness, loss of appetite, headache, nausea and high fever. Epiglottitis (inflammation of the epiglottis) can cause difficult breathing producing soft stridor (a harsh sound during breathing in) and dribbling. Children can be pale, feverish and child. They want to remain upright to assist their breathing.

Meningitis and epiglottitis are often fatal without appropriate treatment. It can be very difficult to differentiate many of the symptoms of Hib infection from those due to other organisms. However, before the introduction of Hib vaccines, epiglottitis was due to Hib in over 95% of cases.

3. Orthodox and Homoeopathic Treatment

To treat meningitis, special antibiotics are required (3rd generation cephalosporins). A lumbar puncture to relieve pressure may be required in non-responsive cases. Infections of the mucus membranes will need different drugs. The drug Rifampicin is used to prevent spread to unimmunised family members and other close contacts.

Homoeopathic treatment would initially revolve around acute remedies like Belladonna, but the patient should always be hospitalised where possible if symptoms progress.

These types of diseases are good examples of where the best in both orthodox and traditional medicine should be used, where available. I believe it is a great mistake for people to refuse to consider either orthodox or traditional treatments simply because of prejudice or ignorance. Both have something to offer us. In some severe diseases, drugs and surgical intervention can and do save lives. In other cases, they are unnecessary, and/or the effects of the drug or surgery can be worse than the effects of the disease. In other words - optimal health requires an open mind!

4. Summary

Hib is a potentially serious disease that is still active in the Australian community, although less since the introduction in 1993 of Hib vaccination. Hib is reasonably well treated if orthodox medical facilities are available, and appropriate treatment is started early. Homoeopathic treatment is possible, depending on the manifestation of the disease.

Prevention is recommended due to continuing activity of Hib in the community, and the potential for serious health effects.

* * * * * * *

9.1.5 Hepatitis A

1. The Organism

Hepatitis A is an acute viral infection of the liver caused by the hepatitis A virus (HAV). The virus survives well in the environment – it can remain on hands for several hours, and in food kept at room temperature for much longer – and is relatively resistant to heat and freezing. Water and food contaminated by sewage or faeces can carry the disease.

HAV is mainly transmitted by the faecal-oral route. Infection may come from a contaminated food item, or contaminated water, or an infected food-handler. The infecting dose is presumed to be low. In regions with poor environmental sanitation and hygiene, HAV infection is 'highly' endemic (always present in the community but with a low incidence). Infections are often asymptomatic in the early years of life. Consequently hepatitis A is an 'invisible' public health issue with few reported cases.

It is more present in low socioeconomic areas, and young children play a substantial role in the spread of the virus. Certain groups of people are regarded as being at high risk both among themselves, and as a source for transmission into to the general community. The high risk settings include: groups of homosexual men; child day-care centres and preschools; facilities for the intellectually disabled; and groups of injecting drug users.

The incubation period of hepatitis A can last up to 50 days. HAV is excreted in faeces for up to 2 weeks before the onset of symptoms and for at least one week afterwards. Hepatitis A patients should be regarded as being infectious for a week following the onset of jaundice.

The diagnosis is made by blood tests showing HAV antibodies during the acute illness, which can last for 3 to 6 months after the acute illness. Antibodies indicate past infection and therefore immunity which may last for life.

2. Clinical Symptoms

In young children HAV usually causes either an asymptomatic infection or a very mild illness without jaundice. Patients with symptomatic illness typically have a 4 to 10 day initial period of systemic symptoms (fever, malaise, weakness and loss of appetite) and gastrointestinal (nausea and vomiting) symptoms. Dark urine is usually the first specific manifestation of acute hepatitis A, followed a day or two later by jaundice and pale faeces.

The initial symptoms tend to lessen with the onset of jaundice, although the loss of appetite and weakness may persist; itching skin and liver discomfort or pain due to an enlarged liver may follow. Once the colour of the stool returns to normal, the end of the disease process can be assumed. The duration of illness varies but most patients feel better and have normal, or near normal, liver function tests within a month of the onset of illness. Complications of hepatitis A are uncommon. Hepatitis A does not usually cause chronic liver disease. However, up to 15% of cases with symptoms can last up to six months, and a similar percentage can be hospitalised.

3. Orthodox and Homoeopathic Treatment

There is no specific orthodox treatment recommended, and hospitalisation is normally avoided unless very severe symptoms manifest in a particular patient. Very careful hygiene measures are essential to prevent the spread of the disease to contacts of the patient.

Homoeopathic treatment can be aimed at the liver itself through what is termed organ "drainage". Presenting symptoms can be treated using the Law of Similars, and the patient's constitutional remedy will provide excellent support.

4. Summary

If hepatitis A is not endemic in the area, then there is no need for prevention. However, if exposure is likely, prevention is preferable to having to treat the disease.

Strict hygiene and "safe" food sources will provide protection, but if they are not possible in a possibly suspect area, then vaccination or the homoeopathic option can be considered.

* * * * * * *

9.1.6 Hepatitis B

1. The Organism

Hepatitis B virus (HBV) is present around the world, but the rate of infection varies considerably between regions, with community infection rates of up to 70% in parts of Asia and Africa (Davies et al, 2001, p.307). In Australia, community prevalence is low, except in Aboriginal groups where the prevalence is relatively high.

Transmission occurs through exposure to blood, tissue fluid, semen and cervical secretions, and saliva (in descending order of risk). People may become carriers of the disease, and although the infection does not cross the placenta, there can be a high level (80%) of infection during or just after birth due to exposure to maternal blood. These children often exhibit few or no acute symptoms, but are very likely to become carriers themselves, and have a higher risk of developing chronic liver disease and liver cancer later in life.

If sensible infection control is used, transmission rates are low. Transmission rates are very high among injecting drug users who share needles, and through unprotected sexual intercourse.

The Victorian Department of Human Services have advised that transmission of the virus occurs via contaminated blood and body fluids, and that this may occur during the following activities: sexual contact; birth; injecting drug use; some household activities such as sharing razors or toothbrushes; invasive procedures in the community such as tattooing or body-piercing, if there has been inadequate infection control; invasive medical or dental procedures if there has been inadequate infection control.

(http://www.health.vic.gov.au/ideas/bluebook/hepatitis_b.htm)

2. Clinical Symptoms

Most children who are perinatally (shortly before and after birth) exposed to hepatitis B develop no symptoms (90%), but many become carriers (90%). Weight loss, loss of appetite, dark urine, light coloured stools, diarrhoea and general lethargy are common symptoms in others in the acute form of the disease. At times a rash, persistent nausea and arthritic symptoms may occur. Jaundice (yellowish colour of skin and eyes) may or may not appear. Around 30% of older persons develop symptoms, but fewer (10%) become carriers.

In some patients severe chronic hepatitis develops. The symptoms may go unnoticed for years. Cirrhosis of the liver (inflammation of the liver associated with liver degeneration and thickening of the surrounding tissue), liver failure and liver cancer may develop in about 20% of carriers.

3. Orthodox and Homoeopathic Treatment

There is no specific orthodox treatment for acute hepatitis B infection. There is use of recombinant interferon-alpha treatment to attempt to clear chronic hepatitis. Immunisation within 24 hours of birth has a high probability of preventing infection of the infant, and Australian new-borns are now being vaccinated routinely unless parents refuse.

Hepatitis B immune globulin is used to prevent hepatitis B infection in unprotected persons who have been exposed to the virus. One dose of hepatitis B immune globulin is generally administered as soon as possible after exposure (within 24 hours after birth for newborns, within 7 days after needle-stick exposure, and within 14 days after sexual exposure), along with the first dose of the hepatitis B vaccine series, followed by the usual schedule of vaccines (Poland G A & Jacobson R M, 2004).

Homoeopathic treatment is available, and the comments relating to hepatitis A apply.

4. Summary

Hepatitis B is often a mild, asymptomatic disease, and protection is not needed unless there are specific risks. However in some individuals it can develop into liver cancer and death.

The disease is mainly acquired through unprotected sexual intercourse with an infected partner and sharing of contaminated needles, both of which can be prevented with suitable care. Infantile infection is unlikely unless the mother is infected. Healthcare workers in potentially risky areas are vulnerable to accidental infection. Prevention is desirable in these circumstances, otherwise it is not essential.

The drive to vaccinate all newborns has attracted both support and questioning within the orthodox community. It would seem to make little sense for most infants unless there was a specific risk due to their mother having the disease, or if they were born into a high risk area where potential contamination was unavoidable.

* * * * * * *

9.1.7 Hepatitis C

1. The Organism

Hepatitis C virus (HVC) is present around the world, but the rate of infection varies considerably between regions, with high community infection rates in Egypt, Japan, southern USA and some Mediterranean countries (Davies et al, 2001, p.315).

While information concerning this virus, especially in children, is still being developed, it is known that transmission occurs principally through infected blood. Sexual transmission is less common. It can also be acquired when infected drug users share straws when they inhale cocaine through the nose. Transmission rates between mother and child, and between monogamous sexual partners, are relatively low.

Many of those with the disease remain symptom free, but around 20 % develop cirrhosis after 10 years, and cancer may develop in some cases. The disease may progress to chronic hepatitis in up to 80% of patients with an acute infection (Mosby, 2002, p. 805).

2. Clinical Symptoms

The classic symptoms are weight loss, lethargy, nausea and jaundice. Abdominal pain is also common.

3. Orthodox and Homoeopathic Treatment

Interferon-alpha is sometimes used in patients with chronic hepatitis C, or combination interferon and ribavirin in serious cases. The side effects of this therapy can be significant.

Homoeopathic treatment can be undertaken in a variety of ways, including liver drainage, symptomatic prescriptions, and constitutional treatment. Naturopathic support can be helpful, especially if the patient is under orthodox treatment.

4. Summary

Avoidance of infection through a careful and “appropriate” lifestyle is the preferred option. If infection does occur, professional help must be sought.

* * * * * * *

9.1.8 Influenza

1. The Organism

Influenza is caused by a group of viruses that are generally classified as types A, B or C based on their antigenic characteristics. Influenza A and B are clinically important in human disease. The influenza A virus can be divided into subtypes based on differences in the surface antigens, whereas influenza B cannot be divided into subtypes. Transmission occurs by respiratory droplets, produced during coughing or sneezing or direct contact with an infected person.

The influenza virus is capable of continual change due to either *antigenic drift* (minor changes that happen annually or every few years), and *antigenic shift* (major changes that lead to national and international pandemics). These changes mean that there is little or no existing antibody defence to the changing strains.

Annual attack rates in the general community are typically 5 to 10%, but may be up to 20% in some years. In households and 'closed' populations such as nursing homes and boarding schools, attack rates may be 2 to 3 times higher.

In most years, minor or major epidemics of type A or type B influenza occur, usually during the winter months. During epidemics, the death rate rises, especially among the elderly and people with chronic diseases, and there are more cases with hospitalisation for pneumonia and aggravation of chronic diseases. Every 10 to 30 years, new subtypes of influenza A emerge through antigenic shift, and cause pandemics in which a quarter or more of the population may be affected over a short period.

2. Clinical Symptoms

Influenza virus causes a wide range of disease symptoms, from asymptomatic infection, to respiratory illness, to wide-ranging complications and death from primary viral or secondary bacterial pneumonia.

The severity of the disease is influenced by the following:

- the patient's age
- prior exposure to a similar influenza virus
- the virulence or strength of the viral strain
- the presence of chronic medical conditions (e.g., heart or lung disease, renal failure and diabetes)
- pregnancy
- smoking

Following a brief incubation period, there is often a sudden onset of chills with a temperature, head and body aches, a dry cough with a sore throat and weak voice. There can be a nasal discharge. The cough and weakness can linger for weeks after the initial symptoms have passed. If the fever lasts for more than 5 days it is very likely that complications will follow, especially pneumonia (viral or bacterial), acute bronchitis, croup, acute otitis media (inflammation of the middle ear), myocarditis (inflammation of the muscular walls of the heart) and pericarditis (inflammation of the sac that encloses the heart).

3. Orthodox and Homoeopathic Treatment

A new family of anti-influenza drugs reduces multiplication of the virus and can be beneficial if administered within 48 hours of onset of symptoms.

Homoeopathic treatment once again is based on symptoms. Each flu season produces a number of homoeopathic remedies that fit the most frequent symptoms presenting. For example, I found that the remedy Eupatorium Perfoliatum fitted many (but not all) of the presenting cases in the 2004 flu season in the region where I live, and has emerged again in the 2010 season in my area. This is called the *genus epidemicus* for the 2004/2010 flu. It may require a different remedy for most cases in other flu seasons. Naturopathic treatment is also available.

4. Summary

Influenza is a treatable disease, especially in reasonably healthy people, and it may be very unpleasant. Influenza may also be a very serious illness in unhealthy people, and in these cases prevention makes sense during the flu season. However, their very health weaknesses make them most susceptible to vaccine damage. The homoeopathic alternative is the ideal option in such cases.

* * * * * * *

9.1.9 Japanese encephalitis

1. The Organism

Japanese encephalitis (JE) is caused by a mosquito-borne virus. It is a significant public health problem in many parts of Asia including the Indian subcontinent, Southeast Asia and China. In recent years, however, the disease has extended beyond its traditionally recognised boundaries with, for example, an outbreak occurring in the Torres Strait, north of Australia, in 1995. To date there have been 5 cases of JE acquired in Australia.

Japanese encephalitis produces a severe infection of brain tissue. Most cases are asymptomatic. Published estimates of the ratio of symptomatic:asymptomatic infections range from 1:25 to 1:1,000. However, the disease can cause very serious symptoms, or be fatal.

2. Clinical Symptoms

The majority of patients exhibit no symptoms. In those who do, the disease begins with chilliness and "shudders". There are headaches, fever, convulsions, neck stiffness, paralysis, weight loss, a lessening of consciousness and coma. It has a high death rate and up to 50% of those who survive the acute symptoms suffer neurological complications.

3. Orthodox and Homoeopathic Treatment

Orthodox treatment is mainly supportive nursing care.

Homoeopathic treatment comprises acute remedies such as Belladonna, Opium (remember, this is in potency, there is no material quantity of opium in the remedy), and Hyoscyamus. Professional treatment is needed.

4. Summary

This is a potentially very serious disease, and if travelling to endemic areas, prevention makes sense. The alternatives for this are discussed in Section 3.6.10.

* * * * * * *

9.1.10 Measles

1. The Organism

Measles is a highly infectious, acute viral illness which is spread by respiratory droplets. It may be transmitted to others from a few days before the rash appears, to 4-5 days after the rash. There is a 10-14 day incubation period. The virus only survives outside the body for a couple of hours.

Maternal antibodies give protection against disease, but are becoming less of a factor because of fewer natural infections as a result of vaccination. In fact, measles is now becoming a disease of teenagers and adults in whom it is potentially more serious than in children.

2. Clinical Symptoms

Measles was a common, relatively benign disease in Australia prior to mass vaccination. Complications from measles are more common and more severe in chronically ill and very young children. This is particularly true in developing countries. The initial stage of measles, lasting 2 to 4 days, is characterised by fever, followed by cough, coryza (nasal discharge) and conjunctivitis (inflammation of the eye). Tiny white Koplik's spots appear on the inner surface of the mouth. The rash follows on the fourth day of the illness, typically beginning on the face and upper neck, and then becoming generalised, or joined together.

In people with chronic health problems, measles may be complicated by otitis media (inflammation of the middle ear) and bronchopneumonia (an acute inflammation of the lungs and bronchioles). Acute encephalitis (inflammation of the brain and its coverings) is said to occur in between 2 and 10 per 10,000 reported cases. Measles encephalitis occasionally causes death, and may leave the patient with permanent brain damage. Subacute sclerosing panencephalitis (SSPE) is a late complication of measles said to occur in about 1 per 100,000 cases. SSPE causes progressive brain damage and is always fatal.

It is worth noting here that orthodox medical references give apparently precise percentage rates of infection. The reliability of these rates is questionable, given that the severity of the disease varies so considerably, depending upon the initial health of the patient. A particular complication rate may be very low in healthy patients and very high in those with weakened immune systems (whether from a chronic illness, or environmental factors such as malnutrition). Very often quoted percentages are used to scare readers. They should always be read with care.

It is also interesting to note that vaccination is contraindicated in children with compromised immune systems, yet they are the ones most at risk from the disease. If such people are exposed, they are given NHIG (normal human immunoglobulin) within 7 days of exposure.

3. Orthodox and Homoeopathic Treatment

Simple nursing care is the front line treatment for measles. Antibiotics are used to treat secondary bacterial infections but are of no use to treat the viral infection. Vitamin A has been shown to reduce deaths and serious reactions to the disease, especially in malnourished children. Doctors used to give Cod Liver Oil which is rich in Vitamin A to treat measles, now parents and naturopaths use it..

Simple and effective homoeopathic treatment exists for the disease. The remedy Pulsatilla is often indicated, but other remedies may be used.

4. Summary

Measles is basically a simple disease to treat in healthy children. It is potentially more serious in adults and in immune compromised people. This is why measles can be a deadly disease in undeveloped countries where children are malnourished with very weak immune systems.

The need for immunisation, either through vaccination or homœoprophylaxis, is questionable in healthy children.

* * * * * * *

9.1.11 Meningococcal disease

1. The Organism

Meningococcal infections are caused by *Neisseria meningitidis* (*N. meningitidis* or meningococcus). There are 13 known serogroups (different sub-types of the organism). Globally, serogroups A, B, C, W135 and Y most commonly cause disease. In Australia, serogroups B and C occur most frequently. There is no consistent relationship between the different sub-types and the intensity of infection.

Serogroup A disease occurs predominantly in developing populations such as those in Africa and Asia, while serogroup B is the major cause of sporadic meningococcal disease in most developed countries. Serogroup C disease has a more cyclic pattern of occurrence, and has been increasing in incidence in the last 10 years in developed populations such as those in Australia, the United Kingdom and North America. In populations with a temperate climate, disease incidence peaks in winter and spring.

Nationally, meningococcal serogroup C disease has accounted for around 30% of all meningococcal disease (over the period 1995 to 2001), with serogroup B around 70%. The incidence of meningococcal disease in indigenous Australians is nearly 6 times that in non-indigenous Australians. However, in indigenous people, serogroup C causes 15% of disease, compared with about 30% in the non-indigenous population.

The highest rates of meningococcal disease occur in children under 5 years of age, and a second peak in incidence occurs in the 15 to 24 years age group.

Asymptomatic respiratory tract carriage of meningococci is present in about 10% of the population, and the prevalence may be higher when groups of people occupy small areas of living space. Risk factors include smoking and living in crowded conditions.

Transmission of the disease takes place through inhalation of an infected droplet from a carrier. The bacteria then gather in the naso-pharynx. After a brief incubation period of 3 or 4 days, the bacteria spread through the bloodstream to the joints, skin, lungs and central nervous system. There may be extensive and disfiguring tissue damage in some cases

Basic hygiene can help prevent meningococcal disease, for example, washing the hands before eating and after coughing and sneezing, covering the nose and mouth when coughing or sneezing, not sharing cutlery, drink containers, or any other item that may be covered with saliva.

It should be remembered that *N. meningitidis* is not the only cause of bacterial meningitis. Other causative agents are *Streptococcus pneumoniae* (causing pneumococcal disease) and *Haemophilis influenzae.*

2. Clinical Symptoms

Neisseria meningitidis can cause meningitis (inflammation of the covering of the brain and spinal cord), septicaemia (the presence of bacteria or their toxins in the blood) or both. Occasionally there may also be pneumonia, arthritis and conjunctivitis. Septicaemia, also called meningococcemia, can be particularly severe. There is a high death rate despite appropriate antibiotic therapy.

Meningitis is characterised by a sudden onset of headache and neck stiffness, plus restlessness. Nausea and vomiting is common. The patient may quickly become delirious and disorientated. High fever, sweating, aversion to light, and pains in the back and joints occur. Hydrocephalus (abnormal accumulation of cerebrospinal fluid in the head, causing enlargement and a variety of symptoms) may develop. Infants may become floppy, irritable when handled, and grunt or moan.

Septicaemia, occurs when the bacteria enters the bloodstream. There is a sudden presence of joint and muscle pain, headache, and a sore throat. Tiny red or purple spots on the skin caused by bleeding of the blood vessels within the skin (called petechiae) will develop, and the spots may enlarge and cover the whole body. The patient will collapse. The pulse and breathing rate is increased. The condition is often fatal if not treated rapidly.

3. Orthodox and Homoeopathic Treatment

Benzylpenicillin or ceftriaxone are given urgently if the disease is expected, and the patient hospitalised and emergency treatment given.

Homoeopathic treatment could be used in conjunction with orthodox treatment. The bottom line is that anyone infected with meningococcal meningitis needs to be immediately hospitalised.

4. Summary

Meningococcal disease is one of the most potentially devastating diseases considered in this book. Patients may die within 48 hours, and some survivors are horribly crippled by the disease. If there is any chance of exposure occurring, then prevention is a vastly superior option to treatment.

It would be interesting to hear the opinions of those few in natural medicine who rigidly believe we should never prevent, and only treat diseases. If any disease shows the folly of such a rigid approach, then meningococcal disease is it.

Prevention is available through vaccination against types A and C, but at the moment there is no vaccine available for type B, even though this is the type that is most prevalent in our community.

Homœoprophylaxis will offer some protection against type B, as well as types A and C.

* * * * * * *

9.1.12 Mumps

1. The Organism

Mumps is caused by a parainfluenza virus. It is rapidly inactivated by heat, the chemical formalin and ultraviolet light. Mumps is reported worldwide, and is a human disease with transmission by the airborne route or direct contact. It is primarily a disease of children, with a peak incidence in the group aged 5 to 9 years, although in communities with widespread vaccination the disease is shifting to older age groups (where typically it does more harm).

The incubation period can be from 12 to 25 days. Patients may be infectious from 6 days before parotid swelling to 9 days after. Maternal antibodies, if present, can give protection up to 12 months of age.

2. Clinical Symptoms

About 35% of infections in children are asymptomatic. About 15% of reported cases occur in adolescents and adults. Permanent long-term complications are rare.

The first signs of mumps are a fever with a headache, followed by parotid swelling (salivary glands below and behind each ear), usually on both sides of the face, but occasionally on one side only. The earlobe may be pushed upward and outward. The swellings may be painful, and there may be tiredness, appetite loss and abdominal pain. Nerve deafness is one of the most serious of the rare complications (1 in 500 hospitalised cases). Orchitis, or inflammation of the testicles (usually one sided) has been reported in up to 20% of mumps cases in older males, but subsequent sterility is rare. Inflammation of other glands and organs has been observed less frequently (pancreas, testes, liver, myocardium, thyroid). Occasional encephalitis and meningitis complications are experienced.

3. Orthodox and Homoeopathic Treatment

As with many acute viral illnesses, bed rest and sensible nursing care are front-line treatments.

Homoeopathically, Pilocarpus Jamborandi is a commonly indicated homoeopathic remedy used in the treatment of mumps.

4. Summary

Mumps is another disease which is typically mild in healthy children. It becomes more potentially serious in adulthood, although the greatest advertised fear, that of sterility in adult males, is relatively rare. A strong case can be made for allowing healthy children to acquire the disease, as this will provide the longest lasting immunity.

* * * * * * *

9.1.13 Pertussis (Whooping Cough)

1. The Organism

Pertussis (whooping cough) is a highly infectious respiratory tract infection caused by the bacterium *Bordetella pertussis*. Some other organisms (such as *Bordetella parapertussis*, *Bordetella bronchiseptica, Mycoplasma pneumoniae* and *Chlamydia pneumoniae*) can cause symptoms similar to whooping cough.

B. pertussis is spread by respiratory droplets or at times through soiled linen. It can infect 70 to 100% of susceptible household contacts and 50 to 80% of susceptible school contacts. The death rate is roughly 10 times higher in infants under 6 months of age, and lessens as the child's age increases.

Epidemics occur regularly every 3 to 4 years. Unlike some viral diseases, maternal antibodies do not protect against whooping cough which is why very young infants can be at risk. There have been a growing number of cases in teenagers and adults, and these people are often the ones who pass the disease on to infants.

2. Clinical Symptoms

Whooping cough typically last for about 6 weeks, and can be divided into 3 stages, each stage lasting about 2 weeks.

(1) There is a hacking, irritating night-time cough with a low-grade fever. The patient is weak, with little appetite and sometimes infected eyes.

(2) The cough develops into recurring, spasmodic bouts that expel sticky, adhesive mucus. This is when the typical "whoop" may occur (although not in every case), during the in-breath following the cough. The tenacious mucus can cause choking and vomiting. The face typically changes colour to blur or red. This is the stage where viral or bacterial complications may occur, especially pneumonia.

(3) The final stage sees all symptoms lessen, although sudden attacks of coughing can occur for months.

3. Orthodox and Homoeopathic Treatment

Hospitalisation is required in severe cases, especially to ensure that breathing does not stop. Antibiotic treatment will not stop the illness, but will prevent transmission to others. Otherwise, careful nursing, rest, and adequate fluids are helpful.

Homoeopathy can greatly reduce the severity of the disease if an exact remedy match is found. There are many possibly useful remedies, and the best choice should be made by an experienced professional to ensure an appropriate match of symptoms. It is also useful when a patient has never been well since whooping cough.

4. Summary

Prevention of whooping cough definitely makes sense for infants. The disease is most dangerous for the very young, and the vaccine is potentially most dangerous at a very young age. This is a perfect example of the value of homœoprophylaxis which can offer significant protection for tiny infants without any risk of toxic damage.

* * * * * * *

9.1.14 Pneumococcal disease

1. The Organism

Pneumococcal diseases is caused by the bacterium *Streptococcus pneumoniae*, also known as *pneumococcus*. To date 90 different antigenic sub-types have been recognised, each producing type-specific immunity. Many people carry some of these sub-types in the upper respiratory tract with any symptoms. Some sub-types, and some are more frequently associated with invasive pneumococcal disease (IPD), which is recognised when *S. pneumoniae* is isolated from a normally sterile site, most commonly blood.

S. pneumoniae is the leading cause of meningitis in children under 5 years of age, with children under one year of age being at the highest risk of pneumococcal meningitis. There is a very high death for pneumococcal meningitis ranges for both children and especially the older patients.

Patients who cannot mount an adequate immune response to different pneumococcal antigens have the highest risk of IPD, including those with heart disease, diabetics, alcoholics, and smokers. A history of recurring ear infections and commencing child-care, point towards a greater risk of IPD in children.

2. Clinical Symptoms

The major clinical symptoms of IPD include pneumonia (acute infection or inflammation of the lung), meningitis (inflammation of the membranes that cover the brain and spinal cord) and bacteraemia (the presence of bacteria in the blood). In adults, pneumococcal pneumonia is the most common clinical presentation of IPD, while in children bacteraemia accounts for more than two-thirds of cases.

Pneumococcal pneumonia often begins with a sudden onset high temperature, accompanied by shaking and chills. There is a painful cough with blood tinged sputum. Weakness and prostration are common. There may be some gastrointestinal problems such as nausea and loss of appetite.

Non-invasive pneumococcal disease includes otitis media (inflammation of the inner ear) and (non-bacteraemic) pneumonia. Diagnosis for these conditions is difficult, because other organisms can cause very similar symptoms.

3. Orthodox and Homoeopathic Treatment

The emergence of antibiotic-resistant strains of this organism has become an increasing challenge for the management of invasive pneumococcal disease. Recent reports in Australia indicate that up to 21% of strains are resistant to 2 or more classes of antibiotics.

Benzyl penicillin (for at least 10 days in meningitis) is usually used during severe childhood infections in high risk groups. Intravenous penicillin or oral amoxicillin are usually used for lobar pneumonia in childhood, and is often used before the actual infection is formally identified.

Homoeopathic treatment once again is symptomatic, and as with meningococcal disease, takes second place to hospitalisation.

4. Summary

Pneumococcal disease is potentially very serious. Even though it is not highly infectious, it is present in the Australian and other communities, and prevention is worth considering, especially if the child is likely be frequently exposed to others (such as with regular child care etc). It is worth noting that it claims more lives in Australia than meningococcal disease, even though the latter claims more public attention.

* * * * * * *

9.1.15 Poliomyelitis

1. The Organism

Poliovirus is an enterovirus (infects the gastrointestinal tract (GIT) and is eliminated in the faeces). There are 3 types of poliovirus; P1, P2 and P3. The virus enters through the mouth, multiplies in the pharynx and GIT and can be passed on in the faeces for 2-6 weeks. This transmission is also possible with the viral material in the vaccine. The virus may then spread to the lymph system, the circulatory system, and finally to the central nervous system causing the paralysis so associated with polio.

Poliomyelitis still occurs in developing countries, particularly in the Indian subcontinent, the Eastern Mediterranean and Africa. The virus can incubate for up to 21 days. The patient is most infectious from 10 days before to10 days after the appearance of symptoms. The virus is spread from faeces to the mouth, usually via unwashed hands.

2. Clinical Symptoms

It is commonly believed that anyone who contracts polio either becomes partially paralysed or dies. The reality is rather different. In fact, most people who are infected with poliovirus present with no apparent symptoms.

Nelson's Textbook of Paediatrics (a standard text) states: "when a susceptible person has had effective contact with polio virus, one of the following responses may occur in order of frequency: (i) asymptomatic infection, (ii) abortive poliomyelitis, (iii) non-paralytic poliomyelitis, (iv) paralytic poliomyelitis" (Vaughan VC, McKay RJ, Behrman RE, Nelson W E, 1979, p.926). Of these four, only the last response involves long term damage.

The NH&MRC suggest that paralysis develops in about 1 in 1,000 children, and 1 in 75 in adults with the disease (NH&MRC, 2003, p. 235).

Volk and Wheeler state that: "In most infections caused by poliomyelitis virus there are no distinctive symptoms . . . undoubtedly the vast majority of such cases are not diagnosed" (Volk W A, Wheeler M F, 1980, p.455).

Dr R Moskowitz suggested that the polio virus was ubiquitous before the vaccine was introduced: "the wild-type poliovirus produces no symptoms whatsoever in over 90% of contactees even under epidemic conditions and, of those who exhibit recognizable clinical symptoms, perhaps only 1 or 2% ever progress to the full blown neurological picture of poliomyelitis with its characteristic lesions in the anterior horn cells of the spinal cord or medulla oblongata"(Moskowitz R, 1985). Dr Moskowitz cites standard references (Burnett M & White D 1976, p. 91; Davis B et al, 1979, pp. 1280, 1290) and others to support his argument.

He concluded that polio requires peculiar conditions of susceptibility in the host, even a specific anatomical susceptibility, and that this is why people with such susceptibility develop paralytic polio from the vaccine (Moskowitz R, 1985, pp. 152, 153).

This view was further supported by studies showing that immune-deficient children were considered prone to paralytic poliomyelitis following oral poliomyelitis vaccine (reported in the British Medical Journal, Vol III, 1975, p. 158).

This idea, however, is not new. In 1936, Dr T M Rivers wrote: "for unknown reasons, most children are much more resistant to Poliomyelitis than are the remaining few". Dr F Klenner concluded that: "this small remaining few is no doubt the ones Salk reported would not or could not make antibodies. Thus it sums up itself so simply. The majority do not need it (the vaccine), and the minority cannot use it if they get it" (Klenner F R, 1955, p. 4).

Further, if you are breastfeeding your child close to the time when the vaccine is administered, it will not work (Strond CE, 1969, p. 438).

Finally, in July 1954, the Department of Health for Scotland (under the UK Ministry of Health) issued a Medical Memorandum on Poliomyelitis, which stated that: "a feature of infection with poliomyelitis virus is the variable degree of the disturbance which it may produce. … Evidence suggests that comparatively few infections go on to develop paralysis . ... Even of the recognisable cases of poliomyelitis, only a small proportion become severely paralysed. Associates of cases of poliomyelitis are frequently infected without showing any clinical evidence of this process . . . yet others infected go on to develop minor illnesses characterised by one or more of the following symptoms: fever, headache, sore throat, listlessness, anorexia, vomiting, constipation, and muscle and abdominal pain. These illnesses usually last for only 24 to 48 hours and are commoner in children than adults. Laboratory studies indicate that for every person with symptoms there may be 10 to 100 infected individuals with no obvious illness and epidemiological evidence suggests that under some circumstances the proportion may be even higher" (Ministry of Health UK, 1954).

As medical studies show, poliomyelitis is normally a mild disease, which occasionally leads to serious complications. Even in serious cases, however, effective treatment is available. This does not in any way diminish the tragedy of suffering that advanced cases of polio can and have caused to thousands of people over time. It highlights the basic problem associated with the entire topic of infectious diseases:

- one never knows in advance if a person will be exposed to a disease
- one never knows in advance whether infection will follow exposure
- one never knows in advance how severe any infection may be
- one never knows in advance how well an infected patient will recover

This is why long-term prevention of potentially serious diseases makes sense for many parents – why take a risk when a non-toxic preventative is available (homœoprophylaxis).

3. Orthodox and Homoeopathic Treatment

An effective means of treating polio (successful in stopping paralysis) was described in 1956 by US physician Dr F Klenner who worked with patients in the polio epidemic at that time. In summary, he suggested the following:

(a) The case must be acute. If paralysis is present, immediate continuous, gentle massage is required.

(b) Give ascorbic acid (vitamin C) intravenously (300-500 mg per kilogram of body weight, diluted with 5D water or saline). Juice or water should be given before and after the injection.

(c) Penicillin or Sulfadiazine should be administered for two days to patients where secondary infection presents a problem.

(d) DCA should also be given daily for three days, concurrently with the days of ascorbic acid therapy.

(e) In certain young patients showing paralysis, Thiamine HCl must be given following the ascorbic acid treatment.

(f) The patient must be made to eat (Klenner F R, 1956).

Obviously the help of a suitable doctor should be sought for this type of treatment; Orthomolecular physicians would be among those competent to provide such assistance.

It is worth mentioning here that homoeopathic treatment for polio has been available for many years, and a number of remedies are frequently cited:

- Drs Kichlu and Bose mention the remedies Aconite, Alumina, Conium, Dulcamarra, Nux Vomica, Rhus Tox, Arnica, Argentum Nitricum, Oxalic Acid, Lathyrus Sativus, Kali Iodatum, Merc. Corrosive, Cuprum Metallicum, Picric Acid, Thalium Anaholinum, and Kali Tartaricum (Kichulu KL & Bose LRN, 1979, pp. 833-835).
- The list presented by Dr Clarke included the remedies shown above, with the addition of Gelsemium, Secale, and Hypericum tincture externally (Clarke JH, 1984, p. 261).
- Dr Ruddock listed Aconite, Belladonna, Gelsemium, Calc. Carb., Nux Vomica, Phosphorous, Rhus Tox, and Lathyrus Sativus (Ruddock EH, 1986, pp. 125-127).

Common to each of these lists are the remedies Rhus Tox and Lathyrus Sativus. In Section 3.2, Lathyrus Sativus is shown to be one of the most effective prophylactics against polio (vaccines included). Note: Treatment should only be undertaken with the assistance of an experienced homoeopathic practitioner.

4. Summary

Polio is a potentially serious disease, even though it is only the relatively few cases that develop the most severe symptoms. Because of the memories of the polio epidemics in the mid 1950's, it is a disease against which many parents seek protection. It is a reasonable position for any parent to take.

* * * * * * *

9.1.16 Rubella

1. The Organism

Rubella is generally a very mild infectious viral disease. The virus is relatively unstable, and is inactivated by extremes of heat and pH, amantadine and UV light. Rubella occurs worldwide and is spread from person to person by airborne transmission of respiratory droplets.

The incubation period is from 2 to 3 weeks, and the patient is contagious from one week before until 4 days after the onset of the rash.

2. Clinical Symptoms

Many cases of rubella are asymptomatic, i.e., the presence of infection is unknown because there are no clear symptoms. Rubella causes a fever, a brief erythematous (congestive redness) rash, swelling of the lymph nodes behind the ears and the back of the neck and, occasionally, joint and muscle pains. Very occasionally neurological and blood disorders may occur. The symptoms are usually brief and can be caused by other viruses, making rubella difficult to diagnose. The rash also does not confirm rubella infection.

The main concern with rubella relates to the infection of pregnant women, and the effect that this may have on the foetus. The NH&MRC make an important statement concerning rubella infection in pregnancy which is worth reading if you have a particular interest in this disease (NH&MRC, 2003, pp. 251-253).

3. Orthodox and Homoeopathic Treatment

Rest and sensible nursing care is generally all that is required to treat rubella. Homoeopathically, remedies such as Pulsatilla and Rhus Tox, as well as the Tissue Salts Ferrum Phos 6x and Kali Mur 6x are frequently indicated.

4. Summary

This is a very mild disease in healthy children. Infection in childhood should give the most certain future protection. If there were no implications of the disease for pregnant women, then rubella vaccination would be considered as unnecessary by many in orthodox medicine. A strategy of allowing the child to acquire the disease, and protect pregnant women with the rubella Nosode if necessary (the remedy is safe during pregnancy), would appear to make most sense.

* * * * * * *

9.1.17 Tetanus

1. The Organism

Tetanus, also called lockjaw, is caused by *Clostridium tetani*, a bacterial organism. Normally transmission is through a puncture wound that is contaminated by dirt or animal (especially dog and horse) excreta containing the organism, or sometimes via burns where the integrity of the skin is destroyed. People who have body piercing, tattoos and injecting drug users occasionally contract tetanus.

The organism can grow without oxygen. *C. tetani* produces a potent toxin which has two components, tetanospasmin (a neurotoxin) and tetanolysin (a haemolysin – a substance that destroys red blood cells). The incubation period varies from 2 days in severe cases to 10 days or more in less severe cases.

2. Clinical Symptoms

If the infection is localised, then spasms and increased muscle tone will be felt near the wound. If the infection spreads throughout the entire body then muscle rigidity, deep tendon contractions and spasms, a low-grade fever with sweating, and involuntary muscle contractions will occur. These latter may occur in the neck and facial muscles giving the grinning "lockjaw" symptom from which the common name is derived. The patient may also arch backward, and convulsions may lead to death from asphyxiation (cannot breath), or heart failure. Other complications may occur.

Tetanus in newborns in the first few weeks of life can result from the unsterile treatment of the umbilical cord stump. It may be indicated by loss of appetite, rigidity, and spasms.

3. Orthodox and Homoeopathic Treatment

Effective wound hygiene is the most effective way to prevent tetanus. However, this is not always possible, for example, with deep puncture wounds that cannot be cleaned. A tetanus booster may be given in such cases. Human tetanus immune globulin is given if the wound is tetanus prone and the patient has not been vaccinated against tetanus.

There appears to be widespread agreement in the medical literature that wound hygiene is of greatest importance in the prevention of tetanus, as shown in the following examples.

(i) Dr H K Bournes wrote, "Thorough wound toilet is the only treatment for a wound, and when it is carried out correctly, antibiotics are not necessary unless either the circumstances under which the wound was obtained or the general condition of the patient make the development of infection either likely or unlikely. Thorough wound toilet makes the use of either tetanus anti-toxin or prophylactic antibiotics undesirable" (Bourns H K, 1964).

(ii) While expressing support for vaccination, Drs Smith, Laurence, and Evans stated that, "Surgical toilet is of prime importance for all wounds and is usually sufficient for tetanus prophylaxis in patients with wounds that are less than six hours old, clean, non-penetrating, and with negligible tissue damage" (Smith J W G et al, 1975)

(iii) Drs Crosslight and Howard, who supported compulsory vaccination despite their own findings, wrote that, "The decline of tetanus as a disease began before the introduction of tetanus toxoid to the general population. This was due in time to accompanying changes in hygiene and sanitation, improved nutritional status, the use of antibiotics and antiseptics, tetanus anti-toxin, wound care and changes in living conditions from a rural to an urban situation for most Australians . . . Avoidance of overimmunization with its possible side effects must also be kept in mind" (Crosslight G M & Howard B, 1978)

It is even acknowledged that the mere presence of the tetanus organism in the body does not automatically place the individual at risk of developing tetanus; for example, "The isolation of C. Tetani from a wound does not necessarily imply that tetanus will develop" (Impulse, 17 April 1978).

Medical literature also suggests that ascorbic acid can play a significant role in the conventional treatment of tetanus. Drs Jahan, Ahmad, and Ali studied two groups of patients with tetanus, one group receiving conventional treatment only and the other group also receiving (intravenously) daily doses of 1000mg of ascorbic acid. Their findings are summarised in Table 1-2 (Jahan K et.al., 1984).

The use of ascorbic acid in the treatment of tetanus was described in detail in 1954 by Dr F Klenner, who used Vitamin C and tolserol with great effectiveness. His essay on the subject began with the statement: The purpose of this paper is to dispel the popular belief that Tetanus is a difficult disease to cure" (Klenner F, 1954).

Table 9-1 Studies on the Effect of Daily Administration of (I.V.) 1000mg of Ascorbic Acid as Supplement to Conventional Treatment on the Recovery of Tetanus Patients

Age Group (years)	**Patients Receiving Ascorbic Acid**			**Patients Not Receiving Ascorbic Acid**		
	Total patients	No. who recovered	% not recovered	Total patients	No. who recovered	% not recovered
1 - 12	31	31	0%	31	8	72.2%
13 - 30	27	17	37%	28	9	67.8%

4. Summary

Tetanus is a potentially serious disease, which is usually easily prevented by effective wound hygiene. There is good reason to treat potentially serious wounds. Effective orthodox treatment is available, as is proven homoeopathic treatment. This gives people the option of not taking preventative options prior to a wound, but only treating if there is a wound.

Clearly, efficient wound hygiene is normally all that is needed to prevent tetanus. When coupled with the ability to successfully treat tetanus (if at all necessary following proper wound cleansing), then the need for the vaccine is questionable. Prior protection (using the Nosode) as well as treatment (using Ledum 30 and/or Hypericum 30) can also be undertaken using homoeopathic remedies if desired (refer Section 4.2.1).

* * * * * * *

9.1.18 Tuberculosis

1. The Organism

Tuberculosis (TB) is caused by *Mycobacterium tuberculosis* complex (M.TB complex). M.TB complex consists of *Mycobacterium tuberculosis*, *M. bovis* and *M. africanum*. *M. tuberculosis* is the cause of TB in Australia, whereas *M. bovis* and *M. africanum* are rare. The organism can settle in the lungs and may cause an acute or chronic illness.

About 1,000 cases of TB are notified to Australian health authorities each year, with the lowest reported 923 cases in 1998. In Australia, most TB (70 to 80%) occurs in migrants, particularly from Asia, Southern and Eastern European countries and the Pacific Islands. Rates of TB are also high in Indigenous people in some parts of Australia. Immunocompromised patients are at high risk of developing active TB if they are infected with *M. tuberculosis*.

2. Clinical Symptoms

After a long incubation period of up to 2 months, most patients remain asymptomatic. However non-specific symptoms may appear, such as loss of appetite and weight loss, weakness and debility, night sweats and a low-grade fever. If the disease is reactivated, it may cause, in addition to these symptoms, haemoptysis (coughing and spitting of blood from any part of the respiratory tract) with infected sputum and chest pains. The severity of the illness depends on the overall state of the immune system, which is why malnourished people, the elderly, alcoholics, and people on immuno-suppresive drugs are most at risk

3. Orthodox and Homoeopathic Treatment

Isolation, rest, and extensive long-term drug therapy is used in orthodox medicine to treat this potentially serious disease. Cases of drug-resistant TB may require special medication.

Homoeopathic treatment has been used extensively, but selection of remedies by an experienced professional is required.

4. Summary

Once again, prevention is much preferred to treatment of this potentially serious chronic disease.

* * * * * * *

9.1.19 Typhoid

1. The Organism

Typhoid fever is caused by the Gram-negative bacillus *Salmonella typhi*. Typhoid is usually spread through food or drink contaminated by faeces or urine from a person with the disease. It passes from the faeces of an infected person, usually via the hands to the mouth. Raw vegetables, salads, shellfish, water or ice, and milk may carry the organism. The bacterium is destroyed by boiling water, cooking food. Sensible personal hygiene can provide effective protection.

There are less than 100 cases of typhoid reported in Australia each year and, most occur in people who have recently travelled to countries in South America, Asia, Africa, and some parts of Southern Europe. A few cases are transmitted by local people with a long-term infection who pass the disease on in food they have prepared.

2. Clinical Symptoms

Symptoms can range from none, to severe enteric fever with progressive spread of intestinal perforation. Enteric (relating to the gastrointestinal tract) fever is characterised by slow onset of a sustained fever, weakness, headache, constipation and loss of appetite.

There also can be bradycardia (abnormal slowness of the heart rate and pulse), splenomegaly (enlargement of the spleen), 'rose spots' and abdominal symptoms of pain, constipation or diarrhoea. If the infection is untreated it can kill up to 20% of sufferers due to bowel perforation, haemorrhage, toxaemia (the presence of body cells or bacteria in the blood) and effects on other organs.

3. Orthodox and Homoeopathic Treatment

Treatment with antibiotics is usually used for invasive infections, but there is an increasing concern regarding the growing resistance to commonly used antibiotics.

Symptomatic treatment using homoeopathic medicines has been used since the 1800's.

4. Summary

The severity of this disease can vary widely. The first line of defence is sensible hygiene and heating food and drinks. The conventional vaccines are not reliable, and thus homoeopathic prevention makes sense if travelling into areas where typhoid or paratyphoid diseases are active.

* * * * * * *

9.1.20 7th Edition Additions

9.1.21 Dengue Fever

1. The Organism

Dengue fever is caused by a virus carried by mosquitos. There are 4 types, and infection with one type does not make the person immune to the other types.

2. Clinical Symptoms

Dengue Fever presents great problems with diagnosis. There may be no obvious symptoms arising from an infection in many young children, then mild to severe fevers, or even fatal conditions such as dengue haemorrhagic fever or dengue shock syndrome.

Commons symptoms include: sudden onset of fever (lasting three to seven days); intense headache (especially behind the eyes); muscle and joint pain (ankles, knees and elbows); unpleasant metallic taste in mouth, loss of appetite, vomiting, diarrhoea, abdominal pain; flushed skin on face and neck, fine skin rash as fever subsides; rash on arms and legs, severe itching, peeling of skin and hair loss; minor bleeding (nose or gums) and heavy menstrual periods; extreme fatigue.

Clinicians in active areas often note that symptoms may be confused with other conditions with similar symptoms.

3. Orthodox and Homoeopathic Treatment

Nursing care with fluid management and pain relief is often the only mainstream treatment possible. The Cuban physicians have developed interesting and effective protocols, which include the use of indicated homoeopathic remedies.

4. Summary

Dengue fever is the next great scourge of the planet according to WHO. Homoeopathy has much to offer if used appropriately.

* * * * * * *

9.1.22 Human Papiloma Virus

1. The Organism

Human papillomavirus (HPV) is the most common sexually transmitted disease (some estimates suggest that 50% of sexually active people will get the virus some time in their lives). There are more than 100 HPV types that can infect the genital areas of males and females. These HPV types can also infect the mouth and throat. Most people who become infected with HPV do not even know they have it, and the virus is naturally cleared from the system within a couple of years in around 90% of infected people.

2. Clinical Symptoms

Because there are so many variants of HPV, there can be a wide range of presenting symptoms. Certain types of HPV can cause genital warts in males and females, and very occasionally warts in the throat. Other HPV types can cause cervical cancer. These types can also cause other, less common but serious cancers, including cancers of the vulva, vagina, penis, anus, tongue, tonsils and throat.

The types of HPV that can cause genital warts are not the same as the types that can cause cancer. There is no way to know which people who get HPV will go on to develop cancer or other health problems. In general, cancer will only occur when the infection persists for more than 2 years.

It is suggested that HPV types 16 and 18 that cause 70% of cervical cancer, but this is suggestive only. Types 31, 33, 35, 39, 45, 51, 52, 56, 58, and 59 are deemed as being high-risk types.

3. Orthodox and Homoeopathic Treatment

Orthodox treatment tends to revolve around physical removal of warts, and the general treatment protocols for cancer (surgery, radiotherapy and chemotherapy) depending on the individual case.

Homeopathic treatment will focus on anti-miasmatic treatment, taking into account the presenting symptoms, as well as the use of appropriate Nosodes.

4. Summary

HPV lends itself to creating fear in the general population, and indeed concern is warranted. Lifestyle choices will not ensure complete protection, but will minimise the chance of being infected, and maximise the chance of the disease naturally clearing from the system. However people who are at risk will of course consider the vaccines on offer, which will be discussed in the next Section and, as will be seen, there are no easy answers.

* * * * * * *

9.1.23 Leptospirosis

1. The Organism

The disease is caused by infection with strains of Gram negative bacterium *Leptospira* spp. It is a water-born zoonotic disease (carried by animals) and is potentially severe in developing countries and the tropics. Human infection usually occurs through contact with the urine of infected animals.

2. Clinical Symptoms

The symptoms are varied, and may be easily confused with other conditions, making diagnosis difficult. They include meningitis, pneumonitis, hepatitis, nepthritis, mastitis, myocarditis, haemorrhagic crisis, and multi organ failure.

3. Orthodox and Homoeopathic Treatment

Orthodox treatment centres on antibiotic use and appropriate nursing care. Homeopathic treatment would be entirely dependent on presenting symptoms, plus appropriate nursing care.

4. Summary

Leptospirosis is a potentially severe and at times fatal disease. Prevention is without doubt better than cure. Physical measures to reduce the spread of water born infections are crucial, including rodent control.

The vaccination and chemoprophylaxis options are compared with homoeoprophylaxis in the next Appendix. However the new material on HP in Cuba in large part describes the campaign against leptospirosis in that country.

* * * * * * *

9.1.24 Rotavirus

1. The Organism

Rotavirus is a double stranded RNA virus. It is extremely common, and most children have been infected at least once with the virus by the age of 5 years. Immunity builds with each infection, and most adults become immune to subsequent infections. There are 5strains of the virus – A, B, C, D and E, of which A is the most common being estimated to cause around 90% of all infections. Transmission is usually via the faecal-oral route. There is an incubation period of 2 days. The virus is stable in the environment, and is difficult to control being present in both affluent and poor countries.

2. Clinical Symptoms

Rotavirus is the most common cause of childhood diarrhoea, and can lead to severe and occasionally fatal gastroenteritis. Symptoms include vomiting, watery diarrhoea and mild fever with abdominal cramps.

3. Orthodox and Homoeopathic Treatment

Orthodox treatment centres around the prevention of severe dehydration in children, and appropriate nursing care. Drips are often used in severe cases. There are typically few associated problems, and well managed cases typically improve.

Homeopathic treatment is possible, and a well conducted trial of treatment was conducted in Nicaragua in 1993 (Jacobs, 1994).

4. Summary

If a child is generally healthy, and if any gastrointentinal symptoms and dehydration are well managed, then the prognosis is excellent. It is a disease which almost everyone reading this book will have had, and will have recovered from without long-term consequences. A number of vaccines are available, and is a homeopathic option.

* * * * * * *

9.1.25 Swine Flu

1. The Organism

Swine flu has generally been considered to be the H1N1 influenza strain which can infect both pigs and humans. However other type A subtypes can be involved, including H1N2, H2N3, H3N1and H3N2. The H1N1 form of swine flu is one of the descendants of the strain that caused the 1918 flu pandemic.

In late April 2009, Margaret Chan, the World Health Organization's director-general, declared a "public health emergency of international concern" under the rules of the WHO's new International Health Regulations when the first two cases of the H1N1 virus were reported in the United States, followed by hundreds of cases in Mexico. The pandemic did not eventuate. A review of the global response to the 2009 H1N1 pandemic was launched on 12th April, 2010.

2. Clinical Symptoms

Symptoms are very similar to those of influenza and of influenza-like illness in general, namely fever, chills, sore throat, muscle pains and severe headaches, coughing, weakness and general malaise.

3. Orthodox and Homoeopathic Treatment

Orthodox and homoeopathic treatment are the same for swine flu as for general seasonal influenza. Each year people die from the flu. Swine flu appears to be no more severe than typical seasonal flu and some have suggested that it is in fact less severe (Belongia EA et.al., 2010).

4. Summary

Readers will know of the of the 2009 pandemic declared by the WHO. The associated fear campaign created billions in sales for the vaccine manufacturers. The WHO response is now being investigated internationally and there is little doubt that examples of inappropriate behaviour and financial dealings will be revealed in high places before the incident is laid to rest.

* * * * * * *

9.2 Appendix to Question 3: The Safety and Effectiveness of Vaccines

NOTE: The ingredients of the current vaccines are outlined in the NH&MRC (2008) *Australian Immunisation Handbook* 9th Edition. (http://www.health.gov.au/internet/immunise/publishing.nsf/Content/Handbook-vaccinesbydisease). September 2010 website entries.

NOTE: The vaccines discussed below contain a range of antigenic (diseased) material, plus the following metals, biological, chemicals and compounds: formaldehyde; aluminium hydroxide; phenoxyethanol; neomycin; aluminium phosphate/hydroxide; yeast proteins; egg protein; borax; aluminium; bovine serum albumin; human serum albumin; thiomersal; kanamycin; gentamicin; polymyxin; gelatin; monosodium glutamate; mouse brain serum protein; lactose; amino acids; sorbitol; mannitol; phenol; streptomycin; anhydrous sodium carbonate; sodium bicarbonate; anhydrous citric acid; sodium citrate; saccharin sodium; raspberry flavour; sodium chloride; sodium phosphate – monobasic; sodium phosphate – dibasic anhydrous; potassium chloride; potassium phosphate - monobasic; calcium chloride; sucrose; sodium taurodeoxycholate; urea; polyalcohols; human diploid cells.

These materials can be researched on the web. They range from the benign Amino acids) to the toxic (aluminium) to the disgusting (mouse brains).

9.2.1 Chicken Pox (Varicella) vaccination

9.2.1.1 The current vaccines

Vaccines against Chicken Pox are relatively new. Two vaccines are currently available in Australia. They are:

Varilix (GSK) – live attenuated Oka strain of the varicella-zoster virus propagated in human diploid cells. Also contains human serum albumin; lactose; neomycin; polyalcohols. No preservative is used.

Varivax (refrigerated) (CSL/MSD) – live attenuated Oka/Merck strain of the varicella-zoster virus. Also contains sucrose; gelatin; urea; monosodium glutamate; residual components of MRC-5 cells; trace amounts of neomycin and fetal bovine serum from MRC-5 culture media. No preservative is used.

Current recommendations are that children up to 14 years receive one dose, and adolescents receive 2 doses. These recommendations are being reviewed. The vaccine is also recommended to be given within 3 to 5 days following exposure.

The efficacy within household outbreaks is estimated at 70-90%. A recent outbreak in a day care centre revealed that "The effectiveness of the vaccine was 44.0 percent against disease of any severity and 86.0 percent against moderate or severe disease. Children who had been vaccinated three years or more before the outbreak were at greater risk for vaccine failure than those who had been vaccinated more recently" (Galil K et al, 2002, p. 1909).

The study by Galil and colleagues stirred up some controversy in the New England Journal of Medicine. This lead to the following revealing comment: "The report by Galil et al. raises a more important issue: reversal of the decision to mandate universal varicella vaccination. The logic behind the initial varicella immunization recommendation was based largely on the assumption of substantial economic benefits from "social cost" savings. All the analyses cited to substantiate this claim assumed only one vaccination, and none found any economic benefit from direct medical cost savings. As Gershon acknowledges, more than one dose is almost certainly required to ensure a reasonable level of immunity. Therefore, the economic arguments for universal immunization must also be revisited and probably discarded. … Let us acknowledge the shaky assumptions underpinning the original decision on immunization and consider a more justifiable policy of voluntary immunization for children and mandatory immunization for non-immune teenagers and adults" (Wack RP, 2003, p. 1405).

The need for more than one dose to ensure the effectiveness of the vaccine was reinforced by Chaves and others where people vaccinated 9 years previously had a 36 greater chance of infection compared to children vaccinated within one year (Chaves SS et.al., 2007).

Adverse events reported in the orthodox literature include:

- Fever up to 39°C in 15% of healthy children. Interestingly a similar percentage was observed in children receiving placebo, suggesting the fever is caused by the other ingredients in the vaccine, and not the viral material.
- Injection site reactions in 7-30% of injected children. These include pain, redness and swelling.
- Rash either around the injection site or generalised in 3-5% of vaccinated children from 5 to 42 days following vaccination.
- Serious adverse events (including encephalitis, seizures and death) were reported in 2.9 per 100,000 distributed doses. (Davies E G, et al. 2001; NH&MRC, 2008, pp. 318).

9.2.1.2 Comment

One real concern relates to the possibility of the vaccine implanting the varicella zoster virus in the cells of the nervous system in the same way that the natural disease sometimes does. This may cause shingles later in life, and who really knows what else?

We don't really know the long-term health consequences of the widespread use of the chicken pox vaccine. We do know there are short-term health consequences. We know that the live virus can persist for life in infected patients. We know that the disease is mild in all except immune compromised children. The question clearly becomes – is this questionably effective vaccine worth the obvious risk?

For those who believe that it is not, but who still wish to protect against chicken pox, then homoeopathic protection may be used.

* * * * * *

9.2.2 Cholera vaccination

9.2.2.1 The current vaccines

One vaccine is currently available in Australia.

Orochol (CSL) – live recombinant oral vaccine. Also contains anhydrous sodium carbonate, sodium bicarbonate, anhydrous citric acid, sodium citrate, saccharin sodium and raspberry flavour.

The effectiveness of the vaccine is not established in randomised trials (in one trial reported protection was not demonstrated). The vaccine is not officially required, or recommended by the NH&MRC.

Being a live, oral vaccine, people who come into contact with a recently vaccinated individual are potentially at risk as the organism is excreted.

9.2.2.2 Comment

If protection against Cholera is required, the homoeopathic alternative has been well tested, is safe and certainly offers a level of protection which would appear to exceed that of the vaccine, based on the orthodox community's own reports.

* * * * * *

9.2.3 Diphtheria vaccination

9.2.3.1 The current vaccines

In September 2010, the Handbook lists 8 different formulations of diphtheria vaccine are available in Australia, including the combination vaccines CDT, dT (ADT), DTPa or adult/adolescent formulation dTpa. The current vaccines are: **Infanrix hexa; Infanrix IPV; Infanrix Penta; ADT Booster; Adacel; Adacel Polio; Boostrix; Boostrix IPV**.

As well as a variety of antigenic material, including Diphtheria toxins, the vaccines included a variety of streptomycin; phenoxyethanol; aluminium hydroxide/phosphate; formaldehyde; polymyxin and neomycin and yeast proteins.

The purpose of the diphtheria vaccine is to stimulate the production of antitoxin, which then is meant to protect against the toxin. Boosters are recommended at mid-teens and at 50 years. It is part of the recommended vaccination schedule, and is recommended for travellers to certain countries in Asia and Eastern Europe.

Adverse events reported in the literature:

- Extensive limb swelling in 2% of children given later booster doses.
- Typical general reactions which are probably due to other ingredients in the combined vaccines (see whooping cough in Section 3.6.13).

9.2.3.2 Comment

Diphtheria, which was a common and fatal disease at the turn of the century, is now virtually nonexistent in countries with adequate sanitation and nursing facilities. It is treatable both homoeopathically and pharmaceutically, but it is still a potentially serious disease where active. It is still a disease to be considered if travelling to or living in an area where outbreaks are common.

The disease was clearly declining prior to the introduction of routine vaccination, which had practically no impact on the rate of decline. It is unlikely that an unvaccinated child in Australia would ever be exposed to an active diphtheria carrier unless a recently returned traveller.

Should an outbreak occur, homoeopathic protection against diphtheria has been scientifically tested for efficacy by French Homoeopath, Dr Paul Chavanon. In using two doses of Diphtherotoxinum 4M, six to eight weeks apart, in 45 persons with positive Schick tests (proving they had no antibodies against diphtheria beforehand), Dr Chavanon found that, in all 45 cases, the Schick test became negative thus indicating immunity (AIH, 1988, p.25). Statistically, this is a significant result. It also clearly demonstrates that highly potentised substances can cause physiological changes in patients.

Neustaedter has spent some pages attempting to discredit the Chavanon findings by pointing out potential problems associated with the Shick test itself causing a negative result (Neustaedter R, 2002, pp. 100-102).

What he showed is that Chavanon's findings may be incorrect. He has not proved that they were. What is even more remarkable is that Neustaedter repeated claims that "no long-term studies have been conducted to evaluate" homœoprophylaxis. The many editions of this book provide clear evidence that Neustaedter is incorrect.

Those who do wish to use protection against diphtheria do have a choice.

* * * * * * *

9.2.4 Haemophilis influenzae type b (Hib) vaccination

9.2.4.1 A brief history of the Hib vaccines

The first Hib vaccine was released in the U.S. in 1985, a "polysaccharide" vaccine (PRP) used in children over 15 months old. It was originally supported by a Finnish trial, which was significantly flawed in its follow-up of vaccine recipients.

Information documenting significant vaccine failures began to appear (Granoff DM et.al, 1986), and after a large study of U.S. children (reported in the Journal of the American Medical Association on 19 August, 1992) showed that only two thirds were protected by the vaccine, the polysaccharide vaccine was largely discontinued.

The next group of vaccines to be produced were "conjugate" vaccines; that is, vaccines combining the Hib polysaccharide vaccine with other types of vaccines. They included:

PRP-D	-	Hib + Diphtheria toxoid.
PRP-DPT	-	Hib + triple antigen vaccine.
PRP-OMPC	-	Hib + outer membrane protein complex of Neisseria meningitidis
PRP-T	-	Hib + tetanus toxoid.
PRP-CRM	-	Hib + CRM mutant Corynebacterium protein (also called HbOC)

Note: PRP = polyribose ribitol phosphate (purified polysaccharide vaccine).

OC = oligosaccharide conjugate.

Other conjugate vaccines have been developed with varying success.

Lederle Laboratories released **HibTITER**, which was widely used in Australia. This PRP-CRM vaccine was recommended for children at two, four, and six months of age, coinciding with their DPT and polio vaccines. For older children, the PRP-D vaccine is often used; alternatively, a booster with PRP-CRM is administered.

Dr Viera Scheibner's study of the medical literature revealed the range of reported efficacy for the PRP-D vaccine as being 45-88%. Interested readers should refer to her heavily referenced book for further details (Scheibner V, 1993). The Canadian Medical Association reported a range of efficacy of the HbOC (PRP-CRM) vaccine of 35-95% (CMA, 1992, p. 1364).

These figures, taken from orthodox medical literature, show clearly that the true efficacy of the Hib vaccines is unknown. Efficacy appears to be high in some situations and low in others. The figures certainly do not support a conclusion that the different vaccines are always highly effective.

Dr P McIntyre stated: "It is important that the immunogenicity and efficacy of Hib vaccines continues to be monitored, as batch to batch variation and reduced immunogenicity over time has been observed" (McIntyre P, 1994).

Dr McIntyre also noted the following disadvantages of the four most common conjugated vaccines:

PRP-D Least immunogenic vaccine.

PRP-OMP Lot-to-lot variations in immunogenicity reported; lower antibody levels; must be reconstituted.

PRP-CRM At least two doses required for protection in infants; three doses under 6 months of age.

PRP-T Limited data from formal vaccine trials; three doses under 6 months of age; must be reconstituted.(McIntyre P, 1994, p.16)

It is generally accepted that the first generation Hib vaccines, consisting of purified polysaccharide (PRP) from the Hib capsule, were not effective in children under the age of 18 months. The second generation Hib vaccines, which consist of PRP chemically linked ('conjugated' or combined) to a variety of carrier proteins, are said to be highly effective (over 95%) in protecting young children from invasive Hib disease. Two or 3 doses may be required to achieve immunity, depending on the type of vaccine used (NH&MRC, 2008, page 135).

The NH&MRC comments are seriously at odds with the other references quoted above. The only conclusion can be that the efficiency of the Hib vaccines is variable. The grand claims that the Hib vaccines were totally responsible for the decline in the disease no doubt have some validity, but the case has yet to be proved beyond any doubt.

This conclusion is reinforced by recent findings that the effectiveness of Hib conjugate vaccines in the UK is falling (McVernon J et al, 2004).

The safety of the Hib vaccines has also been questioned by various medical studies, and a range of safety estimates has been reported. Nevertheless, experience demonstrates that the bottom line with any new chemical vaccine or drug is that the potential side effects are unknown until the substance has been used for many years. The medical scientists' much revered double-blind, placebo-controlled trial does not reveal all side effects, which is why many drugs tested in this way are later withdrawn from use due to complications that (presumably) were not discovered during the trials. However, in the case of the PRT-T vaccine, the trial found that it caused more seizures, distress and fevers in the vaccinated group than in the control group (Vadheim C M et al, 1993).

In 1993, some eight years after its release, the US Institute of Medicine reported that the unconjugated vaccine could cause Hib disease in some children (Stratton K R et al, 1994). Further, the newer vaccines were reported to cause lowering of antibody levels within the first week following vaccination (Daum RS, 1989).

Once again, a familiar list of potentially serious health problems was found to be associated with the Hib vaccine. They included GBS, transverse myelitis (paralysis of the spinal cord), seizures, thrombocytopenia (a blood disorder affecting blood clotting) and diabetes (Neustaedter R, 2002, pp. 191-193).

9.2.4.2 The current vaccines

The following four vaccines are currently available in Australia as at 1/9/2010:

Comvax (CSL/MSD) – PRP-OMP, with HepB and Meningococcal protein. Contains aluminium hydroxide, borax and yeast proteins.

Infarix hexa (GSK) – the "big daddy" of them all, containing the following 6 antigens: diphtheria-tetanus-acellular pertussis-hepatitis B-inactivated poliomyelitis vaccine-*Haemophilus influenzae* type b (Hib). It also contains aluminium hydroxide/phosphate; phenoxyethanol as preservative; formaldehyde, polymyxin and neomycin.

HibTITER (W) - HbOC, conjugated to a non-toxic diphtheria protein.

Hiberix (GSK) - PRP-T; PRP conjugated to tetanus toxoid.

Liquid PedvaxHIB (CSL/MSD) - PRP-OMP, conjugated to meningococcal protein. Contains borax, aluminium hydroxide and aluminium.

Combination vaccines that include both DTPa and Hib: **Infarix Hexa**; **Infarix-Hib**; **Pediacel**; **Poliacel**.

9.2.4.3 Comment

Hib is potentially a very serious disease, and a good case can be made for protecting children and the elderly against this disease. Confident claims have been made regarding the positive effects of the more recent Hib vaccines; however it is still too early to thoroughly assess the real advantages and risks associated with their use. There seems to be a clear protective effect from the vaccines, but their true effectiveness appears to vary considerably.

As is the case with any other vaccine, homoeopathy has an option which parents may wish to consider. Although some homoeopaths are not familiar with the Haemophilis nosode, it has been used for many years. For example, Kichlu and Bose recognised the effect of H influenzae in meningitis twenty years ago, and homoeopaths have used the Hib nosode in the same way that the nosodes of other disease have been used for decades (Kichlu KL & Bose L, 1987, p. 805).

The other factor to consider is that fully breastfed children who do not mix in groups with other infants, such as in child care groups, are much less likely to contract Hib. But of course, only complete isolation can guarantee protection.

* * * * * * *

9.2.5 Hepatitis A vaccination

9.2.5.1 The current vaccines

Eight varieties of Hep A vaccine are currently available in Australia, including **Avaxim; Havrix Junior; Havrix 1440; Twinrix Junior (360/10); Twinrix (720/20); VAQTA Paediatric/Adolescent formulation; VAQTA Adult formulation;** and **Vivaxim**.

As well as the antigenic materials, these vaccines contain formaldehyde; aluminium hydroxide; phenoxyethanol; formaldehyde; neomycin; aluminium phosphate/hydroxide; yeast proteins; borax; aluminium; bovine serum albumin.

Clinical trials of inactivated Hep A vaccines suggest a high level of immunity, over 95%. The length of protection is uncertain, although it is advised that it should last for at least 10 years. However, this has not been verified.

The inactivated Hep A vaccines are prepared in human diploid cells, inactivated by formaldehyde, and adsorbed into an aluminium hydroxide adjuvant. Some vaccines contain a preservative, 2-phenoxyethanol.

Hepatitis A vaccination is generally recommended for travellers to endemic areas, health care workers, patients with chronic liver disease, injecting drug users, sexually active homosexuals, certain Aboriginal communities, sewerage works and some others.

Adverse events reported in the literature include:

- Soreness at injection site – 50% of adult recipients and 20% of children.
- Headaches – 15%
- Malaise and fatigue – 5%

(the NH&MRC suggest that these are probably caused by the aluminium hydroxide adjuvant – NH&MRC, 2008, p.146).

However, a range of very serious adverse events have been reported (Niu MT, 1998, pp. 1475-6), making the hepatitis A vaccine potentially dangerous.

9.2.5.2 Comment

Effective personal hygiene (especially hand washing) and improved sanitation and general living conditions are effective preventatives against hepatitis A.

If the likelihood of exposure to the disease is high, the additional protection is warranted. The hepatitis A Nosode can provide some protection without the risk of toxic damage.

* * * * * * *

9.2.6 Hepatitis B vaccination

Australian vaccination policy

In 1988, Australian authorities began targeting groups at high risk of hepatitis B for vaccination at birth. The program was extended in 1996, and in 2000 a national hepatitis B vaccination program involving injecting newborns commenced. The original blood-based vaccines were replaced by synthetic recombinant vaccine in the mid 1980's to prevent the possibility of infection with the live virus.

9.2.6.1 The current vaccines

There are eleven vaccines currently available in Australia, including adult and infanct variants, as of 1/9/2010:

Engerix-B (GSK) - recombinant DNA hepatitis B vaccine. Both the adult and the paediatric formulations contain aluminium hydroxide and the paediatric formulation contains thiomersal and yeast..

H-B-Vax II (CSL/MSD) - recombinant DNA hepatitis B vaccine. There are three options, all advertised as preservative free, but all contain aluminium hydroxide.

Twinrix (720/20)(adult) **Twinrix (360/10)**(junior) - combination Hep A and Hep B vaccines containing aluminium phosphate/hydroxide; phenoxyethanol; formaldehyde; neomycin; yeast proteins.

Comvax (CSL/MSD) - Hib(PRP-OMP) with Hep B, aluminium hydroxide and borax.

Other combination vaccines including both DTPa and hepatitis B: **Infarix Hep B**; **Infarix Penta**; **Infarix Hexa**.

The vaccine is claimed to be around 95% effective (Koff RS, 2001), however the length of protection is uncertain (maybe 3-10 years). Longer-term protection would certainly require boosters every 5-10 years.

The NH&MRC state that adverse events reported in the media are rare, with the main reaction being 5% of temporary reactions such as soreness, fever, pains, and nausea. Polakoff and Vandervelde reported a rate of adverse reactions of 11% (Polakoff S & Vandervelde EM, 1988, p. 249).

Three product information sheets prepared by Merck Sharp & Dohme for H-B-Vax II vary in their advice. Sheet #409610050 mentions injection site and systemic complaints in 15-17% of injections, sheet #408600050 says 25% incidence, and sheet #404600051 removes the percentage reference altogether.

However, research by Neustaedter shows clearly that potentially serious adverse events are possible. In an excellent piece of research he gives examples of the vaccine causing the following: death, autoimmune reactions, thrombocytopenic purpura, GBS, CNS demyelinating disease, diabetes, arthritis and anaphylaxis (Neustaedter R, 2002). Clearly HBV is not a risk-free vaccine.

His opinions are certainly supported in the orthodox literature. For example, "The Australian Government's Adverse Drug Reactions Advisory Committee (ADRAC) has received 203 reports of suspected adverse reactions occurring in patients who had received recombinant hepatitis B vaccines. In almost all cases, hepatitis B vaccine was administered intramuscularly and was the sole suspected agent. In general, the onset of symptoms occurred within the first week after vaccination and the vast majority of patients had recovered fully at the time of reporting" (ADRAC Warnings, 1990). This report was in 1990. The number of reported adverse reactions had risen to 597 from 1988 to March 1996 (ADRAC Bulletin, Vol. 15, No.2, May 1996). Many more reports will have been received since then, and not all the adverse events were mild. ADRAC was replaced by ASCOM – the Advisory Committee of the Safety of Medicines - in 2010.

The US Vaccine Adverse Events Reporting System (VAERS) has recorded 17,497 adverse reactions to the vaccine from 1990-1998, which included 5,983 life threatening health problems, hospitalisation, disablement and death (from letter to Prof. M. Burgess, 8.5.2000).

Classen reported that juvenile diabetes increased 60 percent following a massive increase in hepatitis B vaccination in New Zealand for babies 6 weeks and older from 1988 to 1991 (Classes JB, 1996, p. 195).

Professor Bonnie Dunbar has been reported as saying that “No basic science research to determine the biological mechanism of vaccine injury or long-term studies into the side effects of this vaccine have ever been conducted in babies or children. In adults, only limited follow-up has been carried out in genetically restricted populations”. In the same article, Fisher reported that “the French government became the first country to end hepatitis B vaccine requirements for schoolchildren” following many reports of adverse events. (Fisher BL, 2000).

The vaccination of newborn infants who are not exposed to hepatitis B has raised concerns with many parents. Even supporters of vaccination question the new policy - “HBV vaccine is most cost-effective when a strategy of screening newborns is combined with routine administration to 10-year-old children” (Bloom BS et al, 1993, p. 298) – in other words, only give vaccine to at-risk infants. In 1996 in the US there were 279 cases of hepatitis B in children under 14 years, but there were reports of 872 serious adverse events including 48 deaths (Association of American Physicians and Surgeons, statement, 3.8.99). Vaccination of children less than 14 years of age once again appears to be counter-indicated.

9.2.6.2 Comment

Hepatitis B is principally a disease passed on through unprotected sex, sharing needles, and rare accidental infections of health care workers. Vaccination of people at high risk of contracting the disease is supportable, as is the use of the homoeopathic alternative in such situations.

Vaccination of infants makes no sense, unless the mother carries hepatitis B. The infant vaccination campaign is clear “overkill”, and the long-term health effects are completely unknown. Time may shown them to be considerable.

* * * * * *

9.2.7 Hepatitis C vaccination

9.2.7.1 The current vaccines

An effective vaccine against hepatitis C is not available, and may be many years away.

9.2.7.2 Comment

I have included hepatitis C in this review because, using the Law of Similars, homoeopathy does have something to offer. The whole tragedy of the matter is that orthodox authorities are not prepared to seriously look at the homoeopathic option.

As with meningococcal B prevention, the medical authorities would rather that people remained unprotected against hepatitis C, than receive some protection by using homœoprophylaxis.

So much for the Hippocratic oath!

* * * * * * *

9.2.8 Influenza vaccination

The Influenza virus is usually classified as type A, B or C depending on their individual protein characteristics. Types A and B are the ones of most concern to humans. The viruses mutate – "shift" and "drift" as it is called – and sub-strains are constantly forming. Every 10 to 30 years new subtypes of Influenza A appear, and cause pandemics which can affect up to one third of the entire population.

9.2.8.1 The current vaccines

The vaccines currently available in Australia are:

Fluad (DC/Nov) - inactivated influenza. Contains thiomersal, neomycin and formaldehyde.

Fluarix (GSK) - inactivated influenza. Contains thiomersal, gentamicin and formaldehyde.

Fluvirin (Md/EHS) - inactivated influenza.

Influvac (SyP) - inactivated influenza. Contains thiomersal.

Vaxigrip (SPPL) - inactivated influenza. Contains formaldehyde, neomycin and egg protein.

Vaxigrip Junior (SPPL) – inactivated influenza. Contains formaldehyde, neomycin and egg protein.

Fluvax (CSL) - inactivated influenza. Contains polymyxin, neomycin and egg protein

All influenza vaccines in Australia are prepared from purified inactivated influenza which has been cultivated in embryonated hens eggs. Most vaccines contain 2 strains of type A virus and one strain of type B virus.

The Influenza is one of the least effective routine vaccines, with estimates of efficacy ranging from 30% to 90% (NH&MRC, 2008, page 188). The crucial points here are old and how infirmed the vaccinated individuals are, and how well the current flu vaccine matches the current viral strain.

Adverse events can be severe in people with allergies to eggs, and the vaccine is not recommended in these people. People with sensitivities to other vaccine components should also not be vaccinated. People who have an acute febrile illness or Guillain-Barré Syndrome (GBS) are advised to delay vaccination. In 1976 in America the flu vaccine caused an outbreak of GBS (Safranek T J et al, 1991), and again in the 1992-4 flu seasons (Lasky T et al, 1998).

Other adverse events reported in the literature include: drowsiness or tiredness, muscle aches, localized pain, redness & swelling at injection site, low grade fever, headaches. In fact this list does not include a side-effect that is known to occur often each year – the flu. Anecdotally, many cases of the flu are reported each year in recently vaccinated people.

McMahon and colleagues examined reported reactions to the influenza vaccine between 1990 and 2003. A small number (166) of reports were received by the US Vaccine Adverse Events Reporting System (VAERS) for infants less than 2 years of age. They included some serious reactions, but were few enough for the Advisory Commission on Immunisation Practices to recommend influenza vaccination of 6 to 24 month old infants. This type of funding illustrates the great weakness in the system – the reliance on VAERS when GPs are notoriously loath to connect any adverse reaction to a recent vaccine (McMahon et al, 2005).

When I searched the VAERS data base for 2009, there were 15,262 adverse reactions reported for various Influenza vaccines out of the yearly total of 50,560 adverse reactions for all vaccines given during 2009.

The Australian Vaccination Network (AVN) has released an *Influenza Information Pack* which is full of reports, mostly from medical journals, concerning the influenza vaccine. Details of how to contact the AVN are shown in the Appendix.

9.2.8.2 Comment

The vaccine is clearly risky, and not nearly as effective as many of the other vaccines available. One reason for this is that the strains of flu virus constantly mutate. This is a problem for many vaccines in general. It is much less of a problem for homoeopathic preventatives, provided the general symptoms of each type of organism are similar.

So the influenza vaccine has a low level of efficacy, and a significant level of adverse reactions. It is a less than ideal procedure. The homoeopathic influenza nosode certainly provides a safe and relatively effective alternative for those who feel they need protection against influenza.

* * * * * * *

9.2.9 Japanese Encephalitis vaccination

9.2.9.1 The current vaccines

There is one vaccine currently available in Australia:

JE-VAX (SPPL) - Japanese encephalitis virus vaccine. Contains formalin, thimerosal, formaldehyde, and mouse brain serum protein.

MOUSE BRAIN SERUM PROTEIN??? And we inject this into people!!

The NH&MRC report that one clinical trial in the 1980's showed that 2 doses of the vaccine given to children 7 days apart had an efficacy of 91%. However, other studies have questioned this.

Adverse events reported in the literature include:

- 20% - tenderness, redness and/or swelling at injection site.
- 10% - fever, headaches, chills, dizziness, aching muscles, nausea, vomiting, generally unwell.
- Rare severe allergic reactions and deaths have been reported.

In May, 2005, the Japanese Health, Labour and Welfare Ministry issued a national order to suspend recommending Japanese B vaccinations for minors because of the potentially serious side-effects. Of concern was the condition acute disseminated encephalomyelitis (ADEM) which has been reported in more than 10 vaccinated individuals since 1994. "Since the vaccine for Japanese encephalitis is made from mice brains, some experts suspect the debilitating side effects might be linked to tiny amounts of brain tissue remaining from production" (The Japan Times, 31/5/05).

9.2.9.2 Comment

This vaccine, being produced as it is in mouse brain serum protein, raises concerns regarding its long term safety. The homoeopathic nosode is available. Protection against mosquitos (if possible) will prevent transmission of the disease.

* * * * * * *

9.2.10 Measles vaccination

9.2.10.1 The current vaccines

Measles vaccine is currently only delivered as part of the MMR (Measles-Mumps-Rubella) vaccine. The MMR vaccines are discussed more completely in Section 9.2.20. Only one vaccine is currently recommended in the Handbook as at 1/9/2010.

Priorix (GSK) - live attenuated measles virus (Schwarz strain), mumps virus (derived from Jeryl Lynn strain), and rubella virus strain (Wistar 27/3 strain). The vaccine includes lactose; neomycin; amino acids; sorbitol and mannitol

Adverse reactions reported in the literature include:

- A rash and weakness for 7-10 days following vaccination, lasting 2-3 days.
- A moderate to high fever.
- A variety of potentially severe reactions, including febrile convulsions, anaphylaxis (an unusual or extreme reaction of the body to a foreign protein or other substance), encephalopathy (any disease or disorder of the brain), thrombocytopenia (a reduction in the number of platelets in the blood) have been reported occurring up to 2-3 weeks following the vaccine.
- An association between MMR vaccine and inflammatory bowel disease and autism has created controversy in the orthodox literature. The official line that there has been no scientific evidence to support this claim and that there is now evidence to contradict it. Many, including myself, remain unconvinced.

The measles component of the MMR vaccine is regarded as being one of the most effective vaccines, with claims of efficacy after 2 doses of up to 99%. The figures certainly support the impact of the vaccine on the disease.

As shown in Figures 3-5, 3-6, and 3-7 concerning the progress of measles in the USA, UK, and Australia during this century, there is a clear suggestion that:

- vaccination does reduce the incidence of the disease
- the death rate from measles was falling well before the introduction of vaccination, which had little impact on the rate of decline in deaths.

Evidence also suggests, however, that during measles epidemics, approximately 60% of all children infected will have been previously vaccinated (Neustaedter R, 2002, p. 203). While this does not mean that 60% of all vaccinated people will contract the disease, it is indicative of the many cases where failures of the measles vaccine have been reported in medical literature. A measles outbreak in Australia during 1994 occurred mainly in vaccinated children. Similar experiences are found in the UK and the USA (Neustaedter R, 2002, pp. 202-204).

However there is also evidence that the field efficacy of the measles vaccine can vary considerably. For example, a vaccine efficacy of 66.9% was reported in a measles outbreak in Ethiopia (Talley L & Salama P, 2003, page 545). Three field studies in India reported rates of 53.1%, 61.7%-75.1%, and 100% (Puri A, 2002, p. 558).

Puri and colleagues make the relevant point "It has been realised that most of the laboratory-based trials on vaccine efficacy are carried out under laboratory controlled conditions, giving results which are unrealistic in the field conditions. Under field conditions immunisation cannot be strictly supervised and many factors affect the subsequent development of protective antibodies. Vaccine efficacy obtained under field conditions, thus realistically assess the protection afforded by the vaccine against the diseases" (Puri A, 2002, p. 559).

9.2.10.2 The severity of the disease vs. the vaccine

Although the incidence of measles has declined significantly following routine vaccination, not all doctors agree that vaccination against measles is our best option. For example, Professor George Dick (referred to in previous sections), who is an internationally respected supporter of vaccination in general, has questioned the use of the measles vaccine in England, except in very selective cases. Once the decision to introduce the vaccine was made, he recommended that the vaccine be given to only three or four year old children in order to minimise the number of adverse reactions (Dick G, 1987, Pages 67 and 70).

In communities where children are severely malnourished and basic hygiene and nursing care are unavailable, measles is often fatal and otherwise serious. This experience cannot be generally extended to Australia, where appropriate nursing care (usually at home) is all that is generally required to manage this rarely serious disease.

Professor Robert Mendelsohn noted that the incidence encephalitis may be 1/1000 for children who live in conditions of poverty and malnutrition, but for just about everyone else the incidence of true encephalitis is probably more like 1/10,000 or 1/100,000, and the majority of these cases will not show evidence of brain damage.

However, it is true that significant complications, including SSPE and sometimes death, do occur in developed countries; a child may also acquire SSPE or die from being vaccinated. The incidence of SSPE is generally quoted as 1/100,000 from the disease and 1/1,000,000 from the vaccine. It is also generally assumed that 1/10,000 children suffer other serious impairments as a result of measles; however, there is disagreement among doctors regarding this figure.

The Victorian Health Department's pro-vaccination brochure states that: "One in every 15 children who catch measles will develop pneumonia, or an ear infection or some other complication. One child in 1000 cases of measles will develop encephalitis (inflammation of the brain) which can cause permanent brain damage. Death may result" (Health Department of Victoria, 1987, p. 2).

This statement clearly exaggerates the potential for damage from the disease for Australian children, as the figures quoted above indicate. The implication that death may result in one in every 1000 cases is grossly misleading. The extent of overstatement in the Victorian campaign is reflected in Table 9-2 following.

Table 9-2 A Comparison of Measles Data

Complications	Health Dept Promotion	Standard Figures
Encephalitis from the disease	1/1,000	1/100,000
Encephalitis from the vaccine	1/1,000,000	1/1,000,000
Other significant complications from the disease	1/15	1/10,000

A growing number of doctors are now questioning the belief that the risks of vaccination are negligible, and that the dangers of the disease far outweigh the risks of vaccination. For example, Dr D Levitt of the Guthrie Research Institute has said of most vaccines and drugs that we use: "We really don't know with certainty what many of their effects are upon the system" (reported by Coulter H L & Fisher B L, 1985, p. 2). Some figures are presented in Section 7 showing the extent of drug damage.

Dr Levitt's statement explains why scores of commonly prescribed drugs (from Thalidomide onwards) are withdrawn from circulation every year. Even though double-blind, placebo-controlled trials are used routinely, they do not reveal all possible problems with a drug. As well, there are issues such as research results only being reported if favourable, researchers having financial links with drugs houses, etc (MJA, June 2005). Only an objective analysis of use through time provides a final test of safety and efficacy.

I believe that the greatest danger associated with vaccination is the subtle, long-term damage to a child which may only appear indirectly in later life, particularly in the form of immune system diseases. The much feared SSPE, for instance, is medically considered to be a 'slow virus'. Dr Moskowitz, among others, has suggested that one of the possible consequences of vaccination is the introduction of slow viruses into a child. Regarding measles specifically, Dr Moskowitz wrote that: "even if the measles vaccine could be shown to reduce the risk of deaths or serious complications from the disease, it still could not justify the high probability of auto-immune diseases, cancer, and whatever else may result from the propagation of latent measles virus in human tissue culture for life" (Moskowitz R, 1985).

One can only speculate how many of the reported cases of SSPE with high measles antibodies are actually related to the disease and how many to the vaccine. Far more statistical data is required to provide complete information concerning measles. Therefore, while doctors who pioneered developments in vaccination believed they were copying the processes of nature to protect their patients, it is clear that vaccination perverts rather than duplicates the process of nature.

Neustaedter thoroughly reviewed the potential complications of the measles vaccine. He said, “The problems caused by the measles vaccine read like a neurologic textbook. Encephalitis, meningitis, autism, subacute sclerosing panencephalitis, seizure disorder, sensorineural deafness, optic neuritis, transverse myelitis, Guillain-Barré syndrome. The human tragedy described in the thousands of reports is staggering. This vaccine is dangerous” (Neustaedter R, 2002, pp. 204-5).

Measles vaccine has also been linked to a threefold increase in the incidence of Chron’s Disease, and a 2.53 times greater chance of Inflammatory Bowel Disease (Thompson NP et al, 1995). One of the authors of this study was Dr A Wakefield, who with colleagues came to prominence over claims regarding the adverse effects of the MMR vaccine (see Section 9.2).

In response to the question, "Are There any Reactions to the Vaccine?", the previously quoted Victorian Health Department booklet stated: "Sometimes, but they are very mild"; to the question, "Is it a Safe Vaccine?" the statement, "Very. Serious complications are as rare as one per every million children immunised" (Health Department of Victoria, 1987, p. 2). Obviously, these answers do not give parents all the facts regarding the risks associated with measles vaccination. In conjunction with the threat of death to children, the HDV promotion is clearly based in fear rather than on fact.

Your doctor may say, "How would you feel if your child acquired SSPE after you decided against having him vaccinated?" (a question every parent should ask themselves). The doctor should also ask, "How would you feel if your child acquired SSPE or an immune disorder after you had him vaccinated?". While the obvious answer to the second question would be, "my doctor told me to have my child vaccinated", this answer would not be acceptable to genuinely concerned parents. If parents decide to vaccinate their children, the decision should be made after weighing up the facts, not just the fears.

Highlighting the need for parents to take responsibility for making informed decisions is a statement by a US doctor who refused to vaccinate his own child against measles, although continuing to vaccinate his infant patients: "As a parent I have the luxury of making a choice for my child. As a physician . . . legally and professionally I have to accept the recommendations of the profession" (Mendelsohn R, 1984, p. 49).

9.2.10.3 Comment

In the case of measles vaccination, as with most vaccines, pro-vaccination campaigns have relied heavily on scare tactics. Parents need to make their decisions factually, rather than fearfully, despite the usual lack of encouragement from conventional health professionals to look beyond the promotional literature.

If parents decide to protect their children against measles, a homoeopathic alternative is available. Unlike the vaccine, the nosode Morbillinum contains no physical quantity of the antigen and is perfectly non-toxic; it may therefore be safely repeated if necessary. If your child does acquire measles, careful diet and nursing care together with indicated treatment using homoeopathic remedies will ensure smooth progress through the stages of the disease.

Note that more material on this vaccine is presented in Section 9.2 on the MMR vaccine.

* * * * * * *

9.2.11 Meningococcal Disease vaccination

Type B disease is the major cause of meningococcal disease in most developed countries, including Australia. Type C is less common, and usually peaks in winter and spring. The highest incidence occurs in children under 5, and people aged 15 to 24. To date, there are no vaccines available in Australia for type B disease.

9.2.11.1 The current vaccines

There are two different types of meningococcal vaccine: (i) tetravalent meningococcal polysaccharide vaccines (4vMenPV) and (ii) meningococcal C conjugate vaccines (MenCCV).

Type (i): tetravalent meningococcal polysaccharide vaccines (4vMenPV)

Mencevax ACWY (GSK) - serogroups A,C,W135 and Y. Contains phenol.

Menomune (AP) - serogroups A,C,W135 and Y. Contains lactose.

Type (ii): meningococcal C conjugate vaccines (MenCCV)

Meningitec (W) - type C conjugated on diphtheria protein. Contains aluminium phosphate.

Menjugate/Menjugate Syringe (CSL/Nov) - type C conjugated on diphtheria protein. Contains aluminium hydroxide.

NeisVac-C (BH) - type C conjugated on tetanus toxoid protein. Contains aluminium hydroxide.

In countries where type C meningococcal vaccines have been introduced, the incidence of this type of meningococcal disease has decreased, while the incidence of type B disease has increased.

Adverse events occur more frequently with type (ii) conjugate vaccines. Pain, redness, and swelling at injection sites, fever, irritability, anorexia and headaches have been reported in more than 10% of cases. A Victorian government information sheet identified local reactions and headaches in up to 30% of vaccinated individuals (Department of Human Services. *Immunisation Information*). The experience in Britain when the vaccine was introduced in 1999 lead to a public outcry, including concerns that four people advising the Government on the vaccine were on the payroll of the manufacturer of the vaccine (Neustaedter R, 2002, p.196).

9.2.11.2 Comment

The use of the homoeopathic nosode Meningococcinum has been tested on some large groups in epidemic situations. The first was during an outbreak of meningitis in Brazil in August 1974. 18,640 children were given the homoeopathic Nosode, and 6,340 were unprotected (Eizayaga FX, 1991). A more recent example occurred during an outbreak, again in Brazil, where 65,826 children were given the homoeopathic preventative and 23,532 were unprotected (Mroninski C, Adriano E, Mattos G, 2001). The nosode was shown to be 95% effective in the first outbreak, and 95% effective after 6 months and 91% effective after 12 months in the second outbreak. These significant results are discussed in Section 4.1.4. They show that a genuine option is available which potentially can cover type B as well as type C disease.

I offered this information to state and federal governments in 2002/3, in the light of no vaccine being available for type B disease. They were not interested. It appears that health authorities prefer that people remain unprotected than consider the use of the homoeopathic alternative! In fact the TGA released a notice on 9/9/2002 warning the community against "Homeopathic meningococcal 'vaccines'". I wonder if the politicians in charge of the health department concerned even got to hear of the possible protection being offered against type B diseases. I suspect not.

* * * * * * *

9.2.12 Mumps vaccination

This disease, which is typically mild in healthy young children, is more serious after puberty; however, the often-quoted dangers of sterility are greatly exaggerated. Contracting the disease in childhood normally confers life-long immunity; the mumps vaccine does not guarantee immunity in later years.

If parents wish to protect children against mumps, the homoeopathic remedy described in Section 3.2 will offer equivalent protection to the vaccine. It may, however, have the same disadvantage as the conventional vaccine in that protection against infection is not guaranteed in later years, since the duration of its effectiveness in preventing infection is currently not established.

Following the general advice given in Section 2.1 for boosting children's general health will certainly help to minimise the effects of the disease. This is particularly relevant for those parents who (very reasonably) choose not to use the mumps prophylactic included in the earlier homoeopathic programs.

9.2.12.1 The current vaccines

In Australia the mumps vaccine is no longer delivered individually, but as part of the MMR vaccine. The MMR vaccine (**Priorix**) is discussed in the above Section on Measles, and in the MMR Section below.

The efficacy of the vaccine is stated as being between 75% and 95%. An examination of three different mumps vaccines in Switzerland showed the following efficacy:

Rubini strain	-	4%
Jeryl Lynn strain	-	78%
Urabe strain	-	87% (Schlegel M, 1999, p. 352).

It is clear that the efficacy of the mumps vaccine is variable, and depends both on the strain(s) used, and the state of health of recipients.

The Institute of Medicine (IOM) stated that the mumps component may be a cause of aseptic meningitis. Cases of diabetes have also been reported following mumps vaccination (IOM, 1994).

9.2.12.2 Comment

The potential risks of the disease and the vaccine have not been adequately compared. However, given that the disease is typically mild, and that the efficacy and the safety of the vaccine are uncertain, it certainly is an option not to vaccinate, or to use the homoeopathic option if protection is required.

* * * * * * *

9.2.13 Pertussis (Whooping Cough) vaccination

Whooping cough (pertussis) is most dangerous in very young children, but administration of the vaccine is possibly least effective and most dangerous for children in this age group.

Studies consistently show that children under one year of age are most at risk; yet, as Professor George Dick stated, "There is very little evidence that the vaccine is effective if given in the first few months of life", and adverse reactions to the whooping cough vaccine can be up to 20 times greater in babies under six months than in older ones (Dick G, 1978, p. 41). While there is general agreement about the lack of vaccine efficacy in very young children, the evidence as to complication rates in this age group varies. Drs Joshi and Phelan have provided figures suggesting that children under nine months are more than ten times as likely to be admitted to hospital with complications as older groups (Joshi W & Phelan P, 1986, p. 726).

Prior to the MMR vaccine, the pertussis component of the triple antigen vaccine was regarded as being the potentially most dangerous of all the vaccines in current use. The pertussis component has been changed (from 1999 in Australia) from a whole cell vaccine to an acellular pertussis-containing vaccine in order to reduce the potential adverse effects of pertussis vaccination.

9.2.13.1 The current vaccines

There are now 10 acellular pertussis vaccines available in Australia, which contain 3 or more purified components of *B. pertussis.* The NH&MRC has claimed that the new acellular pertussis vaccines are much safer than the old whole cell vaccines, with fewer reported adverse events. They also claim that the new vaccines that have 3 or more antigens are also comparably effective with efficacy around 80% (NH&MRC, 2003, p. 207). The 80% efficacy has been confirmed for children following 3 doses of vaccines, which also showed that outbreaks are possible in highly vaccinated populations (Khetsuriani N et.al. 2001).

The following vaccines are currently in use in Australia:

(i) Children less than 8 years of age.

Infarix hexa (GSK) – DTPa + Hep B + IPV + Hib (PRP). Contains neomycin, polymyxin, and phenoxyethanol. Note – IPV = inactivated polio virus (given by injection, not orally).

Infarix-IPV (GSK) – DTPa + IPV. Contains neomycin, polymyxin, and phenoxyethanol.

Infarix Penta (GSK) – DTPa + Hep B + IPV. Contains neomycin, polymyxin, and phenoxyethanol.

(ii) Children older than 8 years, and adults

Boostrix (GSK) – dTpa. Adult formulation with primarily tetanus toxoid. Contains aluminium hydroxide/phosphate; phenoxyethanol; formaldehyde.

Adacel (SPPL) – diphtheria-tetanus-acellular pertussis. Also contains aluminium phosphate; phenoxyethanol; formaldehyde.

Adacel Polio (SPPL) – diphtheria-tetanus-acellular pertussis-inactivated poliomyelitis. Also contains aluminium phosphate; phenoxyethanol as preservative; traces of formaldehyde, polymyxin, neomycin and streptomycin

Boostrix-IPV (GSK) - diphtheria-tetanus-acellular pertussis-inactivated poliomyelitis. Also contains aluminium hydroxide/phosphate; formaldehyde; polymyxin; neomycin.

The following vaccines have been withdrawn from the 9th edition Handbook:

Infarix (GSK) - DTPa. Contains aluminium hydroxide and phenoxyethanol.

Infarix Hep B (GSK) – DTPa + Hep B. Contains aluminium hydroxide, formaldehyde, and phenoxyethanol.

Pediacel (AP) – DTPa + IPV + Hib (PRP-T). Contains aluminium phosphate, bovine serum albumin, streptomycin, neomycin, polymyxin, and phenoxyethanol.

Poliacel (AP) – DTPa + IPV + Hib (PRP-T). Congugated to Quadracel (see next).

Quadracel (AP) – DTPa + IPV. Contains aluminium phosphate, bovine serum albumin, neomycin, polymyxin, and phenoxyethanol.

Tripacel (AP) – DTPa. Contains aluminium phosphate and phenoxyethanol. Contains aluminium phosphate, aluminium hydroxide, and phenoxyethanol.

9.2.13.2 How effective is vaccination against whooping cough?

As discussed in section 3.4.1.1, deaths from whooping cough in USA, UK, and Australia were declining well before vaccination began, with little acceleration in decline following vaccination. On the other hand, notifications did fall after vaccination was introduced.

Ehrengut presented figures indicating similar results in West Germany, which had a policy of avoiding routine whooping cough vaccination; he noted that "the milder course of the disease owes nothing whatsoever to pertussis vaccination" (Ehrengut W, 1978).

A summary of a number of trials of vaccine efficacy is shown in Table 9-3 below. These studies measured 'secondary attack rates' - the percentage of other family members infected as a result of definite exposure to a family member with whooping cough. The figures also report the percentage of infection through secondary attack on vaccinated and unvaccinated people, as well as the efficacy of the vaccine.

The efficacy of a vaccine

$$= \frac{\text{attack rate (unvaccinated children-vaccinated children)}}{\text{attack rate in unvaccinated children}}$$

The figures reporting secondary attack rates are more reliable than general community studies due to the certainty of exposure to pertussis. On average, they suggest that only 72% of children definitely exposed to whooping cough are susceptible to infection; of these, vaccination will protect 71%. The best of these figures are similar to the NH&MRC estimate (above) of around 80% efficacy in fully vaccinated children.

Table 9-3 The Efficacy of Whooping Cough Vaccination

	Attack Rates Among Family Members		
STUDY	**Vaccinated**	**Unvaccinated**	**Efficacy**
Grob et al (1981) UK	19.0	72.0	73.5
Broome et al (1981) USA	30.0	82.0	63.4
PHLS (1982) UK	25.6	63.4	59.6
Brink (1982) USA	13.7	70.4	80.5
Aoyama et al (1985) Japan	15.0	73.1	79.4

The wide divergence of the above results suggests that the reliability of the vaccine is uncertain; however, two general conclusions may be drawn:

- Vaccination is not the major factor in controlling deaths from whooping cough
- Vaccination does offer some protection against infection, but the extent of protection is far from certain.

The figures in Table 9-3 relate to the old whole-cell vaccine. Even more doubts exist about the effectiveness of the newer acellular vaccines.

A trial of 3 vaccines revealed the following efficacy rates - a whole cell (48.3%), a 2 component acellular (58.9%) and a 5 component acellular vaccine (85.2%) (Gustafsson R, 1996). A long-term randomised, double-blind, placebo-controlled clinical trial in Italy showed a range of efficacy for DTPa of 76% to 86% (Salmaso S et al, 2001). Since that time different trials have suggested a range of results, but it is commonly acknowledged that the acellular vaccine represents a trade off between fewer adverse reactions and less efficacy.

In 2003, Cherry stated that "Lessened potency of pertussis vaccines is a legitimate issue. Because of reactogenicity of whole-cell vaccines, vaccine manufacturers manipulated culture techniques in attempts to lessen toxicity. In the 1970's in Sweden these attempts led to an ineffective vaccine in 1979. In the United States it is also known that attempts were also made to lessen reactogenicity. The acellular vaccine trials in Sweden and Italy noted that the Connaught DTP vaccine used in the United States had minimal efficacy. In addition, 2 of the first 4 acellular pertussis component vaccines had poor efficacy"

He commented on the possible causes of the increase in pertussis in the USA over the last two decades – "There have been many suggestions as to the cause of the increased reporting of pertussis. These include: 1) genetic changes in Bordetella pertussis making vaccines less effective, 2) lessened potency of pertussis vaccines, 3) waning of vaccine-induced immunity, 4) greater awareness of pertussis, and 5) the general availability of better laboratory tests". He concluded that "despite the use of many poor vaccines for a 10-year period there is little scientific evidence that this contributed to the "resurgence" of reported pertussis", which Cherry attributed to a "greater awareness of pertussis and in particular the recognition of the occurrence of atypical disease in adolescents and adults" (Cherry J, 2003, p. 406).

It therefore appears that Cherry, a widely published expert in this field, is arguing that the pertussis vaccines are not very effective, and it hasn't really mattered.

Cherry and Olin had earlier expressed concern that the method of testing vaccine efficacy caused a significant overstatement of pertussis vaccine efficacy. They said "The pressure to move rapidly from whole-cell to acellular vaccines seems to have blinded authorities and experts to the outcome of the efficacy trials. It was apparently more important to demonstrate vigour by switching to acellular vaccines than to bother about the possible long-term disadvantage of considering all DTaP vaccines equal. The sad fact, despite the expenditure of millions of dollars, is that the most efficacious vaccine available in the United States today is 1 of the 2 generally available whole-cell vaccines. Our present era of misinformation has many origins including: an oversimplified theory that suggests pertussis is a disease attributable to a single toxin, the failure to accept protective immunity data available 50 years ago, the inability of epidemiologists and statisticians to recognize the magnitude of bias in efficacy trials, and the acceptance of repeated publication of uncritically reviewed data" (Cherry JD & Olin P, 1999).

"Our data suggest that observer compliance (observer bias), can significantly inflate calculated vaccine efficacy. It is likely that all recently completed efficacy trials have been affected by this type of observer bias and all vaccines have considerably less efficacy against mild disease than published data suggest" (Cherry JD et al, 1998).

In 2010 suggestions are emerging that whooping cough is on the rise again in well vaccinated industrialised countries due to new strains emerging which are not covered by the limited number of strains in the modern acelluar vaccines (Kurniawan J et.al, 2010; Zukerman W, 2010). The new "safer" vaccines may result in falling efficacy and increasing disease rates in highly vaccinated populations. W

9.2.13.3 The 1980's British 'epidemic' – a history lesson

In the UK there was a significant drop in the number of children receiving the DPT vaccine from 1974 to 1982. This fall was due to widespread parental fears after repeated reports of vaccine damage to young children. Following the reduction in vaccination levels, several whooping cough 'epidemics' were reported; these can be seen as peaks in the figures for notifications from 1978 to 1983.

This 'epidemic' has been both used and misused by advocates of conventional vaccination to scare parents into having their children vaccinated. It is not uncommon to hear doctors referring to "thousands of cases and hundreds of deaths" from whooping cough in Britain due to parents failing to have their children vaccinated.

One example of official exaggeration was contained in the Statement of the Paediatric Society of New Zealand on Childhood Immunisations - August 1988. This document stated that, "In the United Kingdom in the 1970's, public rejection of the immunisation against pertussis because of concern about vaccine side effects led to a serious fall in immunisation rates, with consequent epidemics of pertussis exceeding 100,000 cases per year, and many deaths". This is not an isolated example.

However, the truth is rather different. In the two worst years of the epidemic, 1978 and 1982, the combined figure of reported cases of whooping cough was approximately 66,000, with 12 deaths in 1978 and 14 in 1982. The number of notifications and deaths reported in other years of the 'epidemic' period were significantly lower. Nevertheless, detailed examination of the UK experience reveals that even notification rates were grossly exaggerated due to a Health Department driven over-reporting of cases unconfirmed by naso-pharyngeal swabs.

Professor Gordon Stewart (Department of Community Medicine, University of Glasgow), stated that figures showing this 'epidemic' were exaggerated owing to "a significant tendency to report coughs in unvaccinated children as whooping cough, and to under-report coughs in vaccinated children", in addition to "fallacious and unrepresentative" optional notifications (Stewart GT, 1984). Similar comments were made earlier by Professor George Dick, who stated: "It is well recognised that there is considerable under reporting of adverse reactions" (Dick G, 1978, p. 40).

During the 1977-1979 outbreaks, there were reports from a number of areas where 35-46% of cases occurred in fully vaccinated children (Stewart GT, 1981). In fact, a comprehensive study of an entire Shetland community revealed that there was virtually no difference in attack rates between vaccinated and non-vaccinated children (Ditchburn RK,).

According to the Epidemiological Research Laboratory in England, who strongly advocate the practice of routine vaccination, "complete protection is not invariable and severe attacks can occur in vaccinated children" (Public Health Laboratory, 1982, p.359).

Close examination of the UK experience between 1965 and 1985 (refer to the Figures in Section 3.4.1.1) reveals two interesting facts:

(i) The seasonal pattern of deaths over time corresponds to the seasonal pattern of notifications over time, as would be expected by most observers, except after 1976.

(ii) The general trend in deaths has continued to fall despite variations in vaccine acceptance rates and notifications; for example, the pre-1975 'epidemic' peaks in deaths occurred in 1967 and 1971, and the post-1975 peaks in 1978 and 1982.

A comparison of these four periods is shown in Table 9-4 following.

Table 9-4 Comparison of Deaths and Notifications

	1967	1971	1978	1982
Deaths	27	26	12	14
Notifications ('000)	33.5	16.9	66.0	65.8
Deaths/Notifications x1000	0.81	1.54	0.18	0.21

Comparing the years 1978/1982 to 1967/1971, notifications had tripled whereas deaths had halved. From these facts, one of two possible conclusions may be drawn:

(i) The disease became, virtually overnight, over five times less lethal in 1978, as shown by the decline in the average ratio of Deaths/Notifications from over 1.00 to around 0.20. It then suddenly returned to its more lethal state after the 'epidemics' were officially over, or

(ii) Professor Stewart's claim of gross over-reporting during the 1978-82 'epidemics' is correct, and the figures for notifications probably should have been less than 10,000, which would have been entirely consistent with the normal cyclical decline of the disease.

It is clear to any unbiased observer that the only sensible conclusion is the second alternative above. Readers are thus totally justified in dismissing the claims concerning the UK experience in support of routine vaccination. Further examples relate to whooping cough 'epidemics' in the US and UK.

- In the 1982 UK 'epidemic', almost 66,000 cases of whooping cough were reported, with 14 deaths. Dr H Barrie of London's Charring Cross Hospital attacked the "campaign of terror" which "poured through television, radio, post and press" and was being grossly overstated. Dr Barrie and Professor G Stewart separately showed that the figures used in this campaign were exaggerated by up to 50% due to overzealous reporting and incorrect diagnoses, and that most of the deaths occurred in children with other medical complications (reported in H L Coulter HL & B L Fisher BL, 1985, pp. 166,167).
- In 1984 and 1985, whooping cough epidemics were reported in several US states, fuelled by alleged shortages in the vaccine arising from huge compensation payouts to parents of vaccine damaged children. The Utah 'epidemic' during the first nine months of 1984 involved only 162 reported cases of which 30 were laboratory confirmed. Of the 162, twelve required

hospitalisation and none resulted in death or serious complications. In addition, 49% of the 162 cases (in children aged three months to six years) had been properly vaccinated. In other states, 'epidemics' followed a similar pattern. Nevertheless, they were used as the basis for an extensive fear-inspiring campaign advising parents to have their children vaccinated (reported in H L Coulter HL & B L Fisher BL, 1985, p. 428).

9.2.13.4 How safe is the pertussis vaccine?

The short term side-effects of the Triple Antigen vaccine are both well known and accepted, and the pertussis component is generally considered to be the one at fault in the majority of cases. Cody and others have identified the following adverse reactions (refer Table 9-5) (Cody C L et al, 1981).

Table 9-5 Adverse Events Occurring Within 48 Hours of DPT Vaccinations

Type of Event	Frequency*
Local Redness	1/3 doses
Swelling	2/5 doses
Pain	1/2 doses
Systemic Fever > 38°C (100.4°F)	1/2 doses
Drowsiness	1/3 doses
Fretfulness	1/2 doses
Vomiting	1/15 doses
Anorexia	1/5 doses
Persistent, inconsolable crying (duration of hours)	1/100 doses
Fever > 40.5°C (105°F)	1/330 doses
Collapse (hypotonic - hyporesponsive episode)	1/1750 doses
Convulsions (with or without fever)	1/1750 doses

* Rate per total number of doses regardless of dose number in DPT series.

In a major review of the risks of whooping cough vaccination, Professor D L Miller and colleagues acknowledged that: "The risks and benefits of pertussis immunization remain controversial" (Miller D L, 1982). In an earlier study, Professor Miller found that "A significant association was shown between serious neurological illness and pertussis vaccine" (Miller D L et al, 1981, p. 1595).

While the majority of children who receive the vaccine are not permanently affected in a readily observable manner, the likelihood of serious damage has been sufficient for respected doctors and medical researchers to warn against its use. As mentioned previously, such warnings led to a fall in vaccine acceptance by parents in the UK, as well as a re-evaluation of its use by the governments of some European countries.

In the USA, Professor Robert Mendelsohn reported that: "In early 1984, stung by the multi-million dollar judgements awarded to vaccine damaged children, Wyeth Laboratories and Connaught Laboratories stopped the manufacture and distribution of DPT (production has since been resumed). Lederle, while still in the field, has raised the cost of the vaccine greatly" (Mendelsohn R, 1986, p. 17).

These types of vaccine-related problems resulted in the American Congress passing its National Childhood Vaccine Injury Act in 1986. Section 312 of the new law called for the Institute of Medicine to review scientific and other information on specific adverse consequences of the Pertussis and Rubella vaccines. The eminent committee which undertook this task was chaired by Professor Harvey Fineberg, Dean of the Harvard School of Public Health in Boston, USA.

One of the committee's findings was that, after more than forty years of routine vaccination, ". . . its extensive review was hindered by insufficient information in the medical literature . . ." and that " . . . research must be intensified" (Institute of Medicine, 1991). So much for the claim that vaccines have been thoroughly researched! A summary of the committee's findings is shown in Table 3-8.

The Project Director, Dr C P Howson, claimed that the study should reassure and not frighten parents. However, he also estimated that two in

100,000 children could have potentially life-threatening allergic reactions, and up to ten in 1,000,000 children could suffer severe brain damage (reported in the Tampa Tribune, 5.7.1991). If Dr Howson's estimates are correct, we could assume that, based on approximately 1,000,000 vaccinations administered in Australia annually, twenty to thirty children die and up to ten suffer severe brain damage as a result of vaccination. While doctors may claim that this is an acceptable risk, it is an unnecessary waste of life in otherwise healthy children. It also represents only the most extreme of permanently-damaging reactions.

In 1986 the US government established an agency to compensate parents of vaccine-damaged children. The payout to 179 claimants up until May 1988 was $US108.2 million. However, in 1991, there were around 4,100 further petitions pending, with a potential payout value of over $US3 billion.

The UK Vaccine Damage Payments Scheme for whooping cough vaccine made 344 awards between 1965 and 1975. The tribunal awards also led to an estimate of brain damage in approximately 1 in 25,000 children who received the vaccine between 1958 and 1981, although other studies have reported various rates (Mediolegal, 1986). Dr H Barrie made a further estimate of 600 awards from 1979 to 1983.

The payouts by 2010 totalled 2 billion dollars – what more evidence does one need that vaccines can cause severe damage? And these cases are the tip of a very large iceberg of chronic illness.

These and other similar figures lead the editors of the prestigious British Medical Journal to warn that "The balance between risks and benefits to the individual tips strongly in favour of the vaccine when acceptance rates are low and the disease is common; it tips the other way as vaccination rates climb and the disease declines" (BMJ Editorial, 1981). Apparently, even strong advocates of routine vaccination acknowledge that there is a cut off point beyond which further vaccination of the population will result in an overall worsening of general health due to the adverse effects of vaccination.

In 1993, a report arising from the national childhood encephalopathy study in Britain concluded that, while supporting vaccination in general,

"Diphtheria, tetanus and pertussis vaccine may on rare occasions be associated with the development of severe acute neurological illnesses that can have serious sequelae" (Miller D L et.al., 1993). These findings were understated due to the failure to recognise adverse reactions beyond seven days. Dr Scheibner (reported in Appendix 1 in Section 3.5.7) clearly showed that the adverse effects of vaccines last well beyond seven days. This is supported by research into the effects of tetanus vaccination (refer Section 2.4.3).

In 1994, Dr Odent and colleagues reported clear evidence that **children who received pertussis vaccine had a 5.43 times greater chance of developing asthma in later years than unvaccinated children**. They also had twice as many ear infections and were likely to be hospitalised for longer periods. These findings provide convincing evidence that the long term risks of vaccination have been understated (Odent M. et.al, 1994b, pp. 592-3).

Other articles have indirectly supported Odent's hypothesis regarding a link between asthma and DPT vaccination. For example, Kemp and colleagues studied 1,265 children in Christchurch, New Zealand born in 1977. The 23 who were not vaccinated against DPT and Polio had no recorded asthma or other allergic illnesses before the age of 10. In the immunised children, 23.1% had asthma, 22.5% had asthma consultations, and 30.0% had consultations for other allergic illnesses. Similar differences were observed at ages 5 and 16 years (Kemp T et al, 1997). My own research reported in Sections 4 and 5 have built on the work of Dr Odent and confirmed and extended his findings.

Finally, in Australia, we find that the medical professionals responsible for administering whooping cough vaccine and urging parents to vaccinate their children are themselves frequently concerned regarding its safety. Even more disturbing is the fact that approximately half of these would administer the vaccine in situations where health authorities and vaccine manufacturers recommend against vaccination due to potentially serious side effects. In a postal survey of 765 randomly-selected Victorian health professionals involved in childhood vaccination, all were found to "have doubts about the safety of the pertussis vaccine". The study also found that 34% of respondents believed that "pertussis vaccine causes permanent brain damage ... 39% believed it causes encephalopathy ... and up to 54% would give DPT when it is clearly contra-indicated." (MacIntyre C R & Nolan T, 1994).

These findings highlight the hypocrisy of health professionals criticising parents who have fought to obtain information about this vaccine and subsequently decided not to have their children vaccinated. When considered in association with the summaries of short-term and long-term side effects of vaccination generally, the information above argues strongly that whooping cough vaccination presents significant dangers.

The above information relates to whole cell vaccines. The claims that the acellular vaccine is much safer are reassuring. For example, Le Saux and colleagues found a much lower incidence of febrile seizures presenting to Canadian hospitals following the introduction of acellular pertussis vaccination on 1977-78 (Le Saux N, 2003). The controlled trial by Gustafsson and colleagues mentioned in Section 3.6.13.2 above found that "the whole cell vaccine was associated with significantly higher rates of protracted crying, cyanosis, fever and local reactions than the other 3 vaccines" (which did not contain whole cell vaccine). The rates of adverse events were similar for the acellular vaccines and the control DT vaccine" (Gustafsson L et al, 1996, p. 349).

However, we have heard it all before when we were told that the whole cell vaccines were safe. Only time will tell how safe the new vaccines really are. Neustaedter reviewed some safety trials of the new vaccines and found that while there were fewer mild aggravations, that serious aggravations still occurred (Neustaedter R, 2002, pp. 231-233). As noted above, the new acellular vaccines may be loosing their efficacy, but of course they are no less toxic. A loose-loose for parents.

9.2.13.5 The alternatives to pertussis vaccines

Homoeopathy offers a simple and safe alternative to routine vaccination against whooping cough. A specific remedy for protection against infection may be used in conjunction with constitutional remedies. In addition, valuable supportive work can be done to enhance a child's general immunity by ensuring that both child and parents have a nutritious and balanced diet, and by using massage to stimulate drainage of toxins from the body. Chiropractic work may also assist general immunity.

The nosode Pertussin can be administered infrequently in high potencies, offering a decided advantage in that it is non-toxic (unlike the conventional vaccine), and therefore can be given safely to very young babies who are most at risk from the both the disease and the vaccination.

The potential value of the nosode Pertussin has even been noted in the British Medical Journal, where Dr A Campbell stated: "In common with other homoeopathic medication, Pertussin is safe and free from side effects but its efficacy as a preventative is uncertain as no clinical trials have been carried out. There is no reason why this form of homoeopathic immunization should not be given to children who are considered unsuitable for the orthodox vaccine, or those whose parents refuse orthodox immunization" (Campbell A, 1986, p. 538).

Although Dr Campbell recommended the homoeopathic nosode in high risk cases, or for infants whose parents have chosen not to vaccinate, there is no reason why it cannot be used for all children. His reference to the "uncertain" effectiveness of the nosode is only true in that the scientific community has so far chosen not to test homoeopathy in general. As previously mentioned, there is a 200 year history of clinical practice supporting the effectiveness of homoeopathy, and the nosode Pertussin itself has also been well tested. As with the conventional vaccine, however, the length of protection afforded is uncertain at this time.

Since the aim of all methods of healing is to provide the patient with the most effective and least dangerous medication possible, homoeopathy should, and could without difficulty, be subjected to unbiased medical research to test its efficacy scientifically.

9.2.13.6 Comment

The information covered in this section may be summarised as follows:

- Vaccination against whooping cough was not responsible for the dramatic fall in deaths from the disease in the UK, USA, and Australia in this century.
- Vaccination against whooping cough does offer some protection against infection, but this cover is by no means certain.

- The procedure of vaccinating young children against infectious diseases carries a number of risks, possibly including subtle, long term changes to their health through damage of the immature immune system.
- While fatality from the disease itself is unlikely in developed countries, whooping cough can be a serious disease in very young children and a distressing one in the case of older children.
- Use of the homoeopathic nosode may provide effective protection against the disease, without the dangers associated with the orthodox vaccine. The efficacy and length of protection offered are not certain, however, extensive practical experience suggests they are no less than that provided by the vaccine. It is a genuine alternative to vaccination.

* * * * * * *

9.2.14 Pneumococcal Disease vaccination

9.2.14.1 The current vaccines

Two different pneumococcal vaccines are currently available in Australia. (1) a 23-valent pneumococcal polysaccharide vaccine (*23vPPV*) for use in older children and adults who are at risk of invasive pneumococcal disease (IPD); (2) a 7 valent pneumococcal vaccine combined with a non-toxic diphtheria toxin (*7vPCV*) for infants and children aged from 6 weeks to 9 years. The vaccines are:

Pneumovax 23 (CSL, MSD) – 23vPPV. Contains phenol.
Prevenar (W) – 7vPCV. Contains aluminium phosphate.

The efficacy of the pneumococcal vaccines is uncertain. Various studies have shown a wide range of results. For example, a meta-analysis of randomized controlled trials of the efficacy of pneumococcal vaccination in adults concluded that "Pneumococcal vaccination appears efficacious in reducing bacteremic pneumococcal pneumonia in low-risk adults. However, evidence from randomized controlled trials fails to demonstrate vaccine efficacy for pneumococcal infection-related or other medical outcomes in the heterogeneous group of subjects currently labelled as high risk" (Fine MJ et al, 1994, p. 2666).

Another trial of the efficacy of the vaccine in different at-risk groups showed a range of efficacy from 57% to 84% (Butler JC, 1993).

The MMWR Weekly, when commenting on the need to conserve doses of Prevenar vaccine, stated that the efficacy of 4 doses is 97%, of 3 doses is 87%, of 2 doses is 94%, and 1-2 doses is 86%. They then said "Because PCV7 is a new vaccine, no long-term data on vaccine effectiveness are available. However, the incidence of invasive pneumococcal disease declines rapidly after 2 years of age, even in unvaccinated children" (MMWR Weekly, 2004).

It certainly appears as though the vaccine has a low efficacy in the elderly, a low efficacy in preventing ear infections, but is effective in preventing pneumonia and IPD in children. As with some other vaccines, only time will tell if mass vaccination will simply result in moving the incidence of IPD to older age groups who are less able to withstand the disease, and less able to be well covered by the vaccine.

The NH&MRC report that about half of recipients of *Pneumovax 23* will experience soreness after the first injection, but only 5% experience severe pain and swelling. A few will experience fevers. 11% of *Prevenar* recipients experience injection site reactions and some fever (NH&MRC, 2008, p.249).

9.2.14.2 Comment

There is variable evidence as to the efficacy of the vaccine, although there is undoubtedly a definite level of effectiveness. The long-term safety of the vaccine has yet to be fully tested. Given that IPD is potentially serious in young children, some prevention is recommended. The homoeopathic option is once again available if required.

* * * * * * *

9.2.15 Poliomyelitis vaccination

Many parents, who reject vaccines for other diseases, still consider using vaccination against polio. This is understandable because the most severe effects of this disease are both obvious and distressing.

It is commonly suggested that polio suddenly became widespread during the 1950's, but was quickly eradicated by the introduction of the Salk vaccine and later the Sabin vaccines. In addition, since the vaccine is administered orally in Australia, some of the drawbacks of injected vaccines are avoided.

While there appear to be strong arguments in support of vaccination against polio, even where other vaccines are not used, parents are again only given a fraction of the facts - usually just the vaccine manufacturer's version of the story.

9.2.15.1 The vaccine

Two types of polio vaccine have been used:

- Salk (IPV - inactivated polio vaccine) derived from killed polio virus grown in a special medium on the kidney tissue of a species of monkey; the virus is killed without destroying its power to stimulate antibody production
- Sabin (OPV - oral polio vaccine), usually trivalent (i.e., containing Types 1, 2, and 3); the vaccine is live, attenuated, and propagated in monkey tissue culture; residual amounts of antibodies may be present in the final preparation which would multiply in the intestinal tract and be excreted in the faeces for two to six weeks.

The vaccines in use are:

IPOL (AP) – IPV, types 1, 2 and 3. The virus is grown on monkey kidney VERO cells, and inactivated with formaldehyde. Also contains neomycin, streptomycin, and polymyxin B.

Combination vaccines that contain both DTPa and IPV (see other Sections) are **Infanrix hexa**; **Infarix IPV**; **Infarix Penta** (these 3 for younger children); **Boostrix IPV**; **Adacel Polio** (for people older than 8 years).

The oral polio vaccine previously used is now no longer used in Australia (**Polio Sabin** (GSK) – OPV types 1, 2 and 3) due to concerns regarding vaccine associated paralytic poliomyelitis (acquired from the vaccine itself), and vaccine derived polio virus (contactees of recently vaccinated individuals).

The most widely publicised medical 'pioneer' in the fight against polio during the 1950's was Dr Jonas Salk. In 1954, the original vaccine Salk produced was demonstrated to be "reasonably safe but ineffective" (The Francis Report, 1955). In 1955, a new, strengthened version was released, but it was obviously less safe because it was withdrawn rather quickly: its aggravation of symptoms resulted in a spate of legal damage suits in the US. During the 1955 US epidemic, for example, three public health experts found that in Idaho:

(a) The disease struck in areas where there had been no previous Polio cases

(b) Only children who had received the vaccine became ill

(c) The first signs of paralysis occurred in the arm where the children were vaccinated

(d) The paralysis developed first in upper extremities, although the disease usually affects the legs first (The United Press, 5 May 1955).

In the infamous "**Cutter incident**", 380,000 children received doses of the Salk vaccine and 40,000 developed abortive polio, 51 were permanently paralysed and 5 died. As well, 113 people in the children's families or communities were paralyzed, and 5 died. Wyeth Laboratories also produced one lot of vaccine that paralyzed and killed several children in the Northeast (Offit P, 2005, p. 1411).

As a result, the Salk vaccine was replaced by the Sabin oral vaccine in a number of countries, including the US, UK, and Australia. In 1977, Dr Salk concluded: "the live virus vaccine is less effective than had been expected. Immunity in the individual is not reliably established because vaccine virus implementation is blocked by the presence of unexplained inhibitors in the intestinal tract" (Salk J & D, 1977, p. 840).

In discussing why only some children were affected by the vaccine, Dr Klenner stated: "that resistant children are able to stand the vaccine while the susceptible children, the ones highly in need of protection, cannot resist the attenuated active virus present in all of the polio vaccines available, and thus promptly come down with the disease" (Klenner FR, 1955, p. 6).

Dr Salk finally admitted that the live virus vaccines are now the principal cause of Polio in the US and other countries (Salk J & D, 1977, p. 840). His comments are still true today.

Furthermore, the vaccine was found to be dangerous to the unborn foetus (Slone D et al, 1973, p. 648). In fact, other serious, long term problems have been attributed to the vaccines. For example, a report of research undertaken by US Dr Eva Snead described an "Immunization Related Syndrome", and included these points:

(a) Hungarian scientists found SV40 virus (a virus similar to AIDS) in excreta of children who had received oral poliomyelitis vaccines.

(b) Russian scientists found similar results.

(c) The virus contaminated the vaccine because the vaccine was produced in kidney tissue of the African Green Monkey, now a known carrier of SV40.

(d) Millions of persons worldwide may be harbouring the virus through taking poliomyelitis vaccine (Snead E, 1987).

Anyone questioning the truth of Dr Snead's findings should ask:

- why the incidence of AIDS in Central Africa is highest in those countries subject to the most intensive WHO polio vaccination programs
- why the only South American country covered by the polio eradication campaign (Brazil) also has the highest incidence of AIDS in that region
- why the WHO tried to suppress these findings being established by the consultant it had hired to investigate the crisis.

Dr John West concluded: "as all live vaccines have been cultured upon monkey cell tissues they all come under the same umbrella! . . . and the whole vaccine manufacturing industry must be held to accountability" (West J, 1988, p. 13).

The SV40 factor appeared again linking OPVC to SSPE in New Zealand. "From 1956 to 1966 the incidence of subacute sclerosing panencephalitis (SSPE) in the northern half of the North Island of New Zealand was approximately one hundred times greater than might be expected. No case was seen before 1956, and none has been seen since 1969. … Mass vaccination of primary school children with Salk vaccine was begun in 1956. The vaccine used is likely to have contained live SV40 virus. Killed measles virus is another possible contaminant. It is believed that the administration of Salk vaccine in New Zealand was related to the appearance of SSPE in the community. The idea that an unusual reaction to measles infection is the sole cause of SSPE is not consistent with the observations in New Zealand" (Baguley DM & Glasgow GL, 1973, p. 763).

SV40 has been more recently linked to the dramatic increase in cases of non-Hodgkin lymphoma (a group of blood born cancers) in the USA from 1970 to 2000. 42% of non-Hodgkin lymphomas tested here contained SV40 DNA sequences. Millions of people in the USA were exposed to live SV40 DNA through contaminated polio vaccine (Mercola J, 2002(a)).

In Australia, it was reported in 2004 that "A federal government agency knowingly released polio vaccine contaminated with a monkey virus in the 1960's that has since been linked to cancers, including mesothelioma. An investigation by *The Age* found that at least four batches of vaccine – almost 3 millions doses – were contaminated with the virus between 1956 and 1962. Two of those batches were released after testing positive to contamination. The other two had been released by the time tests were carried out. An unknown number of earlier batches were also certainly contaminated. Documents from the then government-owned Commonwealth Serum Laboratories show that it decided to release one batch of about 700,000 doses of contaminated vaccine in 1962 on the grounds that 'much vaccine issued in the past was probably similarly contaminated'" … "CSL was aware from its own research that the monkey virus could cause cancer in humans. The research, which was never made public, was carried out in August 1962 while contaminated batches of vaccine were still being released" (The Age, 2004).

Other reports suggest that not only the Salk vaccine was contaminated, but also the oral Sabin vaccine, which could explain "why SV40 has been found in tumours removed from people who had never received the contaminated Salk vaccine" (Carlsen W, 2001).

In 2004, Bookchin and Schumacher published what may become the definitive record on the SV40 contamination of polio vaccine. Anyone interested in studying a carefully documented record of the whole affair would do well to read their excellent book. They conclude; "The story of SV40 invites us to take pause. The decisions of our health policy makers, even when well intentioned, are not always enlightened. And sometimes those decisions are not even well intentioned. Sometimes they are based on bias or inadequate scientific evidence. Sometimes they are influenced by the close relationship between the pharmaceutical industry and the government health officials who are charged with regulating that industry. Moreover, sometimes even the best scientists can make mistakes. The safest medical procedures can have unforseen side effects. Things do occasionally go wrong, sometimes dreadfully wrong, even during the most noble of scientific endeavours. For that reason, individuals, not governments, must maintain the right to control what medical procedures they and their children undergo and what pharmaceuticals they consume. As long as medicine in general, and pharmaceuticals in particular, remain for-profit industries, it may be reasonably asked whether safety isn't, at times, subservient to the bottom line" (Bookchin D & Schumacher J, 2004, p. 284).

The UK Department of Health Medical Memorandum (referred to earlier) stated: "The statistical evidence of a connection between inoculation and the development of paralytic poliomyelitis is strong . . . it is suggested that immunisation schemes in the locality of an outbreak should be postponed and the local practitioners informed"(Ministry of Health (UK), 1954, p. 10).

The Institute of Medicine has acknowledged that OPV can cause both paralytic polio and Guillain-Barré syndrome (Institute of Medicine, 1994). For example, "A recent outbreak of the paralysing viral infection polio in Haiti and the Dominican Republic has been traced to a strain of oral polio vaccine (OPV) that mutated back to virulence, according to international health officials. Based on genetic analysis of viral samples, they believe the outbreak, which struck nearly two dozen children in both countries between 2000 and 2001, arose from one OPV given to one child in 1998-1999" (reported in Mercola J, 2002).

It is no wonder that Australian Drs Kalokerinos and Dettman appealed to Rotarians not to help unleash polio vaccination on helpless Third World residents through their well meaning, but potentially lethal, drive to raise funds to vaccinate the millions (Kalokerinos A & Dettman G, 1987, 1988).

9.2.15.2 The figures relating to polio

As summarised in the Figures in Section 3.1.4.3 for the US, UK, and Australia, polio continued over the 1920's to the mid 1940's, with minor periodic epidemics. While substantial epidemics occurred in the late 1940's and early 1950's, the disease appears to have been virtually eliminated from the 1960's onwards. Two aspects of these figures required specific examination:

Firstly, the figures do not conclusively prove that the vaccine was responsible for ending the epidemic of the 1950's:

- In the UK, the disease peaked in 1947 and 1950 (the vaccine was introduced in 1956)
- In the US, peaks occurred in 1948 and 1952 (vaccine introduced in 1955)
- In Australia, the disease peaked in 1953 (vaccine introduced in 1956)

These figures demonstrate that epidemics in each country were waning before vaccination was introduced; this decline may well have continued with or without the introduction of the vaccine.

Secondly, it would seem that the vaccine did remove the basic pool of polio cases existing before the 1950's, as indicated by the level of notifications and fatalities falling to almost nil from the 1970's onwards. However, doubts have been raised concerning these figures:

According to Dr T C Fry, the 1950's polio epidemic in the USA was further diffused by a statistical 'fiddle' resulting in less likelihood of polio being reported.

Dr Fry stated: "In conjunction with the introduction of the Salk vaccine, new guidelines were established by the Centre for Disease Control for the diagnosis of polio. Not only was paralysis necessary before the polio diagnosis could be made but it had to persist for more than sixty days. This cut the polio cases down to 10 to 15 per year automatically, for that was the extent of the number of cases even before the Salk vaccine. Yet from the publicity you'd think we had 55,000 cases of infantile paralysis a year instead of a few cases with most of the polio symptoms being 'not life threatening and seldom lasting more than two weeks" (Kalokerinos A & Dettman G, 1986).

I personally tested this remarkable assertion by writing to the Centre for Disease Control, Department of Health and Human Services, Atlanta, USA. The Centre replied as follows:

"Since 1958 all States used a case record consisting of a preliminary and a 60-day follow-up form. These changes permitted Centres for Disease Control to analyse only those reported paralytic poliomyelitis cases that can be classified as 'best available paralytic poliomyelitis case count' (BAPPCC). These cases must be clinically and epidemiologically compatible with paralytic poliomyelitis and have a neurological deficit 60 days after onset of initial symptoms, unless death has occurred or the follow-up status is unknown. The BAPPCC excludes paralytic poliomyelitis cases with no residual paralysis at 60 days after onset of initial symptoms, as well as cases of aseptic meningitis (due to poliovirus or other enteroviruses)."(CDC, 1988).

While Dr Fry's statement appears to be correct regarding a 'defining away' of the problem, it is inaccurate as to timing - the new guidelines were not introduced "in conjunction" with the Salk vaccine, but three years later.

Nevertheless, the figures do suggest that the US epidemic was waning (1952-1955) prior to the introduction of the Salk vaccine in 1955, and continued to wane through to the introduction of the Sabin vaccine in

1961, with few cases thereafter. It is, therefore, questionable whether the Sabin vaccine contributed anything to the overall decline since: (i) the decline was already established, and (ii) the new guidelines for notification reduced the statistical likelihood of polio cases being reported.

If the incidence of polio from 1920 to 1957 could be charted using the criteria established in the 1958 guidelines, the argument could be resolved. Since this is not possible, it can only be said that the US statistics cannot be used in full support of either side of the vaccination argument; they certainly don't prove that the vaccine was of value in preventing the disease.

Information generously provided by the UK Department of Health also suggests that the accuracy of the UK 'epidemic' figures relating to Polio are questionable: The Department acknowledged in 1954, at the height of the epidemic: "Many other agents cause an aseptic meningitis that cannot be differentiated from non-paralytic poliomyelitis, except by elaborate laboratory tests . . . it is not possible to make an accurate diagnosis without resort to virological tests, which are, unfortunately, time-consuming, expensive and not readily available" (Ministry of Health (UK), 1954, p. 5). Since it is recognised that diseases tend to be over-reported during an epidemic, this could easily have occurred in the case of polio for the reasons just stated.

An examination of current experience shows many examples of vaccine failure in heavily vaccinated populations - in Oman, Zambia, Brazil, and Taiwan (Salter RW et al, 1991).

Perhaps the last word on figures concerning polio should rest with the late Professor Robert Mendelsohn who, with others, pointed to a similar decline in cases during the European epidemics of the 1950's where vaccination against polio was not used as extensively as elsewhere (Mendelsohn R, 1984, p. 47). His observations support the idea that vaccination was not responsible for the decline.

9.2.15.3 The alternatives to vaccination

Although the majority of children exposed to the poliomyelitis virus will suffer nothing worse than a minor cold, some form of protection is strongly recommended since we do not have prior knowledge of a child's susceptibility. In addition, because exposure to the virus is so common in countries which use the oral vaccine (where the virus may be excreted by the vaccinated child for weeks following the oral dose), and because susceptibility is so disease-specific and intense in susceptible individuals, the general approach of strengthening a child's immune system through excellent diet, environment, and constitutional remedies may be insufficient. While this may be argued, the documented cases of very healthy and stress-free individuals acquiring infectious diseases suggest that disease-specific protection is warranted.

It has been repeatedly confirmed in clinical practice from the late 1800's to the present time that Lathyrus Sativus in the appropriate potency provides relatively effective protection against polio. This is because of the close similarity between the drug proving, to the symptoms of polio itself. It would also be possible to use potentised preparations of the (combined) various strains of the polio virus. Lathyrus Sativus (200) and (10M) form part of the homoeopathic program described in Section 4.2.1.1.

For community groups interested in improving health care in Third World countries, the homoeopathic alternative has many advantages over the standard vaccine, including:

- its proven effectiveness in clinical (if not laboratory) situations for over 200 years
- the extremely low cost involved compared with vaccines (minimising its exploitation for profit)
- it is much easier to administer than vaccines
- it is, most importantly, much safer than vaccines for malnourished children as it does not stress their weakened immune systems (not, as is often the unfortunate result of indiscriminate vaccination, resulting in possible death or permanent damage).

9.2.15.4 Comment

A clear picture of the disease polio emerges:

- it has been present for many years
- it has affected many individuals without causing obvious symptoms
- it is treatable

- the use of vaccines to prevent polio is, at best, only partially effective, and probably causes the disease in highly susceptible individuals - the only ones at real risk of suffering serious complications in the event of infection.

While these conclusions do not in any way detract from the tragedy of fully-developed paralytic poliomyelitis, they do argue against the use of a vaccine that is as likely to cause the disease as prevent it in the hypersensitive individuals who most need protection. For these, particularly the already vulnerable, malnourished children of Third World countries, homoeopathy provides safe, relatively effective, and economical protection.

* * * * * * *

9.2.16 Rubella vaccination

Mass vaccination of girls with rubella vaccine began in 1971. At risk women were also vaccinated. The MMR vaccination program for all adolescents replaced the rubella program for girls in 1993/94.

A discussion of the effects of rubella during pregnancy was given in Section 9.1.16.

9.2.16.1 The current vaccines

Rubella vaccine is usually administered as part of the MMR vaccine (**Priorix MMR** discussed earlier), although the following monovalent vaccine for rubella is available.

Meruvax II (CSL/MSD) – Contains human serum albumin, sorbitol and hydrolysed gelatin.

Two MMR vaccines are available in Australia, and are described in Section 9.2.20 following. The controversy concerning the MMR vaccine is discussed fully in that Section, and will not be repeated here. Suffice it to say that there are genuine concerns regarding the safety of the vaccine.

It is claimed that a single dose of rubella vaccine produces an antibody response in over 95% of vaccinated children and adults, and will persist for at least 16 years in the absence of endemic disease. However, protection does lessen over time, meaning that adults are no longer protected by the vaccine at the age when the disease has potentially serious implications during pregnancy.

Questions regarding the efficacy of the vaccine have been raised in Australia, including the following:

- In 1978, Dr Beverley Allan of the Austin Hospital in Melbourne undertook trials on the effectiveness of rubella vaccination given to army recruits who had demonstrated low immunity to rubella. Within four months of receiving the vaccine, 80% of these recruits contracted rubella while training in a known high-exposure environment (Allan B, 1978). Dr Allan found similar poor efficacy rates in another study she undertook in a psychiatric hospital.
- In 1982, the effectiveness of the vaccine in Australia was again questioned after a number of cases of Embryopathic Rubella were reported despite maternal vaccination (Brott LM, 1982, pp.514-515).

There is growing evidence that the rubella vaccine may lead to rheumatic and arthritic conditions in later years, amongst other problems (refer Table 3-8) for evidence of this link). In addition, evidence of a probable link between the vaccine and glandular fever may well explain why this disease previously occurred far more frequently in school-age girls than in boys of the same age (both sexes are now vaccinated).

Dr A Allen demonstrated scientifically that the vaccine was also the cause of Chronic Fatigue Syndrome, which was first reported in the United States in 1982 (Allen A, 1988). Dr Allen postulated that the cause was a new, more immunologic strain of the live rubella vaccine (RA27/3), which was first introduced in 1979. His findings are supported by Dr A D Lieberman (Lieberman A D,). Their refreshingly honest research and conclusions support earlier concerns regarding the safety of the rubella vaccine.

9.2.16.2 Comment

Rubella is possibly the most mild childhood infectious disease, but the vaccine has definite potentially serious side-effects. Many question whether the risk is worth it. The policy of vaccinating infants makes little sense when all that seems to be happening is that the disease is now shifting to adults.

It is clearly desirable for girls to contract rubella naturally before reaching child-bearing age, since the natural immunity which results is the most certain form of immunity. If protection against rubella is required during pregnancy, the specific homoeopathic nosode described in section 3.2 will provide protection without the risk of those side effects which mean that the vaccine cannot be given during pregnancy.

* * * * * * *

9.2.17 Tetanus vaccination

Tetanus vaccination is considered to be essential by some parents who question the use of other vaccines. Knowing that the tetanus organisms are present everywhere, they believe their children are constantly at risk if injured while playing near rusty iron, dogs, horses, etc. While there is anecdotal evidence of the vaccine saving many lives during the major wars of the 20th century, other writers dispute this claim.

However, there is considerable material which raises questions concerning the value of the vaccine. The figures provided in Section 4 are not helpful in drawing conclusions, as the falling trends in deaths from tetanus are not clearly attributable to any one cause.

9.2.17.1 Tetanus vaccines currently in use

The tetanus vaccines protect the recipient by stimulating the production of antitoxin. A number of combination vaccines incorporating tetanus vaccines are available in Australia. The following have already been discussed:

Infanrix hexa; Infanrix IPV; Infanrix Penta; Adacel; Adacel Polio; Boostrix; Boostrix IPV.

As well, the following adult booster is offered:

ADT Booster (CSL/Statens) - adult diphtheria-tetanus vaccine. Contains aluminium hydroxide.

Two other tetanus-related products are available, to be used following a wound.

Tetanus Immunoglobulin Human (for intravenous use) (CSL) -

This product is prepared from human plasma obtained by the Red Cross from voluntary donors who have been actively immunised against tetanus, and have a high concentration of antibodies to tetanus toxin; no antiseptic is included. The product is used in the management of clinical tetanus.

Tetanus Immunoglobulin (intramuscular injection) (CSL)

This product is also prepared from human plasma obtained by the Red Cross from voluntary donors who have been actively immunised against tetanus, and has a high concentration of antibodies to tetanus toxin; however, Thiomersal 0.01% w/v is added as a preservative.

The product is used for passive protection of individuals who have received a tetanus-prone wound and have either not been actively immunised against tetanus (within the last ten years) or whose immunisation history is doubtful. It can also be used for prevention of neonatal tetanus when newborn infants considered to be at risk are born of mothers who are non-immune to tetanus.

The efficacy of the vaccine is not certain. One pharmacist informed me that in order to render the vaccine safe it has been significantly diluted, thereby making it clinically ineffective, and that improved sanitation and personal hygiene is preventing tetanus.

This view is supported by Professor Robert Mendelsohn, who stated: "The tetanus vaccine over the decades has been progressively weakened in order to reduce the considerable reaction (fever and swelling) it used to cause. Accompanying this reduction in reactivity has been a concomitant reduction in antigenicity (the ability to confer protection). Therefore, there is a good chance that today's tetanus vaccine is about as effective as tap water . . . until the last few years, government statistics admitted that 40 percent of the child population of the US was not immunized. For all those decades, where were the tetanus cases from all those rusty nails?" (Mendelsohn R,). In other words, infection rates declined markedly even while many children were not vaccinated.

However, other studies suggesting that tetanus nearly always occurs in people who have not been fully vaccinated present a picture of a highly effective vaccine (Esdall, 1959).

The NH&MRC have stated that it is common to experience some injection site discomfort or pain which can last for a few days, but that other reactions are rare (NH&MRC 2008, p. 295).

Drs Eibl, Martha and others have presented research showing that a temporary AIDS-like state can be induced in patients following tetanus vaccination. They showed that the ratio of helper-to-suppressor TÄLymphocytes in healthy adults fell after vaccination, the largest drop occurring between three to fourteen days post vaccine. This drop in helper/suppressor ratios is characteristic of Acquired Immune Deficiency Syndrome (Eibl, Martha et al, 1984).

The question this raises is that, if the vaccine causes a significant effect in healthy adults, what effect does it have on the relatively immature immune systems of young children? Certainly, it suggests that a state of 'anergy' (immunologic unresponsiveness) is caused by tetanus vaccination, leading to increased susceptibility to a whole range of diseases. This may further explain the experience of Dr Kalokerinos among Australian Aboriginal children referred to in Sections 2.1, 3.4.2, and 3.5.2.

9.2.17.2 Comments

Immediate and effective wound hygiene is the most important first line of defence against tetanus. The immunoglobulin is available when vaccination is incomplete.

Once again, the homoeopathic alternative to tetanus vaccination is a legitimate option for parents to consider, as well as the routine use of Ledum 30 (3 doses a day for 3 days) following any wound.

* * * * * * *

9.2.18 Tuberculosis vaccination

9.2.18.1 The current vaccines

BCG vaccine (AP) - freeze-dried live vaccine from attenuated strain of Mycobacterium bovis. Contains monosodium glutamate.

Vaccine efficacy has been set between 0 to 80%, depending on the type of vaccine strains and the recipient's age. It is meant to be highly effective in children less than 5 years of age

Adverse events are reported in about 5% of cases. However, the full picture of reactions to this vaccine is not well studied.

9.2.18.2 Comment

The vaccine is not highly effective, except possibly in young children. Certain homoeopathic nosodes are available which can offer some protection against the disease.

* * * * * * *

9.2.19 Typhoid vaccination

9.2.19.1 The current vaccines

The vaccines available in Australia are:

Vivotif Oral (CSL/Berna) (CSL/Berna) - oral live attenuated typhoid vaccine, strain Ty21A Berna.

Typherix (GSK) - purified Vi capsular polysaccharide vaccine. Contains phenol.

Typhim Vi (SP) - purified Vi capsular polysaccharide vaccine. Contains phenol.

Vivaxim (SP) - combination typhoid and hepatitis A vaccines. Contains aluminium hydroxide, formaldehyde, neomycin and bovine serum albumin.

Efficacy is estimated at between 50 and 77% for the Vi vaccines.

The whole cell vaccines are more effective, but carry much higher risks of adverse reactions (Acharya et al, 1987, p. 268; Levine et al, 1990).

Reported adverse reactions include injection site symptoms in 10-20% of cases.

9.2.19.2 Comment

Homoeopaths have been preventing typhoid using potentised remedies for nearly 200 years. This approach would appear to be a superior option to the vaccines, which are not very effective, and which carry various risks of damage.

* * * * * * *

Some additional vaccines considered

9.2.20 Measles, Mumps, Rubella vaccination

Individual vaccines for measles and mumps are no longer available in Australia. A single vaccine is available for rubella. However, the vaccine delivery for these three diseases was almost always carried out using one of two combination MMR vaccines.

9.2.20.1 The current vaccines

In September 2010, one MMR vaccine remains available in Australia, although there is expectation that a MMRV vaccine will soon be available (including varicella or chicken pox with the MMR components). The vaccine is reported in the orthodox literature to be highly effective in clinical trials – 95% after one dose and up to 99% for measles after the second dose (NH&MRC, 2008, p. 183). As has been shown earlier, these claims do not stand up in field trials, where the efficacy varies considerably.

The vaccine currently used in Australia is:

Priorix (GSK) - live attenuated measles virus (Schwarz strain), mumps virus (derived from Jeryl Lynn strain), and rubella virus strain (Wistar 27/3 strain). The vaccine includes lactose; neomycin; amino acids; sorbitol; mannitol.

Adverse reactions reported in the literature include:

- A rash and weakness for 7-10 days following vaccination, lasting 2-3 days.
- Moderate to high fever.
- A variety of potentially severe reactions, including febrile convulsions, anaphylaxis, encephalopathy, thrombocytopenia have been reported occurring up to 2-3 weeks following the vaccine.
- An association between MMR vaccine and inflammatory bowel disease and autism has created controversy in the orthodox

literature. The official claims dismissing these concerns have left many, including myself, unconvinced.

Many doctors used to recommend that children not be vaccinated against rubella - only females approaching child bearing age. However, due to the routine use of the combined Measles Mumps Rubella vaccine, most children of both sexes now are vaccinated against rubella as well as mumps and measles. The forceful use of this vaccine has been publicly attacked by a group of about two hundred Swiss doctors, who raised concerns as to the safety and effectiveness of this vaccine, stating: "The fears expressed against the MMR vaccination campaign concern the complications that may appear in the short term. But of more concern are the consequences in the longer term; complications that occur in each individual or in the natural balance that exists between these viruses and man" (Albonico H, 1990, p. 10).

They continued: "It is thus possible that doctors and parents live in a fool's paradise as to the allegedly rare risks associated with vaccination. This is demonstrated by the East German experience." "In that country, vaccination is compulsory and so too is the obligation to report and compensate cases of vaccination damage. The recorded complication rates are then much higher than the estimates put forward in our country. It remains a difficult task to record the complications due to vaccinations. For example, mellitus diabetes resulting from vaccination against mumps may not appear until quite a few months after the event" (Albonico H, 1990, p. 12).

Some other examples are summarised as follows:

* **In 1993, Japanese health authorities discontinued the use of the MMR vaccine**. One reason was that the vaccine was causing mumps in recipients. Initially, side effects from the vaccine were predicated as 1/100,000-200,000. This was subsequently revised to 1/30,000. In practice, however, reactions were found to be as frequent as 1/300. Japanese authorities directed that children be vaccinated separately for each of the three diseases (Int. Vacn. Newsletter, 1995, p. 18). More recently **payments to parents of children who have died or suffered serious side effects from the MMR vaccine continue to be made** (Japan Times online, 2003). Information gained under Freedom of Information

law shows that the Japanese government has recognised over 1,000 people to be eligible for help as a result of damage caused by the MMR vaccine.

* Roberts and others examined an outbreak of measles and found that the MMR vaccine was not only ineffective, but increased the severity of the disease. "Symptoms were equally common among immunised and non-immunised subjects. However, significantly more immunised boys than non-immunised boys reported fever, rash, joint symptoms, and headache." (Roberts R J, 1995).

* Joyce and Rees cited the example of a twenty year old man who was vaccinated with MMR. He developed post-vaccination transverse myelitis and remained partially paralysed after treatment. Blood tests showed that there was no increase in measles and mumps antibody titres (Joyce A & Reese J E, 1995).

* On 16 September 1992, the New Zealand Health Department withdrew one of the two brands of MMR vaccine used in that country, namely Pluserix. The reason given for this withdrawal was that a British study had found two cases of meningitis in 22,000 doses of the vaccine administered to British children. Canada and Australia had withdrawn this vaccine eighteen months prior, and Britain also withdrew the vaccine. Despite the withdrawal, this vaccine is still registered for use in some of these countries in the event of an emergency should supplies of the other vaccine run out during an epidemic.

In a thorough review of the MMR vaccine, Neustaedter identified the following possible adverse reactions: acute encephalopathy, Guillain-Barré syndrome, deafness, optic neuritis, thrombocytopenia, inflammatory bowel disease, atypical measles, immune system suppression, meningitis, diabetes, acute arthritis, chronic persistent arthritis, central and peripheral nervous system disorders, and autism (Neustaedter R, 2002, pp. 205-210; 213-4; 218-221).

The so called "Wakefield affair" has thrown the MMR vaccine into the spotlight since the late 1990's, when Dr Andrew Wakefield and his team observed that the parents of eight out of twelve children investigated for gastrointestinal symptoms and autism associated the onset of autism with the MMR vaccine (Wakefield AJ et al, 1998).

Dr Tom Heller made some refreshingly honest comments concerning this. He said "My duties as a general practitioner include immunizing babies and small children against a range of common diseases. Recently, I have been increasingly uncomfortable when giving the combined mumps, measles, and rubella (MMR) vaccine. I find myself wondering if I would submit my own children for this immunization if they were currently at that age.

I find it difficult to be certain that the vaccine is as safe as the authorities say that it is. Somehow, the more strident the experts become, the less believable I seem to find them" (Heller T, 2001, p. 838).

He goes on to note some relevant points, including:

(i) authorities emphasize pro-MMR research and avoid referencing anti-MMR research

(ii) weaknesses in pro-MMR research are ignored while weaknesses in anti-MMR research are highlighted in detail

(iii) doctors in the UK are given financial incentives to vaccinate as many children as possible (similarly in Australia)

(iv) many researchers have financial links with pharmaceutical companies who manufacture what they research

Finally, he points out that many GP's have doubts about the vaccine. "A recent survey of health workers in north Wales sought to elicit the knowledge, attitudes, and practices relating to MMR vaccine, particularly the second dose. Only 45% of the professionals (54% of the general practitioners) agreed completely with the policy of giving the second dose of the MMR vaccine (Heller T, 2001, p. 838, quoting Petrovic M et al, 2001).

Heller's second point above is reinforced when it is seen that even strongest critics of Wakefield's findings who have attempted to cover all the weaknesses in pro-MMR trials still present results which are far from convincing.

For example, a recent study claiming to unambiguously support the MMR vaccine stated that "Overall, there was no increase in the risk of autistic disorder or other autistic-spectrum disorders among vaccinated children as compared with unvaccinated children (adjusted relative risk of autistic disorder, 0.92; 95 percent confidence interval, 0.68 to 1.24; adjusted relative risk of other autistic-spectrum disorders, 0.83; 95 percent confidence interval, 0.65 to 1.07). Furthermore, we found no association between the development of autistic disorder and the age at vaccination (P=0.23), the interval since vaccination (P=0.42), or the calendar period at the time of vaccination (P=0.06)" (Madsen KN et al, 2002).

Far from being conclusive, these figures show a range of results (CI's > 1) which could actually support an association between MMR vaccine and autism. Further, their final 3 results showed P>0.05, the orthodox community's cut-off point for confidence, meaning that their results were not statistically conclusive.

Wakefield was not alone. Professor V Singh analysed blood from 140 children, 80 of them with autism, and found antibodies linked to the measles vaccine in 53% of the autistic children, but no antibodies in the non-autistic children (Singh V & Yang V, 1998). Professor John O'Leary revealed at a congressional hearing on 11/4/2000 that he had found measles virus in the guts of 24 out of 25 autistic children who developed epilepsy after a normal infancy.

More recently, a breakthrough study gave one group of monkeys (rhesus macaques) the infant vaccines and compared their mental-emotional wellbeing to another group who were not given the vaccine. The results were remarkable and conclusions self-evident vaccination causes autism:

"**Results:** Compared with unexposed animals, significant neurodevelopmental deficits were evident for exposed animals in survival reflexes, tests of color discrimination and reversal, and learning sets. Differences in behaviors were observed between exposed and unexposed animals and within the exposed group before and after MMR vaccination. Compared with unexposed animals, exposed animals showed attenuation of amygdala growth and differences in the amygdala binding of [11C]diprenorphine. Interaction models identified significant associations between specific aberrant social and non-social behaviors, isotope binding, and vaccine exposure.
Conclusions: This animal model, which examines for the first time, behavioral, functional, and neuromorphometric consequences of the childhood vaccine regimen, mimics certain neurological abnormalities of autism. The findings raise important safety issues while providing a potential model for examining aspects of causation and disease pathogenesis in acquired disorders of behavior and development." (Hewitson L et.al., 2008).

This paper was submitted to Neurology journal, where it was accepted. When the editors realised that Dr Wakefield was one of the authors it was withdrawn, and now it may reappear with his name removed from the authors list. So much for truth in science.

In his address to the American Congress on 19/6/2007, Hon. Dan Burton referred to two other "hard science" pieces of animal research implicating vaccines with autism (one by Dr Hornig using mice, and another by Dr Burbacher on primates). No matter how hard orthodox authorities and pharma-funded skeptics attack this information, and work to discredit the scientists doing the research, facts are facts and the cover will and must fail.

In the years following his original article in the *Lancet* in Feb 1998, Dr Wakefield has been targeted by the orthodox medical establishment. He has been driven from the UK, accused of being a liar, and in Feb 2010 a full retraction of the 1998 paper was published by the *Lancet*. Dr Wakefield has published his reply in a book *Callous Disregard: Autism and Vaccines – the Truth Behind a Tragedy.*

For those of you who are interested in the real story behind this controversy this book is highly recommended, and you can draw your own conclusions. Personally, Big Pharma's record of deceit and corruption is so established that this organised attack on Dr Wakefield provides yet another example of their obsession with destroying any opposition to their products, and yet another example of how their massive financial power can and does corrupt leaders in medicine.

9.2.20.2 Comment

It is clear that there are significant doubts as to the safety and effectiveness of the MMR vaccine. Yet, parents continue to be told that their children are only ever given completely safe vaccines. The Wakefield affair and the comments by other medical practitioners show that we are not dealing with certainty.

The most disappointing aspect of the entire vaccination debate, highlighted by the MMR controversies, is that many intelligent people who do independent research are simply no longer prepared to trust pronouncements by orthodox medical authorities. They have been misled in the past, and are not prepared to vest the sole decision making regarding disease prevention into the hands of people they no longer trust.

This lack of trust is a tragedy. We should be able to have total confidence in the integrity of our national leaders in health. Instead, a growing number of informed parents doubt what they are told by health authorities - for good reason.

The three diseases covered by this vaccine are all mild conditions in healthy children, and very easily treated using homoeopathic medicine. There is every reason not to give the vaccine, or at least delay administration until the child is older (remember the beneficial effects the Japanese government found when delaying vaccination until two years of age. Further, if parents are really concerned about one or all of these diseases, homoeopathic preventatives are available to cover all three diseases.

* * * * * * *

9.2.21 Smallpox vaccination

Smallpox vaccination is often held up as the first great success of widespread community vaccination. It was claimed on 8 May 1980 that vaccination had eliminated smallpox from our planet.

Initially *variolation* was practised - the intentional inoculation of the smallpox virus. After this practice was banned the vaccine was prepared in animals, originally cattle and later sheep. However, there is much more to the issue and quoted figures than we are told.

The following sections analyse the historical experience with smallpox by examining the records of three countries: England (including Wales), the United States, and Germany. While there is a large body of anecdotal evidence concerning the effect of smallpox vaccination in many countries, the summaries below focus on documented facts.

9.2.21.1 Smallpox vaccination in specific countries

(1) England and Wales

1840 Variolation was made illegal.

1853 Compulsory vaccination was introduced.

"Following the introduction of vaccination the decline of the disease was not dramatic. Better social conditions, the control of vagrants, the establishment of workhouses, the setting up of smallpox hospitals and the surveillance and recording of the disease all played a highly important part in its control, as did the cessation of variolation, which eliminated a source of the virus" (Dick G, 1978, page 45).

1871 Vaccination was enforced.

1871 Worst epidemic occurred with 23,062 deaths in one year.

Prior to 1853 the highest smallpox death rate for any two year period was 2,000.

1887 In Sheffield, England, where 97% of her 20,000 inhabitants had been thoroughly and frequently vaccinated for many years, a smallpox epidemic caused 7,101 cases and 648 deaths (McBean E, 1957, p. 13).

1905 Allowed conscientious objection to vaccine.

1914 Less than 50% of children were vaccinated.

1928 Dr R P Garrow reported in the British Medical Journal that the fatality rate among vaccinated cases of smallpox was five times higher than among the unvaccinated, for people over the age of 15 years (Garrow RP, 1928).

1946 Compulsory vaccination was ended.

1951-70 Deaths from vaccination - 101; deaths from the disease - 37.

1972 Doctors were advised to cease vaccination due to potential adverse consequences.

(2) United States

1855/1872 Vaccination was enforced.

1971 Doctors were advised to cease vaccination.

(3) Germany

1870-71 124,948 deaths in highly vaccinated people (96%).

Bismarck, the Chancellor of Germany wrote that "the hopes placed in the efficacy of the cowpox virus as preventative of smallpox have proved entirely deceptive" (Chaitow L, 1987, p. 5).

1871 "Yet after 35 years of this double and triple vaccination, enforced with a rigour unknown in any other country, the mortality from smallpox in Prussia in 1871 was 69,839, equal to a death rate of 2,430 per million living, or 2½ times the smallpox death-rate in England for the same great epidemic year" (The Harbinger of Light, June 1, 1885).

1928 Dr L A Parry wrote "How is it that in Germany, the best vaccinated country in the world, there are more deaths in proportion to the population than in England." (Parry LA, 1928). At that time less than 50% of English children were vaccinated.

(4) Japan

1872 compulsory vaccination was introduced.

1892 steady increase in the disease to 165,000 cases and 30,000 deaths (Neustaedter R, 2000, p. 249).

In Australia, the USA smallpox vaccine **Dryvax**, has been used to vaccinate Australian laboratory personnel working with poxviruses. This vaccine contains vaccinia which produces cross-immunity against variola.

9.2.21.2 Comment

The statement that smallpox vaccination caused the near elimination of the disease is not correct. It is clear that smallpox was actively present in populations where vaccination rates were high, and declined in many populations with low vaccination rates or none at all. The best preventative was adequate standards of sanitation, hygiene and nutrition. The facts are well summarised in the following final two quotes:

"The credit for the decline in the incidence of smallpox could not be given to vaccination. The fact is that its incidence declined in all parts of Europe, whether or not vaccination was employed" (Chaitow L, 1987, p. 6). "Smallpox died out of England as a result of a change in the social, environmental as well as nutritional status of the population as a whole. It appears unlikely that vaccination played a significant part at all in the demise of the disease" (Mowle A, 1981).

It is time that common statements about the "success" of smallpox vaccination be generally acknowledged for what they really are - myths, not facts.

* * * * * * *

9.2.22 7th Edition Additions

9.2.23 Dengue Fever Vaccination

Currently there are no effective vaccines against Dengue Fever. As noted earlier, I am hoping to participate in a trial of homoeopathic immunisation against Dengue, and I have no doubt that if the trial takes place it will return results consistent with homoeoprophylaxis against other diseases, and make it a viable public health option.

* * * * * * *

9.2.24 Human Papiloma Virus vaccination

There are over 200 different types of human papiloma virus (HPV), but only a few typically cause high risk symptoms such as warts (types 6 and 11) and cancers (types 16 and 18). Both males and females can carry the virus. The vaccines provide little benefit to women who have already been infected with HPV types 16 and 18—which includes most sexually active females. Sexual activity is the transmission route for the potentially serious strains.

9.2.24.1 The Current Vaccines

There are 2 HPV vaccines registered for use in Australia.

- **CERVARIX** – GlaxoSmithKline (HPV types 16 and 18), plus aluminium hydroxide, 3-O-desacyl-4'-monophosphoryl lipid A [MPL], sodium chloride, sodium dihydrogen phosphate dihydrate.

- **GARDASIL** – CSL Biotherapies/Merck & Co Inc (HPV types 6, 11, 16 and 18), plus aluminium hydroxyphosphate sulphate, sodium chloride, L-histidine, polysorbate and sodium borate. May also contain yeast proteins.

The efficacy of the vaccines is variable, and has not been fully established for the 2 valent vaccine. No efficacy trials for children under 15 have been performed. Duration of vaccine efficacy is not yet fully established by rigorous methodologic trials. **Cervarix** efficacy is proven for 7.4 years with published data through 6.4 years while **Gardasil** efficacy is proven for 5 years.

There is also no certainty that HPV is the only cause of cervical cancer, nor that the vaccines will protect against types that can lead to cancer.

In the light of these uncertainties, the potential risks associated with the vaccines, especially **Gardasil**, must be considered. Orthodox sources acknowledge a significant percentage of skin reactions at the injection site, but little else. This is a disturbing omission by health authorities, because there have been numerous published reports of significant adverse effects of these vaccines.

These adverse reactions are not fictional. Australia has a very poor vaccine adverse event reporting system, unlike in the USA which has VAERS (vaccine adverse events reporting system). The information is publically available at http://vaers.hhs.gov/index.

According to NVIC Health Policy Analyst Vicky Debold, RN, Ph.D "The most frequent serious health events after GARDASIL shots are neurological symptoms. These young girls are experiencing severe headaches, dizziness, temporary loss of vision, slurred speech, fainting, involuntary contraction of limbs (seizures), muscle weakness, tingling and numbness in the hands and feet and joint pain. Some of the girls have lost consciousness during what appears to be seizures." Debold added "The manufacturer product insert should include mention of syncopal episodes, seizures and Guillain-Barre Syndrome so doctors and parents are aware these vaccine adverse responses have been associated with the vaccine."

VAERS reports also indicate the doctors are administering GARDASIL to girls and women at the same with Tdap, DT, meningococcal (Menactra), hepatitis A, and other vaccines, even though the Merck product insert states that, with the exception of hepatitis B vaccine, "Co-administration of GARDASIL with other vaccines has not been studied." There is no publicly available information about how many of the 9 to 15 year old girls in Merck's pre- licensure clinical trials received GARDASIL simultaneously with hepatitis B vaccine (Medical News Today, 2007).

In the USA in 2009 alone there were 32,817 reported adverse vaccine reactions. **Gardasil** was implicated in 3,305 reactions. These reactions included 194 deaths, of which **Gardasil** was implicated in at least 16. These figures provide a slight glimpse into the world of official statistics, and represent the tip of a potentially ugly iceberg.

In India in 2010, public pressure from citizens groups have stopped an HPV vaccination program because of severe side effects including death. It has been reported that "According to the extensive documentation compiled by the fact finding mission, of the 14,000 girls vaccinated, there have been 4 deaths and 120 reports of serious adverse reactions including, epileptic-like seizures, severe stomach ache, severe headaches, mood swings, early onset of menstruation, heavy bleeding and severe menstrual cramps." (Erikson N, 2010).

The Indian project received substantial finance from the Bill and Melinda Gates Foundation. I have no doubt that Mr and Mrs Gates would be shocked if they ever learned the extent to which their great generosity has been misused, and the suffering caused by the programs they have funded. The tragedy is that if only a fraction of their donations had been put to using homoeopathic immunisations, considerably more people could have been protected without any risk of toxic damage.

The US Government's own Centre for Disease Control reported in 2010 that "As of January 31, 2010, there were 15,829 VAERS reports of adverse events following **Gardasil** vaccination in the United States. Of these reports, 92% were reports of events considered to be non-serious, and 8% were reports of events considered serious." (CDC, 2010). The serious reactions included Guillain-Barré Syndrome, blood clots, and 49 deaths. Unsurprisingly, the CDC thought that none related to the vaccine even thought they occurred following the vaccine. But then, the CDC is the principal government proponent of vaccination in the world.

Once again, there is so much more data about **Gardasil** in particular that it could, and in time no doubt will fill a book of its own. I have treated severe reactions in my own clinic, and have heard of many more first hand accounts. I suspect that in time **Gardasil** will rank with the MMR vaccine in terms of adverse consequences for a product of questionable need.

9.2.24.2 Comment

Orthodox authorities recommend that women continue to have cervical screening, such as Pap smear testing, even after receiving the vaccine, and these recommendations have not changed for females who receive the HPV vaccine. Without continued screening, the number of cervical cancers preventable by vaccination alone is less than the number of cervical cancers prevented by regular screening alone (Harper D, 2009).

Given the potential for damage caused by the vaccine, the availability of a homoeopathic option, and the questionable effectiveness of the vaccine against cervical cancer, it is reasonable to conclude that the use of the vaccine in non-sexually active females is highly questionable, and is still doubtful in sexually active women.

* * * * * * *

9.2.25 Leptospirosis vaccination

9.2.25.1 The Current Vacines

The Finlay Institute, one of the main scientific institutes in Cuba, has produced the only three-valent Leptospirosis vaccine available on the market (vaxSpiral®). It is a whole cell inactivated vaccine with an efficacy of 78.1%. It proved to be of limited value in the 2007 and 2008 epidemics in Cuba due to the time needed to gain full coverage against the changing serotypes experienced in different outbreaks.

9.2.25.2 Comment

Due to the urgent need to protect the population of the three worst hit (eastern) provinces following severe hurricanes in 2007 and 2008, the Finaly Institute homoeopathically immunised 2.4 million and 2.2 million people in each year. The intervention was highly successful. It is described in detail in Section 4.1.8.

* * * * * * *

9.2.26 Rotavirus vaccination

9.2.26.1 The Current Vaccines

In Australia, Rotavirus immunisation was included on the National Immunisation Program (NIP) from 1 July 2007.The NIP will provide free rotavirus vaccine to all children born on or after 1 May 2007.
Two rotavirus vaccines are licensed for use in Australia:

- **Rotarix®** (GlaxoSmithKline); and
- **RotaTeq®** (CSL Limited/Merck and Co, Inc).

Both vaccines are live attenuated vaccines and must be given orally:

- **Rotarix®** is presented in a powdered form. Reconstitution with the provided diluent makes a 1mL oral dose.
- **RotaTeq®** is presented as a 2mL oral dose.

Both vaccines have claimed a similar efficacy against rotavirus gastroenteritis of any severity of around 70%. The efficacy against severe rotavirus gastroenteritis and against hospitalisation for rotavirus gastroenteritis is claimed to be higher, ranging from 85 to 100% in clinical trials in many different countries.

	Number of Doses	**Age of routine adminis-tration**	**Age limits for dosing**			**Min. interval between doses**
			1st dose	2nd dose	3rd dose	
Rotarix® (GlaxoSmithKline)	2 oral doses (1mL/Dse)	2 and 4 months	6–14* weeks	10–24* weeks	None	4 weeks
RotaTeq® (CSL Biotherapies /Merck & Co Inc)	3 oral doses (2 mL/Dse)	2, 4 and 6 mths	6–12† weeks	10–32† weeks	14–32† weeks	4 weeks

According to *The Australian Immunisation Handbook*, "The vaccine viruses replicate in the intestinal mucosa and can be shed in the stool of vaccine recipients, particularly after the first dose. Vaccine virus shedding is more common with Rotarix and is detected in the stool a week after vaccination in up to 80% of first dose recipients, and in up to 30% of second dose recipients. RotaTeq is only shed after the first dose (in up to 13% of recipients). There have been no studies to assess the implications of shedding for horizontal spread to contacts."(NH&MRC 2008, p.266).

As with the oral Polio vaccines, this means people who come into contact with recently vaccinated infants can be infected when the organism is shed in the stool. The concerns regarding the shedding of the vaccine strain in more than 50% of vaccine recipients after the first dose of **Rotarix** (and thus possibly infecting contactees) are discussed in the orthodox literature (Glass RI, Parashar UD, 2006).

Although orthodox sources assure us that these vaccines are safe, as shown in Section 3.5.2, the Rotavirus vaccines have had a poor safety record. Current controversies continue in 2010.

For example CNN reported on 22/3/2010 "U.S. federal health authorities recommended … that doctors suspend using **Rotarix**, one of two vaccines licensed in the U.S. against rotavirus, saying the vaccine is contaminated with material from a pig virus". The **Rotarix** vaccine, which is made by GlaxoSmithKline and was approved by the FDA in 2008, has already been given to about 1 million U.S. children along with 30 million worldwide. The vaccine was found to contain DNA from porcine circovirus 1. "The FDA learned about the contamination after an academic research team using a novel technique to look for viruses in a range of vaccines found the material in GlaxoSmithKline's product and told the company," FDA Commissioner Dr. Margaret Hamburg told CNN." (Mercola J, 2010).

9.2.26.2 Comment

Simple illnesses are part of life. As parents, we don't want to see our children becoming sick. Rotavirus is everywhere and most people become infected, fall ill, and then become immune. If you have access to reliable healthcare and your child is robust, then the risks of serious problems from the disease are very low. The vaccines have a poor safety record, and whilst it is claimed that recent developments may have made them safer this is questionable as the 2010 controversy noted above demonstrates. It is worth asking whether the risk is worth it, especially when a safe and comparably effecitive homoeopathic immunisation is available.

* * * * * * *

9.2.27 Swine Flu vaccination

Let's start with a news item in the Australian, August 19, 2010. "***EUROPE and the US have banned an Australian-made flu vaccine for young children, after a surge in febrile fits in Australian children.***

The US Advisory Committee on Immunisation Practices has taken stronger action than Australia's Health Department, by recommending that children younger than nine not be vaccinated with ***CSL's*** *seasonal flu vaccine.*

Europe has followed Australia's decision to suspend the CSL vaccine only for the under-fives.

Shares in CSL yesterday fell nearly 3 per cent after the Australian pharmaceutical giant reported an 8 per cent fall in net profit, to $1.05 billion, for 2009-10.

Profits plummeted despite CSR's $121 million contract with the federal government to supply the nation's stockpile of 21 million doses of swine flu vaccine.

Australian health authorities suspended the use of CSL's seasonal flu vaccine, Fluvax, for the under-fives in April, after it was found to trigger febrile fits at nine times the normal rate.

Queensland's Coroner is investigating the death of a Brisbane toddler who died within hours of her seasonal flu jab."
(http://www.theaustralian.com.au/business/industry-sectors/europe-us-ban-csl-kids-flu-shot/story-e6frg97f-1225907050340).

In fact the Australian Government was accused of having too close a relationship to CSL, and thus having made poor decisions regarding the CSL vaccine (Anderson B, 2010)

Vaccination is not a risk free procedure, and we have a great propensity NOT to learn from history - it has all happened before..

> On February 5, 1976, a US army recruit died and four of his fellow soldiers were later hospitalized. Two weeks after his death, health officials announced that the cause of death was a new strain of H1N1 swine flu.
>
> Considerable fear was generated by public health officials, and President Gerald Ford ordered that every person in the U.S. be vaccinated for the disease.
>
> On October 1, 1976, immunizations began and elderly people died soon after receiving their injections leading to mass panic about the vaccination program. Overall there were 25 deaths and 1,098 cases of Guillain-Barré Syndrome (GBS) recorded nationwide by CDC surveillance, 532 of which occurred after vaccination and 543 before vaccination. This lead to the program being cancelled and President Ford loosing the next election.

There has been considerable media attention on the 2009/10 Swine Flu pandemic, and on the actions of the WHO. In fact the Parliamentary Assembly of the Council of Europe, a 47 nation body encompassing democratically elected members of parliament, began hearings in January 2010 to investigate whether the H1N1 swine flu pandemic was falsified or exaggerated to generate the tens of billions of dollars in sales of the untested vaccine.

In June 2010 the verdict was returned, and the Council of Europe issued the following press release 455(2010):

"PACE Health Committee denounces 'unjustified scare' of Swine Flu, waste of public money

Strasbourg, 04.06.2010 – The handling of the H1N1 pandemic by the World Health Organization (WHO), EU agencies and national governments led to a "waste of large sums of public money, and unjustified scares and fears about the health risks faced by the European public", according to a report by the Social, Health and Family Affairs Committee of the Parliamentary Assembly of the Council of Europe (PACE) made public today in Paris.

The report, prepared by Paul Flynn (United Kingdom, SOC) and approved today by the committee ahead of a plenary debate at the end of this month, says there was "overwhelming evidence that the seriousness of the pandemic was vastly overrated by WHO", resulting in a distortion of public health priorities.

Presenting his report, Mr Flynn told the committee: "this was a pandemic that never really was", and described the vaccination programme as "placebo medicine on a large scale.

In its adopted text, the committee identifies what it calls "grave shortcomings" in the transparency of decision-making about the outbreak, generating concerns about the influence of the pharmaceutical industry on decisions taken. Plummeting confidence in such advice could prove "disastrous" in the case of a severe future pandemic, it warns.

In particular, the WHO and European health institutions were not willing to publish the names and declarations of interest of the members of the WHO Emergency Committee and relevant European advisory bodies directly involved in recommendations concerning the pandemic, the parliamentarians point out.

However, attending the meeting was Fiona Godlee, the Editor-in-Chief of the British Medical Journal, who told the parliamentarians that, according to an investigation by her journal, scientists who drew up key WHO guidelines on stockpiling flu vaccines had previously been paid by drug companies which stood to profit.

The WHO has been "highly defensive", the committee said, and unwilling to accept that a change in the definition of a pandemic was made, or to revise its prognosis of the Swine Flu outbreak.

The committee sets out a series of urgent recommendations for greater transparency and better governance in public health, as well as safeguards against what it calls "undue influence by vested interests". It also calls for a public fund to support independent research, trials and expert advice, possibly financed by an obligatory contribution of the pharmaceutical industry, as well as closer collaboration with the media to avoid "sensationalism and scaremongering in the public health domain".

The report is due to be debated by parliamentarians from all 47 Council of Europe member states on Thursday 24 June during PACE's summer session in Strasbourg."

Mr Flynn's full report is available online at http://assembly.coe.int/CommitteeDocs/2010/20100604_H1N1pandemic_E.pdf.

The U.S. Public Health Emergency for 2009 H1N1 Influenza expired on June 23, 2010. On August 10, 2010, the World Health Organization International Health Regulations (IHR) Emergency Committee declared an end to the 2009 H1N1 pandemic globally (http://www.cdc.gov/h1n1flu/).

Books will be written about this entire episode, which has shed further light on the corrupting influence of vaccine manufacturers on the most senior health officials in the world. Whilst much more could be written here, the above account will suffice, as will the full report on the alternative to the billion dollar vaccine – the homoeopathic immunization of 9.8 million people against swine flu in Cuba, reported in Section 4.1.8.

9.2.27.1 The Current vaccines

CSL ***PanvaxH1N1*** is the current H1N1 vaccine used in Australia. There is also a "junior" vaccine. The vaccine comes in single and multidose vials. CSL state that the ingredients include (see their website: http://secure.healthlinks.net.au/content/csl/cmi.cfm?product=cscpanval1209)

Active ingredients: Purified, inactivated virus fragments from influenza type: Pandemic (H1N1) 2009 influenza virus strain, 15 micrograms (0.5 mL dose) or 7.5 micrograms (0.25 mL dose).
The multi-dose vial contains thiomersal as a preservative. Pre-filled syringes are thiomersal-free. Multi-dose vials and pre-filled syringes do not contain latex.
Other ingredients: * Sodium chloride; * Sodium phosphate – monobasic; * Sodium phosphate – dibasic anhydrous; * Potassium chloride; * Potassium phosphate -Monobasic; * Calcium chloride. The vaccine may also contain trace amounts of egg proteins, neomycin, polymyxin, sucrose and detergent (sodium taurodeoxycholate).

9.2.27.2 Comment

We know that this is a potentially dangerous vaccine against a disease which has proved to be milder than the normal seasonal flu. There is a homoeopathic alternative available, which has been used on millions of people. Intelligent people can make their own informed decision.

* * * * * * *

9.3 Additional Data Supporting Homoeoprophylaxis

9.3.1 Historical use of Homoeoprophylaxis

1801 Dr S Hahnemann, *Lesser Writings*. (Jain, p. 369 ff).

"Who can deny that the perfect prevention of infection from this devastating scourge, and the discovery of a means whereby this divine aim may be surely attained, would offer infinite advantages over any mode of treatment, be it of the most incomparable kind soever?

"The remedy capable of maintaining the healthy uninfectable by the miasm of scarlatina, I was so fortunate as to discover."

Hahnemann then describes his use of Belladonna to prevent Scarlet Fever. From his essay, *The Cure and Prevention of Scarlet Fever*.

1849 Dr C M F von Boenninghausen, *Lesser Writings*. (Jain, 1986) (reprint).

"Although the circumstance that thousands of men have through the use of these homoeopathic prophylactics escaped cholera, as has been actually proved, does not incontestably prove that these afford an absolute protection, since it might have been that these very persons might have been the ones who would in any case not have been touched by the disease, nevertheless these facts speak at least very much for the probability of such a salutary action".

[From the essay, *Brief Instructions for Non-Physicians Concerning the Prophylaxis and Treatment of Asiatic Cholera*, p. 303].

1884 Dr J C Burnett, *Vaccinosis and its Cure by Thuja; with Remarks on Homœoprophy*laxis. (W H L, 1992 (reprint), pp. 114, 115).

"It seems to me that the requirement of the age is to systematise the prevention of disease according to the law of similars, and in dynamic dose."

"Strewn about in literature there are examples of small-dose homœoprophylaxis; see Hahnemann's little essay on *Belladonna* for example, at the very birth of Hahnemannian Homoeopathy.

"The vaccine 'lymph' - pus - has been dynamised more homoeopathico and given as a prophylactic against small-pox in epidemic times, and apparently with effect. Thuja Occidentalis has been used in like manner by more than one homoeopathic practitioner, and they claim that it is effective ... Speaking for myself, I have for the last nine years been in the habit of using vaccine matter, in the thirtieth homoeopathic centesimal potency, whenever small-pox was about, and I have thus far not seen any one so far treated get variola."

1900 Dr J T Kent, *Lectures on Homoeopathic Philosophy*. (Jain, 5th Edition, 1954, p. 229).

"We must look to homoeopathy for our protection as well as for our cure."

"Now you will find that for prophylaxis there is required a less degree of similitude than is necessary for curing. A remedy will not have to be so similar to prevent disease as to cure it, and these remedies in daily use will enable you to prevent a large number of people from becoming sick."

1907 Dr C W Eaton, *Variolinum*, [a paper read before the American Institute of Homoeopathy].

Dr Eaton gives the results of the experience in the smallpox epidemic of a number of Iowa physicians. His instructions to his colleagues were precise. The paper "really gives the basis of what is known as 'Homoeopathic vaccination' which was upheld by the supreme court of Iowa".

"I trust that reference to your case book, ledger, and other records will enable you to make your figures on these three points definite and exact. May I ask that in any uncertain cases, such ones be omitted from your report, to the end that the figure be conservative, and an understatement rather than an overstatement".

Dr Eaton collected the following figures (from which he deliberately excluded his own experience):

Persons given Variolinum 30	2806
Definite exposures after taking Variolinum 30	547
Smallpox cases after taking Variolinum 30	14
Efficacy	97.5%

Dr Eaton concluded:

"We must not do Homoeopathy the injustice of giving this, one of its most successful and useful outgrowths, a partial and equivocal recognition, just because it happens to be strange to us. This splendid piece of practice is not new, it has its roots in the past, though we may not have known it. And we must not injure the cause by refusing to recognise its value just because we happen not to have been conversant with it".

1920 Dr S Close, *The Genius of Homoeopathy*. (Jain, 1991, p. 20).

"Homoeopathy is opposed to the methods of vaccine and serum therapy, although it is claimed by many that these methods are based upon the homoeopathic principle. It has been proven experimentally and clinically that such methods are unnecessary, and that the results claimed by their advocates can be attained more safely, more rapidly and more thoroughly by the administration of the homoeopathically indicated medicines in sub-physiological doses, through the natural channels of the body, than by introducing it forcibly by means of the hypodermic needle or in any other way."

1967 Dr Dorothy Shepherd, *Homoeopathy In Epidemic Diseases*. (Health Science Press, 1981 (reprint), p. 15).

"Inoculation with any type of serum in any of these infectious diseases is harmful and can easily and safely be replaced by a remedy or remedies, proved according to our Law of Similars that "likes cures like" on healthy individuals. Nosodes or disease products of the actual disease are often most active preventatives".

Dr Shepherd gives many practical examples of how HP reduced attacks of infectious diseases in boarding schools which she attended, and other examples from her long and distinguished career.

1972 Dr P Sankaran, *Prophylactics in Homoeopathy*. (The Homoeopathic Medical Publishers, 1961).

"Though the efficacy of the Homoeopathic prophylactic remedies for various conditions has not been proved by controlled studies and statistical records, yet generations of homoeopaths have used these remedies to prevent these conditions and they claim to have done it successfully. So their efficacy may be accepted on the basis of this experience even if it is not proved."

Referred to in Chapter 1, this booklet is a very thorough literature review sourcing 92 practitioners and hundreds of examples of HP.

1974 Dr D Castro & Dr G G Nogueira, Use of the Nosode Meningococcinum as a preventative Against Meningitis. *J.A.I.H.* 68: 1975; pp. 211-219.

In August 1974 (Guarantingueta, Brazil) there was an epidemic of meningitis. 18,000 children under the age of 15 were given Meningococcinum 10CH, and 6,340 children of similar ages were not covered. The following results were obtained:

18,000 protected homoeopathically	4 cases
6,340 not protected	10 cases.

1976 Dr M Blackie, *The Challenge of Homoeopathy.* (Unwin, 1981, p. 184).

"The same is true of the homoeopathic oral flu vaccine. Clinical experience proves that protection is given in individuals, yet there is no increase in antibodies to the influenza virus. ... One cannot ignore clinical observation but we have no way of measuring true reasons - it just works. The results, therefore, of Homoeopathy in preventative medicine are justifiably based on experience rather than experiment."

1976 Dr K N Mathur, *Principles of Prescribing.* (Jain, 1987 (reprint), pp. 50, 53).

"Dr Hahnemann found that remedies can act as prophylactic medicines, when the homoeopathic remedy in its provings brings out symptoms similar to a particular disease. It was experienced that the genus epidemicus when given to the members of the family were not suffering from the epidemic disease were protected from developing the disease."

Dr Mathur then quoted Dr Pierre Schmidt from an address given in Geneva on HP:

"The most noble role of medicine is unquestionably prophylaxy. There homoeopathy asserts its superiority over the existing methods. It can prevent disease without endangering the organism, without incurring the disappointments of the prevailing school of medicine."

1978 Dr P Sankaran, *Some Notes on the Nosodes.* (The Hom. Medical Publishers, p. 5).

"The broad general indications of the nosodes are given hereunder. 10. For the prophylaxis of infectious diseases. Wheeler recommends that in epidemics, the corresponding nosode in the 30th potency will protect for at least a fortnight. Others like Grimmer recommend one dose in high potency, once a year."

Dr Sankaran gives various examples of HP when discussing different Nosodes.

1982 L J Speight, *Homoeopathy and Immunisation.* (Health Science Press, p. 3).

"In homoeopathy there is no immunisation as such, but there are remedies that can build up immunity to infections. They can also act as curative agents where a disease has developed. These remedies carry no risk of detrimental effects, they are absolutely safe.

"Dr A. Pulford wrote 'No disease will arise without an existing predisposition to that disease. It is the absence of the predisposition to any particular disease that makes us immune to it. Homoeopathy alone is capable of removing these predispositions'".

Ms Speight then gives examples of HP in nine common diseases.

1989 Dr Andrew Lockie, *The Family Guide to Homoeopathy.* (Guild Publishing, p. 17).

"Homoeopathic immunisation against the graver diseases of childhood is not usually offered unless a child is particularly at risk; most homoeopaths prefer to take the route of boosting general resistance to disease, rather than exposing a child unnecessarily to the influence of powerful disease organisms. That said, homoeopathic immunisation has never damaged anyone".

1991 Dr F X Eizayaga, *Treatise on Homoeopathic Medicine.* (E Marecel, Buenos Aires, pp. 282-286).

"An ideal socio-medical system should assist all individuals before they contract any disease, whether acute or chronic ... In acute diseases: with the remedy of the epidemic genius and with the aetiological nosode of the disease." In homoeopathy, with the nosode of each of the acute diseases we could fulfil a job similar to the one achieved by the vaccines which are known, without any of their inconveniences. While the non specific resistance of an individual to an infection is increased with the homoeopathic remedy, a higher specific immunity against a given germ is obtained with the nosode."

Dr Paul Chauvanon (Paris, 1932) mentions in his book, *La Diptherie*, the immunisation of 45 children with Diphtherotoxinum 4M and 8M, one dose by mouth, some needing a second dose of 4M:

"Chauvanon demonstrated that as regards Schick's reaction, the nosode negatives it or makes it inactive during a first period, as well as immunising without the presence of antitoxins or antibodies. After a short time, one to two months, antitoxins which can be measured in the blood appear and a real vaccination exists ... the respective immunisation lasts just the same as the one provoked by the antitoxin in substance, without any of its disadvantages".

Dr H Roux repeated these same experiences in 1946 and obtained like results.

Dr Eizayaga then quotes his own substantial and successful experience with HP.

1991 Dr B Sethi, *Homoeo Prophylactic Remedies*. (Jain, pp. 22, 47, 56, 78).

"Diphtherinum. Allen says that he had used it for 25 years as a prophylactic and has never known a second case of diphtheria to occur in a family after it has been administered. He challenges the profession to test it and publish the failures. ...Tyler writes that for nearly three years, Diphtherinum in high potency has been used in the London Homoeopathic Hospital to protect nurses and patients exposed to the infection, with perfect success."

"Morbillinum. As a prophylactic given to those who are, or may be, exposed to infection."

"Lathyrus Sativa. Homoeopathic physicians are satisfied that they have a really safe and better polio preventative in Lathyrus Sativa when properly given".

Amongst the many examples of HP given by Dr Sethi, he

then quotes the experience of Drs Smith, Grimmer, Bond, and Foubister:

"Whooping Cough. Dr John H Clarke strongly recommended Pertussin in whooping cough. In practice the results of Pertussin have been verified by Dr Dorothy Shepherd. Children who were given this medicine escaped the disease."

1993 Dr C B Lessell, *The World Traveller's Manual of Homoeopathy*. (C W Daniel Co Ltd, page 14).

"Those nosodes utilised for immunisation, correctly given, are immensely safe, virtually free from side effects, and may be given in pregnancy and lactation. Alternatively, a remedy other than a nosode may be given preventively which would be used to treat the disease in question (e.g., malaria). Such remedies are also generally very safe. Safety and lack of side-effects thus characterise the homoeopathic method. Homoeopathic remedies would seem to work by actively stimulating the immune system of the body in some way. The manner in which this occurs, however, has not been totally elucidated."

Dr Lessell follows with numerous examples of the use of HP remedies against diseases which travellers may face.

9.3.2 The earlier homœoprophylaxis programs, 1986, 1991, and 1993

The first program I developed and used in 1986 was based (i) on a literature review of available information both in the homoeopathic and orthodox journals and texts, (ii) on an understanding of the then current vaccination schedule and the belief by many parents that they were the diseases against which protection was most needed, and (iii) a desire to provide an option for parents (including myself) that could be used instead of the orthodox vaccination schedule.

As shown below in Tables 8-5, 8-6 and 8-7, the 1986 program used mainly single doses of an M potency. It did use a variety of other remedies in the supplementary program given to provide additional protection if required.

The first major change in the schedule in 1991 was based on experience with a whooping cough outbreak in a closed community which showed me that the homoeopathic method was a viable option, but also that if it was not administered correctly, or the remedies were accidentally antidoted, then it would not be effective. My experience was presented to the homoeopathic community at the time (Golden I, 1991). Some changes to the remedies offered were made.

This experience led me to introduce the use of an initial single dose of a 200 potency (to test the sensitivity of the recipient), followed by triple doses (3 doses in 24 hours) over a number of years of a 200, M, and 10M potency (unless sensitivity was established, in which case the program was modified). One purpose of the triple dose was to minimise the chance of an accidental antidoting of the remedies, another was to strengthen the long-term effect of the dose.

The 1997 survey of the first two major protocols showed that this purpose was achieved.

The minor change in 1993 involved adding a remedy for Hib into the program. Only an M potency was used because at the time the 10M was not available, but a triple dose of the M potency was still used.

Tables 8-3, 8-4 and 8-5 show the 1993 program, which is similar to the 1991 program except for the introduction of the Hib remedy (remedy "H").

The change made in 2004 has been discussed in Section 4.2.1. It involved a major change in both the remedies offered and the structure of the program. Triple doses were still used, initially of a 200 potency (following the initial single dose of 200), and later of a 10M potency. The aim was to make the program more current, as well as less likely to cause reactions (even though the level of these was already very small).

The following material simply presents the 1986 and the 1993 programs for the information of interested readers. There is no need to study them to understand and use the present program.

9.3.3 The 1993 long-term HP program

Table 9-6 Basic Program for Protection from Birth (1993)

Age given	REMEDY	Age given	REMEDY
1 month	Pertussin (200)	17 months	Haemophilis*
2 months	Pertussin*	19 months	Parotidinum (200)
3 months	Lathyrus Sativus (200)	20 months	Parotidinum*
5 months	Lathyrus Sativus*	22 months	Diphtherinum*
6 months	Haemophilis (M)	24 months	Tetanus Toxin*
7 months	Haemophilis*	26 months	Lathyrus Sativus*
9 months	Diphtherinum (200)	28 months	Haemophilis*
10 months	Diphtherinum*	32 months	Pertussin*
11 months	Tetanus Toxin (200)	41 months	Tetanus Toxin*
12 months	Tetanus Toxin*	46 months	Haemophilis*
13 months	Pertussin*	50 months	Diphtherinum*
14 months	Morbillinum (200)	54 months	Morbillinum*
15 months	Morbillinum*	56 months	Lathyrus Sativus*
16 months	Lathyrus Sativus*	60 months	Tetanus Toxin*

* = Triple doses to be used.

Note: The disease-remedy relationship (including possible substitutions) is as follows:

- Whooping Cough - *Pertussin* Cuprum Metallicum
- Diphtheria - *Diphtherinum* Gelsemium
- Measles - *Morbillinum* Pulsatilla
- Poliomyelitis - *Lathyrus Sativus* Lathyrus Sativus
- Tetanus - *Tetanus Toxin* Hypericum
- Mumps - Parotidinum Rhus Tox
- Rubella (German Measles)- *Rubella* Pulsatilla
- Hib - *Haemophilis* Arsenicum Album.

A supplementary program described in Table 8-3 was available to be used in conjunction with the basic program. The reason for using both programs is that, although successful use of the remedies in the basic program has been established, *no system of protection can be guaranteed 100% effective*. In the event of definite exposure to a source of infection, parents could give their child additional protection at that time. These two programs comprise the third Homoeopathic Kit, which was first released in 1993.

Table 9-7 Supplementary Program for Protection When Exposed to Infection

DISEASE	ADMINISTRATION OF REMEDY
Whooping Cough	Pertussin (200) twice weekly for 3 weeks after contact with carrier
Tetanus	Three doses of Ledum Palustre (30) daily for 3 days after breakage of skin
Diphtheria	One dose of Diphtherinum (200) weekly for 4-6 weeks during an outbreak of Diphtheria
Measles	Morbillinum (200) weekly during an outbreak, for 3 weeks
Mumps	Parotidinum (200) weekly during an epidemic or after contact with carrier.
Rubella (German Measles)	As natural immunity is the most certain, it is better to allow healthy children to acquire this mild disease. If protection is required, the Rubella Nosode (200) or Pulsatilla (30) may be used twice weekly for two weeks.
Haemoph-ilis (Hib)	Haemophilis (M) every 2 weeks during an outbreak

Table 8-5 shows the actual remedies supplied in the 1993 program (which covers both the main program and supplementary program).

Table 9-8 Remedies used in the 1993 program

Code	Medicine	Pills	Code	Medicine	Pills
A1	Pertussin (200)	30 pills	D1	Diphtherinum (200)	30 pills
A2	Pertussin (M)	6 pills	D2	Diphtherinum (M)	6 pills.
A3	Pertussin (10M)	6 pills	D3	Diphtherinum (10M)	6 pills
B1	Tetanus Toxin (200)	30 pills	E1	Morbillinum (200)	30 pills
B2	Tetanus Toxin (M)	8 pills	E2	Morbillinum (M)	4 pills
B3	Tetanus Toxin (10M)	8 pills	E3	Morbillinum (10M)	4 pills
C1	Lathyrus Sativus (10M)	30 pills	F1	Parotidinum (200)	30 pills
C2	Lathyrus Sativus (10M)	8 pills	F2	Parotidinum (M)	2 pills
C3	Lathyrus Sativus (10M)	8 pills	F3	Parotidinum (10M)	2 pills
			H	Haemophilis (M)	30 pills
			M	Ledum Palustre (30)	30 pills

9.3.4 The Original 1986 program

Tables 8-5, 8-6 and 8-7 show the original 1986 program.

Table 9-9 The 1986 Main Program

MEDICINE	AGE ADMINISTERED (Months)						
A Pertussin (M)	1	2	10	22	32	-	-
B Tetanus Toxin (M)	3	6	12	18	30	42	56
C Lathyrus Sativus.(200)	4	9	20	36	48	60	-
D Diphtherinum (M)	5	16	28	40	-	-	-
E Morbillinum (M)	13	25	-	-	-	-	-
F Parotidinum (M)	14	26	-	-	-	-	-
G Rubella (M)	12	14 (years of age)					

Table 9-10 The 1986 Supplementary Program

CODE	MEDICINE	Current Epidemic
L	Pertussis (30)	Whooping Cough
M	Ledum Palustre (30)	Tetanus
N	Lathyrus Sativus (30)	Poliomyelitis
O	Diphtherinum (30)	Diphtheria..
P	Pulsatilla (6)	Measles/Rubella
Q	Morbillinum (30)	Measles
R	Parotidinum (30)	Mumps
S	Pilocarpine (12)	Mumps
T	Arsenicum Alb. (12)	Colds/Influenza

Table 9-11 Remedies Used in the 1986 Program

Code	Medicine	Pills	Code	Medicine	Pills
A	Pertussin (M)	10 pills	**M**	Ledum Palustre(30).	12 pills
B	Tetanus Toxin (M)	14 pills	**N**	Lathyrus Sativus (30)	10 pills
C	Lathyrus Sat. (200)	12 pills	**O**	Diphtherinum (30).	18 pills
D	Diphtherinum (M)	8 pills	**P**	Pulsatilla (6).	30 pills
E	Morbillinum (M).	4 pills	**Q**	Morbillinum (30).	10 pills
F	Parotidinum (M)	4 pills	**R**	Parotidinum (30).	10 pills
G	Rubella (M)	4 pills	**S**	Pilocarpine (12)	30 pills
L	Pertussis (30)	30 pills	**T**	Arsenicum Alb. (12)	30 pills

10 A Word About God

My preference would be to begin this book with a word about God, but as this would upset some readers - atheists, scientific rationalists, members of the Skeptics Society, etc - I have decided to "leave the best to last", where it can be ignored by the materialists if they prefer.

I believe that everything - from galaxy to planet to smallest organism - is governed by Natural Law. Further, I believe in the continual presence of a creative force (which in simple terms, many of us call 'God'), and that this creative force brought Natural Law into being.

Some readers may accept the existence of Natural Law without believing in God, and this would be sufficient to follow my propositions. Without belief in Natural Law, how can you explain what causes our heart to beat without us thinking about it, our skin to heal after a cut, the sun to rise, rain to fall, seasons to change, grass to grow, etc.? If you reply, 'physics' and 'biology', then I would affirm that the laws which govern these 'sciences' are precisely what is meant by Natural Law.

In examining health topics, we find that it is Natural Law which causes us to function, to physiologically renew, to heal both internally and externally. The old healers, such as Hypocrites and Paracelsus, knew that if they assisted the organism to cooperate with Natural Law, the organism would heal itself, and that if the organism existed in conflict with Natural Law, 'dis-ease' would result.

Dr Samuel Hahnemann, the founder of homoeopathy, stressed that the cause of disease (leaving aside acute accidents and injuries) initially occurred on the inner energy level, affecting what Hahnemann called the 'vital force', which then caused changes to the physical body, termed 'diseases' by modern medicine.

Nature uses infinites (i.e. energy) to cause changes in the body, and heals with infinites. This is why homoeopathically-potentised substances can both heal and prevent infectious diseases.

The extensive use of pharmaceutical medicine is a direct attack on these facts. Drugs for the most part force physiological changes to the body, whether or not the body's superior intelligence deems such changes to be desirable. One of the most common actions of drugs is **suppression** - suppression of skin rashes, fevers, mucus discharges and, at the other end of the scale, of emotions and feelings.

There are times - in some acute situations, in surgery and in a few chronic conditions - when the use of drugs is life saving, and no sensible person would deny their value in such circumstances. However, in most health conditions this is not the case.

In fact, we find epidemics of chronic disease in societies where pharmaceutical medicine controls the bulk of health care. In Australia, for example, a survey conducted by the Commonwealth Government in 1977/78 found that 45% of all Australians suffered from at least one chronic disease, including about 70% of Australians over the age of 45 (A.B.S., 1979). In 1989-90, this had blown out to an alarming 66.2% of all Australians, including 25% of all children under five, and over 90% of all our citizens over the age of 45 (A.B.S., 1991). This **is** an epidemic!

I believe that this epidemic has been caused, in large part, by the suppressive effects of drugs.

The pharmaceutical industry represents one of the greatest and most powerful forces of suppression on this planet. It actively suppresses anyone who publicly disagrees with its position, any therapy which it cannot control and which threatens its financial base, and even the opinions of doctors who are unhappy with the system. One does not need to resort to conspiracy theories to prove this assertion - merely history.

Because of the deeply destructive nature of most pharmaceutical products, including vaccinations, we are really looking at a force which eventually threatens the existence of our society as we know it, and certainly our physical health and peace of mind. In so many ways, this force is directly opposed to our Creator's Law. Dr Harris Coulter has written directly to this point (Coulter H, 1990).

Let us use the best of technology, where appropriate, but let us not become servants of technology, or those who financially control it.

This is not just a contest between natural therapists and drug companies: it is a contest between enlightenment and repression - some would say, between good and evil. That is why I now finish with the statement:

To someone whose who god is science, vaccination makes sense. But to someone whose god is God, it is appalling.

11 REFERENCES AND BIBLIOGRAPHY

The first part shows references used directly in the book, including the Section where the reference was used. The second part shows general references.

Reference	Section
Access Economics (2010) The National Institute of Complementary Medicine. *Cost effectiveness of complementaryMedicines*. September.	5.4
Anderson B (2010) Government 'too cosy with flu vaccine maker'. *ABC News Online* Investigative Unit. Updated Wed Apr 28, 2010.	9.2.27
Australian Bureau of Statistics (1999) Health – Mortality and Morbidity: Asthma. *Australian Social Trends, 1999.* Canberra.	4.2.3.3
Australian Bureau of Statistics (2003) Summary of Results, Australia. *National Health Survey, 2003.* Publication 4364.0. Canberra.	4.2.3.3
ADRAC Warning (1990) Reactions to hepatitis B vaccines CT Alert, *Current Therapeutics*. October; p. 115.	3.6.6.1
Age (2004) Infected vaccine put a generation 'at risk'. *The Age.* 23.10.04.	3.6.15.1
Albonico H et al, (1990) Medical Considerations on the Continuation of the MMR Vaccination Campaign in Switzerland, March 1990.	3.6.20.1
Allan B (1978) *Australian Nurses Journal*, May.	3.6.16
Allen A (1988) Is RA27/3 a Cause of Chronic Fatigue? *Medical Hypothesis*, Vol 27, pp. 217-220.	3.6.16
Asthma Foundation of Victoria (2004) http://www.asthma.org.au/Default.aspx?tabid=35	1.2.1
Australian Bureau of Statistics (1979) *Australian Health Survey 1977-78 - Chronic Conditions.*	7.10

Catalogue No. 4314.0. Canberra.	
Australian Bureau of Statistics (1991) *1989-90 National Health Survey - Summary of Results.* Catalogue No. 4364.0. Canberra.	7.10
Australian Institute of Homoeopathy (AIH) 1988 *Vaccination.* Sydney. p. 25.	3.6.3.2
Baguley DM & Glasgow GL, (1973) Subacute Sclerosing Panencephalitis and Salk Vaccine The Lancet, October 6; pp. 763-765.	3.6.15.1
Barham-Floreani J (2009) *Well Adjusted Babies.* Vitality Productions Pty Ltd, Mt.Macedon, Victoria. Australia. 2nd Edition.	2.1.1 2.1.4
Bedford H & Elliman D, (2000) Concerns about Immunisation *British Medical Journal*; 320: 22 January; pp. 240-243.	3.1
Belkin M (2000) Scientific fraud and conflict of interest in vaccine research, licensing and policymaking. Presented at the *2nd International Public Conference on Vaccination*, Arlington, Virginia	3.5.4
Bellavite P and Signorini A (2003) *Emerging Science of Homoeopathy: Complexity, Biodynamics and Nanopharmacology.* North Atlantic Books. Berkeley, California.	
Belongia EA et.al. (2010) Clinical Characteristics and 30-Day Outcomes for Influenza A 2009 (H1N1), 2008-2009 (H1N1), and 2007-2008 (H3N2) Infections. *JAMA.* 2010;304(10):1091-1098. doi:10.1001/jama.2010.1277	9.1.25
Beneviste J et al, (1988) *Nature*, Vol 333, 30 June, pages 816-819.	4.1.1
Biesel WR (1985) Single Nutrients and Immunity. *Journal of American College of Nutrition*, Vol 4; pp. 5-16.	2.1.2
Blackie M (1976) *The Challenge of Homoeopathy* Unwin Paperbacks. London. 1981 reprint; p. 184.	4.1.3
Bloom BS et al, (1993)	3.6.6.1

A reappraisal of hepatitis B virus vaccination strategies using cost-effectiveness analysis *Medicine and Public Issues*, Vol. 118(4); pp. 298-306.	
Boenninghausen CMF von (1848) Concerning the Curative Effects of Thuja in Small-pox. *Lesser Writings*, p. 3. B. Jain Publishers Pty Ltd. New Delhi. 1986 reprint.	
Boenninghausen CMF von (1849) Brief Instructions for Non-Physicians Concerning the Prophylaxis and Treatment of Asiatic Cholera. *Lesser Writings*, p. 303. B. Jain Publishers Pty Ltd. New Delhi. 1986 reprint.	4.1.3
Bookchin D & Schumacher J, (2004) *The Virus and the Vaccine; The true story of a cancer-causing monkey virus, contaminated polio vaccine, and the millions of Americans exposed.* St Martins Press, New York.	3.6.15.1
Bourns HK (1964) *British Medical Journal*, August.	1.1.17
BMJ Editorial (1981) Pertussis Vaccine *British Medical Journal*, Vol 282; pp. 1563-1564.	3.6.13.3
BMJ Editorial (2003a) Safety and efficacy of combination vaccines *British Medical Journal*, Vol 326, May 10; pp. 995-996.	3.2
BMJ Editorial (2003b) Medical errors: a common problem *British Medical Journal*, Vol 322, March 3; pp. 501-502	7.0
BMJ reference (1992) Pertussis and brain damage *British Medical Journal,* Vol. 304; 27/6/92; p. 1652.	3.5.4
Bracho G, Varela E, Fernández R, Ordaz B, Marzoa N, Menéndez J, García L, Gilling E, Leyva R,Rufín R, de la Torre R, Solis R, Batista N, Borrero R, Campa C. (2010). Massive Application of Highly Diluted Bacteria as Homeoprophylactic Formulation for Leptospirosis Epidemic Control. *Homeopathy*. 99, 156-166.	4.2.3.1
Braun-Fahrlander C et al, (2002) Environmental exposure to endotoxin and its relation to asthma	1.2

in school-age children. *New England Journal of Medicine*. 347; pp. 869-887.	
Brott LM (1982) Congenital Rubella After Successful Vaccination. *Medical Journal of Australia*, Vol 1; pp. 514-515.	3.6.26
Burnett JC (1884) *Vaccinosis and its Cure by Thuja; with Remarks on Homœoprophylaxis.* W H L 1992 reprint	4.1.3 4.1.4
Burnett M & White D, (1981) *The Natural History of Infectious Disease* Cambridge, England.	1.1.15
Butler JC et al, (1993) Pneumococcal polysaccharide vaccine efficacy. An evaluation of current recommendations. *JAMA*. Vol. 270; No. 5. 15th Oct.	3.6.14.1
Buttram HE & Hoffman JC (1982) *Vaccinations and Immune Malfunctions.* Humanitarian Publishing Co., PA; p. 47.	3.5.2
Buttram HE (1987) Personal communication to the author, 27 March 1987.	3.5.2
Campbell A (1986) *British Medical Journal*, Vol 292; p. 538.	3.6.13.5
Campa C, Bracho G, Cruz R, Menendez J, Martinez R, Gilling E, Wella R. (2008). Homoeoprophylaxis: Cuban Experiences on Leptospirosis. *Nosodes 2008*, International Meeting on Homoeoprophylaxis, Homoeopathic Immunisation and Nosodes Against Epidemics. Havana, Cuba. 10-12th December 2008.	4.2.3.1
Canadian Medical Association (1992) *Journal of the Canadian Medical Association*, Vol 146(8); p. 1364.	3.6.4.1
Carlsen W (2001) New documents show the monkey virus is present in more recent polio vaccine. *San Francisco Chronicle*, 22/7/2001.	3.6.15.1
Castro D & Nogeira G.G (1975) Use of the Nosode Meningococcinum as a preventative against Meningitis. *J Am Inst Hom* 68: 211-219	4.1.4
Centre for Disease Control (CDC) (1988) Personal communication to the author.	3.6.15.2

EIS Officer, Division of Immunization, Center for Disease Control, Department of Health and Human Services, USA dated 26 August.	
Centre for Disease Control (CDC), (2010) Reports of Health Concerns Following HPV Vaccination. January, 2010.	9.2.24.1
Chaitow L (1987) *Vaccination and Immunization.* C W Daniel Co Ltd, London.	3.6.21.2 8.9.1
Chandra RK (1980) *Immunology of Nutritional Disorders*. Edward Arnold.	2.1.2
Chandra RK et al, (1982) Nutritional and Immunocompetence of the Elderly. Effect of Short Term Nutritional Supplementation on Cell-Mediated Immunity and Lymphocyte Subsets. *Nutritional Resources*, Vol 2; pp. 223-232.	2.1
Chandra RK (1985) Trace Element Regulation of Immunity and Infection. *Journal of American College of Nutrition*, Vol 4; pp. 5-16.	2.1
Chaves SS et.al. (2007) Loss of Vaccine-Induced Immunity to Varicella over Time. *NEJM.* Vol. 356: No. 11. Pp.1121-1129 15/3/2007.	9.2.1.1.
Cherry J et al, (1988) Report of the Task Force on Pertussis and Pertussis Immunisation. *Paediatrics* (Supplement); pp. 972, 973.	8.3.1
Cherry JD et al, (1998) The Effect of Investigator Compliance (Observer Bias) on Calculated Efficacy in a Pertussis Vaccine Trial *Pediatrics* Vol. 102 No. 4 October 1998; pp. 909-912.	3.6.13.2
Cherry JD & Olin P, (1999) COMMENTARY: The Science and Fiction of Pertussis Vaccines. *Pediatrics* Vol. 104 No. 6 December; pp. 1381-1383.	3.6.13.2
Cherry J (2003) The science and fiction of the "resurgence" of pertussis *Pediatrics*, Vol.112; August 2; pp. 405-406.	3.6.13.2
Clarke JH (1984) *The Prescriber.* B Jain Publishers, 1984 reprint.	1.1.15
Classen JB (1996) Childhood immunisation and diabetes mellitus	3.6.6.1

New Zealand Medical Journal, May 24; 109(1022); p. 195.	
Close S (1920) *The Genius of Homoeopathy* Jain Publishers, New Delhi. 1991 reprint; p. 20.	4.1.3
Cochi SL et al, (1986) Primary invasive Haemophilis influenzae type b disease: a population-based assessment of risk factors. *Journal of Pediatrics*, 108: pp. 887-896.	1.1.4
Cody CL, Baraff LJ, Cherry JD, Marcy SM, Manclark CR (1981) The Nature and Rate of Adverse Reactions Associated with DPT and DT Immunisation in Infants and Children. *Paediatrics*, Vol 68; pp. 650-660.	3.5.2 3.6.13.2
Cookson WO & Moffatt ME (1997) Asthma: An epidemic in the absence of infection? *Science*, Jan 3;275(5296); pp. 41-42.	1.2
Coulter H (1975) *Divided Legacy* North Atlantic. Berkeley. Vol III. p. 268.	
Coulter HL & Fisher BL (1985) *DPT - A Shot in the Dark.* Warner Books, New York.	3.5.2; 8.2 3.6.10.2 3.6.13.3
Coulter H L (1990) *Vaccination, Social Violence and Criminality: The Medical Assault On the American Brain.* North Atlantic Books.	3.5.2 4.1.4 7.10 8.9.1
Cribb J (1992) Was this science's biggest blunder? *The Weekend Australian Review*. 25-26 April, 1992.	8.6.2
Crosslight GM & Howard B (1978) Tetanus Immunization Status in Sydney Adults. *Medical Journal of Australia*, 23 September, Vol 2; pp. 313-316.	1.1.17
Cucherat M et al, (2000) Evidence of clinical effectiveness of homoeopathy. A meta-analysis of clinical trials. *Eur. J Clin Pharmacol* Apr; 56(1): pp. 27-33.	4.1.1
Dahl M et al, (2004)	1.2

Viral-induced T helper type 1 responses enhance allergic asthma by effects on lung dendritic cells. *Nature Immunology*, DOI:10; p.1038/ni1041.	
Daum RS et al, (1989) Decline in serum antibody to the capsule of *Haemophilis influenzae* type b in the immediate postimmunization period *Journal of Pediatrics*; 1114: pp. 742-747.	3.6.4.1
Davies EG et al, (2001) *Manual of Childhood Infections*. W. B. Saunders. London. 2nd ed	1.1.1; 1.1.6,
Davis B et al, (1979) *Microbiology* (2nd ed). Harper.	3.6.15.1
Department of Health and Ageing (2008) Vaccine Preventable Diseases and Vaccination Coverage in Aboriginal and Torres Strait Islander People, Australia, 2003 to 2006. Communicable Diseases Intelligence Volume 32 Supplement - June 2008.	2.4
Deyo RA, Patrick DL (2005) *Hope or Hype: The Obsession with Medical Advances and the High Cost of False Promises.* Amacom, New York	7
Dick G (1987) *Immunisation*. Update Books, London.	3.5.2; 3.6.10.2 3.6.13.2.4 3.6.21.2
Ditchburn RK Whooping Cough After Stopping Pertussis Immunization *British Medical Journal*, Vol 1, pages 1601-1603.	3.6.13.2
Dossetor J, Whittle H.C., and Greenwood B.M. (!977) Persistent Measles Infection in Malnourished Children. *British Medical Journal*, ii; pp. 1633-1635.	2.1
Douglas WC, (1987) WHO Murdered Africa. *Health Freedom News*, September.	8.7.2
Dudgeon (1853) Lectures on the Theory and Practice of Homoeopathy B.Jain Publishing Pty Ltd. New Delhi; pp 541, 542.	
Dutta AC (1983) *Homoeopathy in the Light of Modern Science.* Jain Publishing Co. New Delhi; pp. 18,19.	

Dwyer J (1993) Homoeopathic vaccine is causing concern. *Australian Doctor*, 22.1.93.	4.2.1.1
Eaton CW (1907) Variolinum. A paper read before the American Institute of Homoeopathy. *J Am Inst Hom*	4.1.3 4.1.4
Eber MR et.al. (2010) Clinical and economic outcomes attributable to health care-associated sepsis and pneumonia. *Arch Intern Med.* Feb 22;170(4):347-53.	7
Ehrengut W (1978) Whooping Cough Vaccination. *Lancet;* pp. 370-371.	3.6.13.1
Eibl, Martha et al, (1984) Abnormal T-Lymphocyte Subpopulations in Healthy Subjects after Tetanus Booster Immunizations. *New England Journal of Medicine*, 19 Jan., Vol 310 (3), pp. 198-199.	3.6.17.2
Eisenberg DM et al, (2001) Perceptions about complementary therapies relative to conventional therapies among adults who use both: results from a national survey. *Ann Internal Medicine*, 135(5); pp. 344-151.	7.0
Eisfelder HW (1957a) Oral immunization of anterior poliomyelitis - a preliminary report. *Homoeopathy* 7(9): pp. 144-147	
Eisfelder HW (1957b) Oral immunization of anterior poliomyelitis – a two year report. *J Am Inst Hom* 51; pp. 9-10.	
Eisfelder HW (1958) Oral immunization of anterior poliomyelitis – a final report. *J Am Inst Hom* 54: pp. 166-167.	
Eizayaga FX (1991) *Treatise on Homoeopathic Medicine* E Marecel, Buenos Aires; pp. 282-286.	3.6.11.2 4.1.3
English JM (1987a) Pertussin 30 - preventative for whooping cough? A Pilot Study *Br Homeopath J* 76: pp. 61-65.	4.1.4 8.6.4
English JM (1987b) Symptoms and Treatment of Whooping Cough *Br Homeopath J* 76: pp. 66-68.	4.1.4

Enriquez R et.al. (2005) The relationship between vaccine refusal and self-report of atopic disease in children. *Journal of Allergy and Clinical Immunology*. Vol.115, Issue 4, April, pp. 737-744.	1.2.1
Erikson N (2010) Organisations in India Successfully halt HPV vaccination program. Examiner.com. 7/4/2010.	9.2.24.1
Fine MJ et al, (1994) Efficacy of pneumococcal vaccination in adults. A meta-analysis of randomised controlled trials *Archive of Internal Medicine*. Dec 12-26; 154(23); pp.2666-77.	3.6.14.1
Fisher BL (2000) Shots in the dark. *Mercola Newsletter*. www.mercola.com/2000/oct/15/vaccines.htm; p. 4	3.0 3.6.6.1
Fisher P (1990) Enough nonsense on immunisation (E). *Br Homoeopath J* 79: p. 198.	8.6.4
Fox DA (1987) Whooping cough prophylaxis with Pertussin 30 *Br Homoeopath J* 76(2); pp. 69-70.	4.1.4
Fletcher RH & Fletcher SW (1979) Clinical research in general medical journals: a 30-year perspective. *N Engl J Med*. 301; pp. 180–83.	
Furber S et al, (1993) Whooping Cough in the North Coast Region. *NSW Public Health Bulletin*, July, Vol 4, No 7, pages 83, 84.	8.6.6
Gaier H (1991) Thorsons Encyclopaedic Dictionary of Homoeopathy. Thorsons. London; pp. 290-309.	
Galil K et al, (2002) Outbreak of Varicella at a Day-Care Center despite Vaccination *NEJM*, Volume 347: No. 24; December 12; pp. 1909-1915.	3.6.1.1
Gallo R (1987) *The London Times*, 11 May 1987	3.5.2
Garrow RP (1928) Fatality rates of smallpox in the vaccinated and unvaccinated. *British Medical Journal*, 14 January, Vol 74.	3.6.21.2

Glass RI, Parashar UD (2006) The promise of new rotavirus vaccines. *N Engl J Med.* 354: pp. 75-77.	9.2.26.1
Golden I Neustaedter R (1996) In defence of homœoprophylaxis and Response to Golden article. *Resonance* Mar-Apr;18(2); pp. 26-28.	8.4
Golden I (1986) Vaccination – A Homoeopathic Perspective. *Nature & Health.* Vol. 7, No. 3; pp. 67-70.	
Golden I (1987) A Discussion Paper on a Possible Mechanism of Homoeopathic Prophylaxis. *Aust. Hom. Assn* June; pp. 3-10.	4.1.2
Golden I (1989a) A possible mechanism of homeopathic prophylaxis. *J Am Inst Homeopath* 82(2); pp. 69-76.	4.1.2
Golden I (1991) A Report of a Pertussis Outbreak and Prevention in Unvaccinated Children. *Similia* – the Journal of the Australian Homoeopathic Association, July, Vol 5, No 2; pp. 72-82.	8.8
Golden I (1997) *Homœoprophylaxis – A Ten Year Clinical Study* Isaac Golden Publications, Gisborne, Australia.	
Golden I (1998) *Vaccination? A Review of Risks and Alternatives* Isaac Golden Publications, Gisborne, Australia. Revised 5th ed.	4.1.4
Golden I (2001) *Homœoprophylaxis – A Practical and Philosophical Review* Isaac Golden Publications, Gisborne, Australia. 3rd edition.	4.2.3
Golden I (2002a) Attitudes to and use of Homœoprophylaxis by Australian Homoeopaths. *Similia* Vol 14 No.2; pp. 26-29.	4.4
Golden I (2002b) *Homoeopathic Treatment Of The Energy Bodies: Traditional Strategies And New Developments* Isaac Golden Publications, Gisborne, Australia.	4.1.2
Golden I (2004a) *Homœoprophylaxis s – A Fifteen Year Clinical Study*	3.5.5 4.1.5;

Isaac Golden Publications, Gisborne, Australia.	4.3
Golden I (2004b) A New Program of Long-Term Homœoprophylaxis. *Similia*. Vol 16, No. 2. December; pp. 36-41.	4.5.1
Golden I (2004c) The Safety of Long-Term Homœoprophylaxis – Research Findings. *Homoeopathic Links*. Vol.17 (4).Winter; pp. 261-263.	4.2.3
Golden I (2005) *The Potential Value of Homœoprophylaxis s in the Prevention of Infectious Diseases, and the maintenance of General Health in Recipients.* Swinburne University Press, Melbourne.	4.2.2.2
Golden I (2008) *Vaccine Damaged Children – Treatment, Prevention, Reasons*. Isaac Golden Publications. Gisborne. Australia.	3.5.6
Golden I, Bracho G (2009) The Adaptability of Homoeoprophylaxis. *Homeopathic Links*, November. Vol 22, No.4. pp.211-213.	4.2.3.1.
Golden I, Bracho G. (2010) The Homoeopathic Prevention of Leptospirosis in Cuba. *J.Am. Institute of Homeopathy*. Summer. 2010.	
Granoff DM et al, (1986) Haemophilis Influenzae type b disease in children vaccinated with type b polysaccharide vaccine. *New England Journal of Medicine*, Vol 315; pp. 1584-1590.	3.6.4.1
Greb E (2010) Strong Growth Predicted for Global Vaccine Market Aug 26, 2010. ePT--the *Electronic Newsletter of Pharmaceutical Technology*. http://pharmtech.findpharma.com/pharmtech/Drug+Delivery/Strong-Growth-Predicted-for-Global-Vaccine-Market/ArticleStandard/Article/detail/684403?contextCategoryId=35097	3.0
Gustafsson L et al, (1996) A Controlled Trial of a Two-Component Acellular, a Five-Component Acellular, and a Whole-Cell Pertussis Vaccine *NEJM*. Volume 334: Number 6; Feb 8; pp. 349-356.	3.6.13.2 3.6.13.4
Gutman W (1963) Homoeopathic oral vaccine against influenza	4.1.4

Homoeopathy 13(12); pp. 185, 187.	
Hahnemann S (1801) The Cure and Prevention of Scarlet Fever. *Lesser Writings* B Jain Publishers, New Delhi; pp. 369-385.	4.1.2 4.1.3
Hahnemann S (1828) *Chronic Diseases.* B Jain Publishers, New Delhi .	
Hahnemann S (1830) *Materia Medica Pura Vol II* B Jain Publishers, New Delhi. 1988 reprint; p. 401.	
Hahnemann S (1843) *Organon of the Healing Art* B Jain Publishers, New Delhi. 6th edition.	8.6.4
Harper, D. (2009) Current prophylactic HPV vaccines and gynecologic premalignancies. *Current opinion in obstetrics & gynecology* **21** (6): 457.	9.2.
Heller T (2001) Ethical Debate. *BMJ*; 323: October,; pp. 838-840.	3.6.20.1
Health Department of Victoria (1987) Measles Isn't Child's Play. Health Promotion Unit, July; p. 2.	3.6.10.2
Herald Sun (1996) Infections may help. Herald Sun, 26/3/96; p. 21.	1.2
Hewitson L et.al, (2008) Pediatric Vaccines Influence Primate Behavior, and Amygdala Growth and Opioid Ligand Binding Friday, May 16, 2008: IMFAR.	9.2.20.1
Hindle RC (1991) Immunisation and Homoeopathy. *New Zealand Medical Journal*, 24 April; p. 171.	8.4 8.6.4
Hoover TA (2001) Homeopathic prophylaxis: fact or fiction. *J Am Inst Homeopath* 94 (3); pp. 168-175.	
Hulley SB, ET AL Eds. (2001) *Designing clinical research: an epidemiologic approach*, 2nd edn. Baltimore: Lippincott Williams and Wilkins.	
Institute of Medicine (1991) Press release.	3.5.2 3.6.13.3

National Academy of Sciences, Washington DC, 3.7.1991.	
International Vaccination Newsletter, (1995) September.	3.6.20
Jacobs J. et.al (1994) Treatment of Acute Childhood Diarrhea With Homeopathic Medicine: A Randomized Clinical Trial in Nicaragua. *Pediatrics* Vol. 93 No. 5 May 1994, pp. 719-725	9.1.
Jahan K, Ahmad K, Ali MA, (1984) Effect of Ascorbic Acid in the Treatment of Tetanus. *Bangladesh Medical Research Council Bulletin*, June 1984, Vol X, No. 1; pp. 24-28.	1.1.17
JAMA Special Communication (1994) Adverse Events Associated with Childhood Vaccines Other Than Pertussis and Rubella. *JAMA*, Vol. 271; pp. 1602-1605.	3.5.2
Japan Times online (2003) Families win lawsuit over MMR vaccine. 14.3.2003.	9.2.20.1
Johnston et al, (1985) Impact of Whooping Cough on Patients and their Families *British Medical Journal*, Vol 290; pp. 1636-1638.	3.6.13.4
Jonas WB (1999) Do homeopathic nosodes protect against infection? An experimental Test. *Alternative Therapies in Health and Medicine* 5 (5); pp. 36-40.	
Joshi W & Phelan P (1986) Pertussis Vaccination *Medical Journal of Australia*, Vol 144; p. 726.	3.6.13.4
Joyce A & Reese JE (1995) Transverse myelitis after measles, mumps and rubella vaccine *British Medical Journal*, Vol 311; p. 422.	3.6.20
Julian OA (1980) *The Treatise of Dynamised Micro-Immunotherapy* Jain Publishing Co, India, 1980.	4.1.1
Kalokerinos A (1974) *Every Second Child.* Thomas Nelson Ltd., Australia.	2.1; 3.4.2; 3.5.2; 8.7.2
Kalokerinos A & G Dettman G (1986)	3.6.15.4

Is Polio Vaccine a Health Hazard? Orthomolecular Corner *Toorak Times*, 17 December 1986.	
Kalokerinos A & G Dettman G (1987, 1988) Reported in Orthomolecular Corner *Toorak Times*, 26 August 1987 and 27 April 1988.	3.6.15.3
Kelsey et al, (1986) *Methods in Observational Epidemiology* Oxford University Press. New York; pp. 286-288.	
Kemp T et al, (1997) Is infant immunization a risk factor for childhood asthma or allergy? *Epidemiology*. Nov; 8(6); pp. 678-80.	3.6.13.4
Kent JT (1900) *Lectures on Homoeopathic Philosophy* B Jain Publishers, New Delhi. 5th Edition; p. 229.	4.1.3
Khetsuriani N et.al. (2001) Pertussis outbreak in an elementary school with high vaccination coverage. *Pediatr Infect Dis J.* Dec 20, (12) pp.1108-12.	9.2.13.1
Kichlu KL & L Bose L (1987) *A Text Book of Descriptive Medicine with Clinical Methods and Homoeopathic Therapeutic.* B Jain Publishers, New Delhi. (2nd ed); p. 805.	1.1.15 3.6.4.3
Kleijnen J. et al, (1991) Clinical Trials of Homoeopathy. *British Medical Journal* 302; pp. 316-23.	4.1.1
Klenner F (1954) Recent Discoveries in the Treatment of Lockjaw With Vitamin C and Tolserol. *Tri State Medical Journal*, July.	1.1.17
Klenner FR (1955) Polio Vaccine - Brodie V's Salk. *Tri State Medical Journal*, July.	1.1.15 3.6.15.1
Klenner FR (1956) Poliomyelitis - Case Histories. *Tri State Medical Journal*, September.	1.1.15
Koff RS (2001) Hepatitis vaccines. *Infectious Disease Clinics of North America*. 15(1); pp 83-95.	3.6.6.1
Kotok A (2000)	

The history of homeopathy in the Russian Empire until World War I, as compared with other European countries and the USA: similarities and discrepancies. http://www.homeoint.org/books4/kotok/index.htm.	
Kuhn TS (1970) *The structure of scientific revolutions.* 2nd Edition. University of Chicago Press, Chicago; p. 210	
Kune G (2002) Private communication with Golden, 7.7.02. Melbourne.	
Kurniawan J et.al. (2010) Bordetella pertussis Clones Identified by Multilocus Variable-Number Tandem-Repeat Analysis. In *CDC Emerging Infectious Diseases.* Volume 16, Number 2–February 2010.	9.2.13.2
Kyle WS (1992) Simian retroviruses, poliovaccine, and origin of AIDS *The Lancet*, March 7; 339; pp.600,601.	8.6.2
Lancaster et al, (1996) A.I.H.W. National Perinatal Statistics Unit. ABS Cat. No. 3304.0	
For example refer: *Lancet*, 30.4.1988.	3.4.3
Lasky T et al, (1998) Guillain-Barré syndrome and the 1992-1993 and 1993-1994 Influenza vaccines. *New England Journal of Medicine*; 339; pp. 1797-802.	3.6.8.1
Le Saux N (2003)	3.6.13.4
Lessell CB (1993) *The World Traveller's Manual of Homoeopathy* C W Daniel Co Ltd, Saffron Walden, UK; p. 14.	4.1.3
Lieberman AD, The Role of the Rubella Virus in the Chronic Fatigue Syndrome. *Clinical Ecology*, Vol 7, No. 3; pp. 51-54.	3.6.16
Linde K et al, (1997) Are the clinical effects of homoeopathy placebo effects? A meta-analysis of placebo-controlled trials. *Lancet.* 350; pp. 834-43.	4.1.1
Little D (2000) Prophylaxis in Homoeopathy – The Origin of	4.6.3

Homœoprophylaxis. *http://www.simillium.com/Thelittlelibrary/Homoeopathicphilosophy/* prophylaxis.htm	
Lockie A (1989) *The Family Guide to Homoeopathy.* Guild Publishing, Aylesbury, Bucks, England; p. 17.	4.1.3
Lovett L (1990) *Immunity - Why Not Keep It?* Published by the author, Melbourne.	2.4
Ludtke R, Rutten AL (2008) The conclusions on the effectiveness of homeopathy highly depend on the set of analyzed trials. *Journal of Clinical Epidemiology*. 61(12):1197-204.	4.2.4
MacIntyre CR & Nolan T (1994) Attitudes of Victorian Vaccine Providers to Pertussis Vaccine. *Medical Journal of Australia*, 5 September, Vol 161; pp. 295-299.	3.5.2 3.6.13.3
MacLeod G (1974) Coli-bacillosis of calves, or scour in calves and the rational approach to treatment and prevention. *Homoeopathy* 24; p. 30-31	
MacLeod G (1994) *Pigs: the homoeopathic approach to the treatment and prevention of Diseases.* C.W. Daniel Company Ltd, Saffron Walden, UK.	
Madsen KM et al, (2002) A Population-Based Study of Measles, Mumps, and Rubella Vaccination and Autism. *NEJM* Volume 347: Number 19; November 7; pp. 1477-1482.	3.6.20.1
Maggini S, Wenzlaff S, Hornig D (2010) Essential role of vitamin C and zinc in child immunity and health. *J Int Med Res.* 2010 Mar-Apr;38(2):386-414.	2.1
Mathur KN (1979) *Principles of Prescribing.* Jain Publishers, New Delhi. 2nd edition (1987 reprint); pp. 50, 53	4.1.3
Matricardi PM et al, (2002) Hay fever and asthma in relation to markers of infection in the United States. *J Allergy Clin Immunol.* 110; pp. 381-387.	1.2
McBean E (1957)	3.6.21.2

The Poisoned Needle. Health Research.	
McGauran N, Wiesler B, Kreis J, Schuler Y, Kolsch H, Kaiser T (2010) Reporting bias in medical research – a narrative review. *Trials*, 11:37. http://www.trialsjournal.com/content/11/1/37.	3.1.2 4.2.4
McIntyre P (1994) Vaccines against invasive Haemophilis influenzae type b disease. *Journal of Paediatric Child Health*, Vol 30; p. 15.	3.6.4.1
McIntyre P, Gidding H, Gilmour R, et al, (2002) Vaccine preventable diseases and vaccination coverage in Australia, 1999-2000. *Communicable Diseases Intelligence*;26:S111. http://www.cda.gov.au/pubs/cdi/2002/cdi26suppl/vpd99_00.htm	3.3
McVernon J et al, (2004) T helper cells and efficacy of Haemophilis influenzae type b conjugate vaccination *Lancet Infectious Diseases*. 4(1); January; pp. 40-3.	3.6.4.1
Medical News Today (2007) HPV Vaccine Mandates Risky and Expensive. 3/2/2007. http://www.medicalnewstoday.com/articles/62176.php	9.2.22.1
Mendelsohn R (1986) More on Immunizations. *Australasian Health & Healing*, Dec-Feb; p. 17.	3.6.13.3
Mendelsohn R (1984) The Medical Time Bomb of Immunization Against Disease. *East West Journal*, November; pp. 49, 84.	3.6.10.2 3.6.15.2
Mendelsohn R (1990) *How to Raise a Healthy Child ... In Spite of Your Doctor* Contemporary Books, Chicago.	8.9.1
Mendelsohn R, *The People's Doctor*, Vol 8, No. 12.	3.6.17.2
Mediolegal (1986) *British Medical Journal*, Vol 292; pp. 1264-1266.	3.6.13.3
Mercola J (2002(a)) Vaccine confirmed as source of polio outbreak. Reported in the *Mercola Newsletter*, 1/4/02. Quoting *Sciencexpress*, March 14, 2002; 10.1126/science. 1068284.	3.6.15.1
Mercola J (2002(b)) Polio vaccine linked to lymphoma. Reported in the *Mercola*	3.6.15.1

Newsletter, 1/4/02. Quoting *The Lancet*, March 9, 2002.	
Mercola J (2010) The FDA Shuts Down Common Infant Vaccine After Startling Discovery. April 17 2010. www.mercola.com	9.2.26.1
Miller DL et al, (1981) Pertussis Immunization and Serious Neurological Illness in Children. *British Medical Journal*, Vol 282; p. 1595.	3.6.13.3
Miller DL et al, (1982) Whooping Cough and Whooping Cough Vaccine: The Risks and Benefits Debate. *Epidemiological Review*, Vol 4; p. 21.	3.6.13.3
Miller DL et al, Pertussis Immunisation and serious acute neurological illnesses in children. *British Medical Journal*, 6 November, Vol 307; pp. 1171-1176.	3.6.13.3
Ministry of Health (UK), (1954) Department of Health for Scotland, Medical Memorandum 93222/7/63, July 1954; pp. 3, 5, 6 and 10.	1.1.15 3.6.15.2
MMWR Weekly (2004) Updated recommendations on the use of pneumococcal conjugate vaccine: Suspension of recommendations for third and fourth dose. *MMWR Weekly*; 53(08); 5/3/04; pp. 177-78.	3.6.14.1
Morgan OWC (2004) Following in the footsteps of smallpox: can we achieve the global eradication of measles? *BioMed Central Abstract*. Published online 17/3/04.	1.2
Morrell P (2000) Letter to the Editor. *British Medical Journal*; 321:8 July; p. 108.	8.6.4
Mosby (2002) *Mosby's Medical, Nursing & Allied Health Dictionary* – 6th Edition. Mosby Inc, Missouri. USA.	1.1.7
Moskowitz R (1985) Immunisations - A Dissenting View. Printed in *Dissent in Medicine - Nine Doctors Speak Out*; Contemporary Books Inc; pp. 133-166.	1.1.15 3.5.2 3.6.10.2
Mowle A (1981) Infectious Diseases. *Australasian Nurses Journal*, May.	3.6.21.3
Mroninski C, Adriano E, Mattos G (2001) Meningococcinum: Its protective effect against meningococcal	4.1.4

disease. *Homoeopathic Links* Winter Vol 14(4); pp. 230-4.	
NACA (National Asthma Council of Australia) (2010) Asthma mortality in Australia 1960-2008. Prepared by A/Professor Elizabeth Comino. 12th April, 2010	1.3
Nakatani H, Sano T, Iuchi T (2002) Development of Vaccination Policy in Japan: Current Issues and Policy Directions. *Jpn. J. Infect. Dis*. 55, pp.101-111.	8.3.1
National Health and Medical Research Council (NH&MRC) (2008) *The Australian Immunisation Handbook, 9th Edition.* Commonwealth of Australia, Canberra.	4.6 4.2.3.1
Nemours Foundation (2001) http://kidshealth.org/parent/infections/lung/measles_p3.html	
Neustaedter R (1990a) Measles and Homœopathic Vaccinations *The Homeopath* 10.2; p. 31.	8.4
Neustaedter R (1990b) Measles and Homoeopathic Immunizations. (a review of relevant medical literature). *The Homoeopath*, June 1990, Vol 10, No 2; pp 31 ff.	3.6.10.1
Neustaedter R (1995) Homeopathic prophylaxis - is it valid? *Resonance* Nov-Dec;17(6):12-14; p. 30.	3.6 8.4
Neustaedter R (2002) *The Vaccine Guide: Risks and Benefits for Children and Adults* North Atlantic Books, Berkeley, California.	3.6.21.1 8.9.1
Odent M et al, (1994a) Atopic Eczema. *Lancet*. 344; p.140	
Odent M et al, (1994b) Pertussis vaccination and asthma: Is there a link? *JAMA*. 272; pp.592-3.	3.6.13.3
Odent M et al, (1994c) Pertussis Vaccination and Asthma: Is There a Link? *British Medical Journal*, Vol 272; pp. 592-3.	3.5.2
Offit PA (2005) The Cutter Incident, 50 Years Later *NEJM*, Volume 352: 14; April 7; pp. 1411-1412.	3.6.15.1
Parry LA (1928)	3.6.21.2

Fatality rates of smallpox in the vaccinated and unvaccinated. *British Medical Journal*, 21 January 1928, Vol 116.	
Pawankar R et.al (2008) State of World Allergy Report 2008: Allergy and Chronic Respiratory Diseases. *World Allergy Organization Journal.* Volume 1(6) Supplement. June 2008pp S4-S17.	1.2
Pearson K (1937) *The grammar of science.* 3rd Edition. London; p. 357.	
Petrovic M, Roberts R, Ramsay M, (2001) Second dose of measles, mumps and rubella vaccine: questionnaire survey of health professionals. *BMJ*; 322; pp. 82-85	3.6.20.1
Popper KR (1960) *The logic of scientific discovery.* Hutchinson, London; p. 479.	
Preblud SR (1986) Varicella: complications and costs. *Paediatrics*; 78(supp); pp.728-735.	1.1.1
Polakoff S & Vandervelde EM (1988) Immunisation of neonates at high risk of hepatitis B in England and Wales: national surveillance. *British Medical Journal.* Vol 297; 23 July; pp. 249-253.	3.6.6.1
Poland GA & Jacobson RM (2004) Prevention of Hepatitis B with the Hepatitis B Vaccine *NEJM*, Volume 351: 27; December 30; pp. 2832-2838.	1.1.6
Public Health Laboratory Service (1982) Efficacy of Pertussis Vaccination in England. *British Medical Journal*, Vol 285; p. 359.	3.6.13.2
Puri A et al, (2002) Measles Vaccine Efficacy Evaluated by Case Reference Technique. *Indian Pediatrics*. 39; pp. 556-560.	3.6.10.1
Rappenport J (1988) The AIDS-Vaccine Connection. *Australasian Health and Healing*, Vol 7 No 2, Dec-Feb; pp. 25-29.	3.5.2
Roberts RJ et al, (1995) Reasons for non-uptake of measles, mumps and rubella catch up immunisation in a measles epidemic and side effects of the vaccine. *British Medical Journal*, Vol 310:1629.	3.6.20
Roden J (1993) Immunisation: A Natural Part of Health? Reprinted in	8.6.4

yImmunisation/Communicable Diseases, October; pp. 17-26.	
Rothman KJ & Greenland S. (1998) *Modern Epidemiology*. 2nd Edition. Lippincott, Williams and Wilkins.	
Ruddock EH (1986) *The Diseases of Infants and Children* (8th ed) B Jain Publishers, 1986 reprint.	1.1.15
Runciman WB et al, (2003) Adverse drug events and medication errors in Australia *International Journal for Quality in Health Care*, 15; pp. 149-159.	7.0
Rutten AL, Stolper CF (2008). The 2005 meta-analysis of homeopathy: the importance of post-publication data. *Homeopathy*. 97(4):169-77.	4.2.4
Safranek TJ et al, (1991) Reassessment of the association between Guillain-Barré syndrome and receipt of swine influenza vaccine in 1976-1977: results of a two-state study. Expert Neurology Group. *American Journal of Epidemiology*; 133(9): pp. 940-51.	3.6.8.1
Salk J & D (1977) Control of Influenza and Poliomyelitis. *Science*, 4 April, Vol 195.	3.6.15.2
Salmaso S, (2001) Sustained efficacy during the first 6 years of life of 3-component acellular pertussis vaccines administered in infancy: the Italian experience. *Pediatrics*. Vol. 108; No. 5; November; pp. 81-ff.	3.6.13.2
Salter RW et al, (1991) Outbreak of paralytic poliomyelitis in Oman: evidence for widespread transmission among fully vaccinated children. *Lancet*, Vol 338, 21st September; pp. 715-720.	3.6.15.2
Sanchez P (1993) Immunisation implicated in infants' apnoea. *Australian Doctor*, 12 November 1993.	3.5.3
Sankaran P (1961) *Prophylactics in Homoeopathy* The Homoeopathic Medical Publishers, Bombay.	4.1.1 4.1.3 4.1.4
Sankaran P (1978)	4.1.3

Some Notes on the Nosodes. The Homoeopathic Medical Publishers, Bombay.	
Schleqel M, et.al. (1999) Comparative effectiveness of three mumps vaccines during disease outbreak in eastern Switzerland: cohort study *Br Med J* August 7.	3.5.3
Scheibner V (1990) *Cot Death as Death Due to Exposure to Non-Specific Stress and General Adaptation Syndrome: It's Mechanisms and Prevention.* Association for Prevention of Cot Death (178 Govetts Leap Road, Blackheath NSW 2785), Oct.	3.5.3 8.9.1
Scheibner V (1993) *Vaccination: The Medical Assault on the Immune System* Chapter 6.	3.6.4.1
Scheibner V (2004) Dynamics of critical days as part of the dynamics of non-specific stress syndrome discovered during monitoring with Cotwatch breathing monitor. *J. Aust. Coll. Nutr. & Env. Med.* Vol 23, No. 3; December; pp. 10-14.	3.5.7
Schlegel M et al, (1999) Comparative efficacy of three mumps vaccines during disease outbreak in eastern Switzerland: cohort study *BMJ.* 319: August 7; p. 352.	3.6.12.1
Sethi B (1991) *Homoeo Prophylactic Remedies* Jain Publishers, New Delhi; pp. 22, 47, 56, 78 reprint.	4.1.3
Shang A, Huwiler-Müntener K, Nartey L, et al. (2005) Are the clinical effects of homoeopathy placebo effects? Comparative study of placebo-controlled trials of homoeopathy and allopathy. *Lancet* ; **366**: 726-732.	4.2.4
Shepherd D (1967) *Homoeopathy in Epidemic Diseases* C.W. Daniel Company Ltd, Saffron Walden, UK; pp. 15, 51, 81	3.1 4.1.3
Silfverdal SA et al, (1997) Protective effect of breastfeeding on invasive Haemophilis influenzae infection: a case-control study in Swedish pre-school children. I*nternational Journal of Epidemiology*, 26(2); pp. 443-50.	1.1.4

Silfverdal SA et al, (1999) Protective effect of breastfeeding: an ecologic study of Haemophilis Influenzae meningitis and breastfeeding in a Swedish population. *International Journal of Epidemiology*, 28(1); pp. 152-6.	1.1.4
Singh V & Yang V, (1998) Serological association of measles virus and human herpes virus-6 with brain antibodies in autism. *Clinical Immunology and Immunopathology*, 88(1); pp. 105-108.	3.6.20.1
Slone D et al, (1973) *Clinic. Pharmac. Ther.*, p. 14.	3.6.15.3
Smith JWG, Laurence DR, Evans DG. (1975) *British Medical Journal*, 23 August, Vol 3; pp. 453-455.	1.1.17
Snead EL (1987) AIDS Immunisation Related Syndrome. *Health Freedom News*, Vol 6 No 6, July.	3.5.2 3.6.15.2
Society of Homoeopaths (1990) *Vaccination - A Difficult Decision.* January 1990.	8.4
Speight LJ (1982) *Homoeopathy and Immunisation.* Health Science Press, London; p. 3.	4.1.3
Srugio I et.al (2010) Pertussis Infection in Fully Vaccinated Children in Day-Care Centers, Israel. *Emerging Infectious Diseases.* Vol. 6, No. 5, September–October. pp.526-529.	8.4.10
Stewart GT (1981) Whooping Cough in Relation to Other Childhood Infections in 1977-79 in the U.K. *Journal of Epidemiology and Commonwealth Health*, Vol 35; pp. 139-45	3.6.13.2
Stewart GT (1984) Letter to the Editor. *American Journal of Epidemiology*; pp. 119-135.	3.6.13.2
Strachan DP (1989) Hay fever, hygiene, and household size. *BMJ* **299** November, (6710): 1259–60.	1.2
Stratton KR et.al. (1994) Adverse events associated with childhood vaccines other than Pertussis and rubella. *JAMA*. 25 May, Vol 274, No. 20; pp.	3.6.4.1

1602-1605.	
Strond CE (1969) *Practitioner*, 203.	1.1.15
Sulfaro F et al, (1994) Homoeopathic vaccination, what does it mean? *The Medical Journal of Australia*, 5 September, Vol 161; pp. 305-307	8.6.8
Talley L & Salama P (2003) Short Report: Assessing Field Vaccine Efficacy For Measles In Famine-Affected Rural Ethiopia. *Am. J. Trop. Med. Hyg.*, 68(5); pp. 545-546.	3.6.10.1
Taylor-Smith A (1950) Poliomyelitis and prophylaxis. *Br Hom J* XL; pp. 65-77.	4.1.4
The Francis Report (1955) *Tri-State Medical Journal*, June.	3.6.15.2
Thompson NP et al, (1995) Is measles vaccination a risk factor for inflammatory bowel disease? *Lancet*, April 29; 345(8957); pp. 1071-4.	3.6.10.2
Vadheim CM (1993) Effectiveness and safety of an *Haemophilis influenzae* type b conjugate vaccine (PRP-T) in young infants *Pediatrics*; 92: pp. 272-279	3.6.4.1
Vaughan VC, McKay RJ, Behrman RE, Nelson WE (Ed), (1979) *Textbook of Pediatrics* (11th ed). WB Saunders Co, 1979; p. 926.	1.1.15
Vickers AJ & Smith C (2001) Homoeopathic Oscillococcinum for preventing and treating influenza and influenza-like syndromes (Cochrane Review). *The Cochrane Library* Issue 3, Oxford: Update Software; pp. 5-7.	
Vithoulkas G (1980) *The Science of Homoeopathy*. Grove Press Inc, New York, 1980.	3.1 4.2.3
Volk WA & Wheeler MF (1980) *Basic Microbiology* (4th ed). J B Lippincott Co.	1.1.15
Von Mutius E (2007) Allergies, infections and the hygiene hypothesis--the epidemiological evidence. *Immunobiology.* 2007;212(6):433-9. Epub 2007 Apr 30.	1.2

Wack RP (2003) An Outbreak of Varicella despite Vaccination. *NEJM*, 348:14; pp. 1405-1407.	3.6.1.1
Wakefield AJ et al, (1998) Ileal-lymphoid nodular hyperplasia, non-specific colitis, and pervasive developmental disorder in children. *Lancet*; 351(9103): Feb 28; pp. 637-641.	3.6.20.1
Wakefield AJ, Montgomery SM (2000) Measles, mumps, rubella vaccine: through a glass, darkly *Adverse Drug React Toxicol Rev*; 19; pp. 265-283.	3.6.20.1
Wakefield AJ (2010) *Callous Disregard: Autism and Vaccines – The Truth Behind a Tragedy*. Skyhorse Publishing. New York.	9.2.20
Walach H (2003) Reinventing the wheel will not make it rounder: controlled trials of homoeopathy reconsidered. *The Journal of Alternative and Complementary Medicine*. 9:1; pp.7-13.	
WDDTY (1991) *The WDDTY Vaccination Handbook*. The Wallace Press.	1.1.4
West J (1988) *The AIDS Time Bomb*. Veritas Press, Australia.	3.6.15.3
Wharton R & Lewith G (1986) Complementary medicine and the general practitioner. *Brit. Med. J.* 292; p.1498.	
Wilson G (1967) *The Hazards of Immunisation*. The Athlone Press, London.	3.5.2 4.1.4
World Health Organisation (2007) WHO Global Atlas of Traditional, Complementary and Alternative Medicine. Produced by the WHO Kobe Centre. Bodeker, G., Ong, C.K., Grundy, C., Burford, G., Shein, K.	
Zukerman W (2010) Why whooping cough's making a comeback. *New Scientist*. 11:55 12 February 2010.	9.2.13.2

BIBLIOGRAPHY (not included in References)

Adams QM (1956). Infectious diseases and their nosodes - Morbillinum. *Br Homoeopath J* 45: 263

Agrawal YR (1987). Prophylactics in Homoeopathy. Vijay Publications Delhi

Agrawal YR (1994). Plague prevention, Phosphorus and postponement. *Advent Hom* Oct-Dec;11(4):12-13

Anonymous (1915a). Prevention is better than cure (E). *Br Homoeopath J* 5: 337

Anonymous (1915b). Prevention of infectious diseases (E). *Br Homoeopath J* 5: 436

Anonymous (1961). Polio prevention. *Homoeopathy* 11(6): 81-83

Anonymous (1986). Homoeo-prophylaxis - testimony from masters. *Indian J Homoeopath Med* 21(4):18-20

Arul M (1996). Homoeopathic way of immunisation. *Homoeopath Heritage* Dec; 21(12):707-709

Attena F, Toscano G, Agozzino E, Del Giudice N. (1995). A randomized trial in the prevention of influenza-like syndromes by homoeopathic management. *Revue d Epidemiologie et de Sante Publique* 43: 380-2

Australian Bureau of Statistics (2002). *Occasional Paper: Vaccination Coverage in Australian Children.* ABS Statistics and the Australian Childhood Immunisation Register. Publication 4813.0.55.001. Canberra.

Australian Bureau of Statistics (2003a). Population by Age and Sex – 2001 Census Edition – Final. Publication 3201.0. Canberra.

Australian Bureau of Statistics (2003b). Australian Demographic Statistics – 2001 Census Edition – Final. Publication 3101.0. Canberra.

Australian Bureau of Statistics (2003c). *Breastfeeding in Australia*, Electronic delivery. Publication 4810.0.55.001. Canberra.

Australian Bureau of Statistics (2003d). Health and Communicable Diseases. Year Book of Australia, 2003. Publication 1301.0. Canberra.

Bell et al (2004). Individual differences in response to randomly assigned active individualised homoeopathic and placebo treatment in fibromyalgia: Implications of a double-blind optional crossover design

J Alternative & Complementary Medicine, 10, pages 269-283.

Boyson WA (1966b). Thirty years as clinical research and confirmations of the intestinal nosode Sycotic co. *J Am Inst Homeopaths* 59(7). 238-40.

Bradburn NM, Rips LJ, Shevell SK (1987). Answering autobiographical questions: The impact of memory and inference on surveys. *Science* 236:157-61.

Bungetzianu G (1988). The results obtained by the homeopathical dilution (15 CH) of antiinfluenzal (Anti-Flu) vaccine. *Proc 43rd LMHI Congr*, Athens, Greece:143

Burnett JC (1938) Nature of homoeoprophylaxis (contd). *Homoeopathy* 7(7): 214-218,171-172

Chand H (1950). Prophylaxis in poliomyelitis epidemics (L). *Br Homoeopath J* 40; 310

Chand H (1986). Prophylaxis in poliomyelitis epidemics. *Hahnemann Glean* 53(5):150

Clarke JH (1908). Internal or homoeopathic vaccination: the victory in Iowa. *Homoeopathic World* 43(11): 489-501

Coates J (1992). Vaccination horror - homeopathic success. *Homeopathy Today* 12(6):8-9

Concon AA (1967). Homeo Prophylaxis. *The Indian Homoeopathic Gazette* April

Cook T (1997). Malaria: homeopathic prophylaxis and treatment. *J Am Inst Homeopath* Summer;90(2):76-77

Cook T (1999). Malaria: homoeopathic prophylaxis and treatment. *Homoeopath Int* 12(3):12-3

Curtis S (1994). *A handbook of homoeopathic alternative to immunisation.* Winter Press, London.

Day CE (1987). Isopathic prevention of kennel cough - is vaccination justified? *Int J Vet Homoeopath* 2(1):45-50, also Vol 2 Nov 87, p57-58

Diamantidis S (1990). *Homoeopathic Medicine – Theory, Methodology, Applications*. S.A. Dimantidis. Athens.

Dietz V Jacobs J (1997). Vaccination: attitudes and practices of physicians who use homeopathy. *Alternat Complement Ther* Dec;3(6):414-418

Engineer SJ Engineer LS Vakil AE (1990). Antibody formation by Baptisia tinctoria in experimental animals. *Br Homoeopath J* 79: 109-113

English JM (1995). The rights and wrongs of measles vaccination. *Br Homoeopath J* Jul; 84(3):156-163

Everitt DW (1969). Oral vaccines. *Homoeopathy* 19(4): 44-45

Fausel SL (1998). Debate regarding vaccination procedures and homeopathy. *J Am Vet Med Assoc* 213(6):798-799

Gibson DM (1958). Nosodes and prophylaxis. *Homoeopathy* 8(7): 111-112

Golden I (1988). A Survey of the Effectiveness of a Homoeopathic Prophylactic Kit. *J Aust Fed Hom* Vol. 1, No. 8; 1-6.

Golden I (1989b). Immunisation – A Survey of the Homoeopathic Alternative. *Nature & Health* Vol. 10, No. 1; 37-39

Golden I (1999). Homoeopathic Disease Prevention. *Homoeopathy Online*. Sept.

Golden I (2002b). Meningococcal Disease and Homoeopathic Prevention. *Informed Choice* Spring 43-45

Griggs WB (1967). Clinical research with confirmations of the intestinal nosode

Sycotic co. *J Am Inst Homeopath* 60(5): 152-3

Grimmer AH (1954). Homoeopathic prophylaxis. *Homoeopathy* 4(7):142-145

Hamilton J (1943). Homoeopathy, positive health and prevention of disease. *Br Homoeopath J* 33: 3

Harling ME (1974). Thoughts on prophylaxis. *Br Homoeopath J* 63: 161

Head CJ (1999). *An educated decision: one approach to the vaccination problem using homeopathy.* Lavender Hill Publishing, London.

Henneckens CH, Buring JE (1987). Epidemiology in Medicine. Little Brown and Company ed. Mayrent SL.

Hindle RC (1991). Immunisation and homoeopathy. *N Z Med J* 104(910):171

Ipsen J, Olsen J (1984). Estimating sensitivity and specificity in order to correct for misclassification. *Scand J Soc Med* 12:111-4

Kanji Lal JN (1987). Can homoeopathy allow vaccination ? *Hahnemann Homoeopath Sand* 11(3):65-73

Kanjilal ST (1979). Is vaccine of today homoeopathic nosode of yesterday. *Hahnemann Glean* 46(4): 166-167

Lee F (1991). Attitude to vaccination. *Br Homoeopath J* 80 : 70

Lewith G, Brown PK, Tyrell DA (1989). Controlled study of the effects of a homoeopathic dilution of influenza vaccine on antibody titres in man. *Complement Med Res* 3(3):22-4.

Maceoin D, Cope E (1988). A hearing for an alternative approach to vaccine. *Guardian* Oct; 19

Macnish D (1912a). Vaccine therapy in homoeopathic practice. *Homoeopathic World* 47((8): 363-374

Macnish D (1912b). Vaccine therapy in homoeopathic practice. *Br Homoeopath J* 2: 368

Margutti VM (1976). Homoeopathic methodology in disease prevention. *J Am Inst Homeopath* 69(3): 145-148

McAusland S (1963). Oral influenza vaccines (L). *Br Homoeopath J* 52: 72

Mitchell GR (1957). Infectious diseases and their nosodes. *Br Homoeopath J* 46: 46

Pulford A (1937). Vaccination, smallpox and homoeopathy. *Homoeopathy* 6(7): 225

Pulford A (1994). Are serums, vaccines, etc. homoeopathic? *Homoeopath Heritage* Feb;19(2):87-91

Rawat PS (1998). How to prevent non-virus polio. *Homoeopath Heritage* 23(1):45-7

Rosenthal C (2001). A drop of nature: homeopathic approach to vaccination in Israel. *Homoeopathic Links* 14 (4): 229-230

Sankaran P (1978). *Some Notes on the Nosodes*. The Homoeopathic Medical

Publishers

Sarangi AP (1994). Plague - its homoeopathic treatment and prevention. *Homoeopath Heritage.* Dec;19(12): 769-70/

Schmidt P (1959). Homoeopathic Prophylaxis. *J of Homoeopathic Medicine.* 1(1)

Schmidt P (1994). Homoeopathic prophylaxis against malaria - caveat emptor! *Homoeopath Links* Winter; 7(4):41

Severyn K (1996). Vaccination update. *J Am Inst Homeopath* Win;89(4):217-221

Shafran B (1999). The use of injectable homeopathic preparations in flu prophylaxis. *Biomed Ther.* Jan;17(1):30

Smith AT (1950). Poliomyelitis and prophylaxis. *Br Homoeopath J* 40: 65

Stratton K, Gable A, Shetty P, McCormick M, eds. *Immunization safety review: measles-mumps-rubella vaccine and autism*. Washington, D.C.: National Academy Press, 2001.

Sulfaro F Fasher B Burgess MA (1994). Homoeopathic vaccination. What does it mean? *Med J Aust* 161:305-307

Taylor SM Mallon TR Green WP (1989). Effectiveness of a homoeopathic prophylaxis against experimental infection of calves by the bovine lungworm Dictyocaulus viviparous. *Vet Rec* Jan 7;124(1):15-7

Traub M (1994). Homeopathic prophylaxis. *J Naturopath Med* 5(1):50-61,

Ullman D (1991a). The International homoeopathic renaissance. *Berlin J. Res. Homoeopathy* 1(2): 118

Ullman D (1991b). *A Condensed History of Homeopath.*
http://www.homeopathic.com/articles/intro/history.php

Ullman D (1995). *The Present Status of Homeopathy Internationally.* Homoeopathic Educational Services. Berkeley, CA.

Underhill E (1982) The common cold Prophylaxis and treatment. *Homeotherapy* 8(5): 135-138.

Vakil P (1997). A proving of pertussis vaccine. *Proc. 52nd LMHI Congr.*, Seattle, USA, 100-103.

Wagner H (1997). Herbal immunostimulants for the prophylaxis and therapy of colds and influenza. *Eur J Herbal Med,* Spring; 3(1):22-30.

Wheeler CE (1911). Experiment in prophylaxis. Br Homoeopath J 1: 544.

Wheeler CE (1912). Scientific basis of vaccine therapy as a homoeopathic procedure. *Homoeopathic World* 47(9): 374-379,395-401.

Zaheer Rozina A (2001). Virionum, the nosode of HIV: as remedy and as vaccine! *Homoeopathic Links,* 14 (4): 235-238.

12 Index

About the Author

Dr Isaac Golden Ph.D, D.Hom., N.D., B.Ec(Hon)

Head of School, School of Holistic Medicine, Endeavour College

Isaac Golden has been a homoeopathic practitioner since 1984. Prior to that his career was in financial accounting and taxation following an Honours degree in Economics in 1972.

Isaac was President of the Victorian branch of the Australian Homoeopathic Association - Australia's largest national organization of professional homoeopaths - from 1992 to 1998.

In March 1999 he was awarded the Association's Distinguished Service Award for his "many years of service to the Australian Homoeopathic Association and for his significant contributions to the homoeopathic profession in Australia"

Isaac is the Business Manager Academic Operations at Endeavour College of Natural Health.He has been teaching homoeopathy since 1988. He founded the Australasian College of Hahnemannian Homoeopathy in 1990, offering correspondence and internet courses in homeopathy and natural medicine.

Isaac is a regular contributor to local and international academic journals, and is the author of ten books on Homoeopathy, including –

- *Vaccine Damaged Children: Treatment, Prevention, Reasons.*
- *Vaccination & Homoeoprophylaxis? A Review of Risks and Alternatives* (6th edition)
- *Homoeoprophylaxis - A Fifteen Year Clinical Study*
- *Homoeoprophylaxis - A Practical and Philosophical Review* (4th edition)
- *Homoeopathic Body-System Prescriber - A Practical Workbook of Sector Remedies* (2nd edition)
- *Australian Homoeopathic Home Prescriber –Part 1: The Treatment of Simple Everyday Conditions* (3rd edition)
- *Australian Homoeopathic Home Prescriber –Part 2: A Simple Materia Medica of Common Remedies with Repertory*

- *Australian Homoeopathic Home Prescriber –Part 3: A Simple Introduction to Homoeopathic Medicine*
- *Homoeopathic Treatment of the Energy Bodies – Traditional Strategies and New Developments.*
- *Homoeoprophylaxis - A Ten Year Clinical Study*

In his own practice, Isaac specialises in treating patients suffering from chronic disease using constitutional and anti-miasmic homoeopathic treatment. He also specialises in the treatment of vaccine-damaged children.

Isaac is a world authority on homoeoprophylaxis - the use of homoeopathic medicines for specific infectious disease prevention, and has undertaken the world's largest long-term study of parents using such a program. In 2004 he completed a PhD research program at the GSIM, Swinburne University, Melbourne, studying homoeoprophylaxis. This was the first time a mainstream Australian University granted a PhD for research on a homoeopathic topic.

Vaccination & Homœoprophylaxis?
A Review of Risks and Alternatives - 7th Edition

The first edition of this book was published in 1989, containing the author's research using orthodox medical references, as well as the first results from studying responses from parents whose children used his homœoprophylaxis program. Over the years the research program has grown, the evidence questioning the long-term safety of vaccination has grown, and significant new data about the safety and effectiveness of homœoprophylaxis has been included in the new edition.

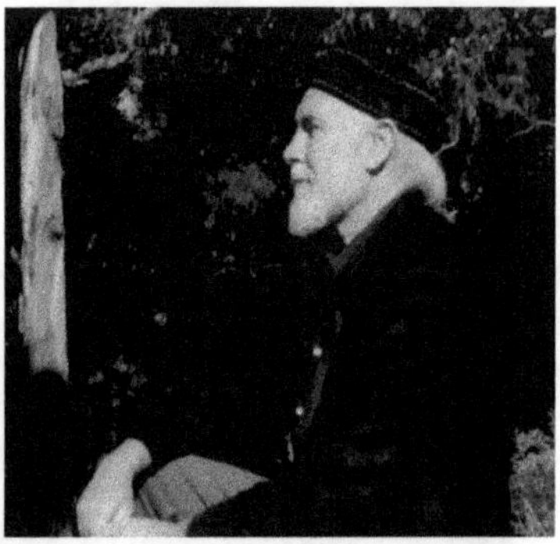

This is the most comprehensive international reference book on this controversial topic, with referenced data substantiating the effectiveness and safety of homœoprophylaxis, as well as the safety and effectiveness of vaccines. This permits a scientific comparison of the two methods, something which is not seen in the orthodox literature. It is a book of facts, not supposition.

The author calls for the use of both methods of immunisation to be freely available within the mainstream health-care system, something which would increase national coverage against targeted diseases, at a reduced cost to government, as well as reducing the incidence of vaccine-induced chronic disease; a win-win for all except multinational pharmaceutical companies and their dependents. A book for parents and politicians, as well as practitioners.

Dr Isaac Golden was the first person to be awarded a PhD from a mainstream Australian university for research in a homoeopathic topic. The rigorous scrutiny of the data presented in this book can give readers confidence in the rigor and objectivity of the evidence supporting homoeoprophylaxis, and the balance of the recommendations.

www.ingramcontent.com/pod-product-compliance
Lightning Source LLC
Chambersburg PA
CBHW070006010526
44117CB00011B/1446
* 9 7 8 0 9 5 7 8 7 2 6 7 7 *